SKILLS AND TECHNIQUES FOR
THE
NEW NURSING
ASSISTANT TEXTBOOK

7th Edition

Written by
Barbara Gillogly, Ph.D., Ed.

Revised and Updated by
Molly Conley, R.N., M.S.N.

FOR REORDERING INFORMATION PLEASE CALL:
(714) 891-1443   (800) 877-1443

www.medcomRN.com

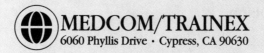

MEDCOM/TRAINEX
6060 Phyllis Drive • Cypress, CA 90630

Production Management by Tina Armstrong.
Edited and revised by John Shannon.
Book design and layout by Patty Mago.
Art by George Dimichina.
Photography by Ross Olson.

About the Author

Barbara Gillogly is the Director of the Gerontology Program at American River College in Sacramento, California.

Dr. Gillogly received her education at California State University, Sacramento, and the University of California, Davis with degrees in Psychology, Gerontology, and Human Development. Dr. Gillogly would like to thank Ann Jasper, R.N. for her invaluable advice and expertise.

Seventh Edition

Advice and technical expertise for the completion and updating of the 7th edition of this manual have been provided by Molly Conley, RN, MSN. Ms. Conley is a California Director of Vocational Nursing and is responsible for renewal of the Certified Nursing Assistant and Home Health Aide programs. She teaches at the North Orange County Regional Occupational Program in Anaheim, California. She has completed post-graduate work in nursing at SUNY-Buffalo, and in nursing education at California State University, Long Beach, California State University, Fullerton, and California State Polytechnic University, Pomona.

Dedication

To the nursing assistant, the most important hands-on care giver in the long term care profession. Without your sincere dedication, devotion to your patients and desire to promote high quality care, it would be impossible for us to satisfy the social consciousness of the nation toward our frail and elderly patients.

TABLE OF CONTENTS

SECTION I

WORKING IN A LONG-TERM CARE FACILITY

THE ROLE OF THE NURSING ASSISTANT

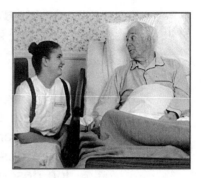

In this chapter... you will learn about:

▶ The duties of a nursing assistant.

▶ The personal qualities needed in a nursing assistant.

DEFINITIONS

Activities of Daily Living (ADL):	Common daily tasks such as dressing, eating grooming or bathing.
Ambulation:	To walk in upright position, or assist someone to walk.
CNA:	A Certified Nursing Assistant who has successfully completed an approved certification training program including a written and/or manual skills test, and who has received a certificate by the state.
Compassion:	Sorrow for the suffering of others with the desire to help.
Empathy:	Ability to experience the feelings and thoughts of another person.
Nursing Assistant:	Member of the healthcare team who provides care to a resident, meeting his or her physical, psychosocial and individual needs.
Policy:	An official statement of what will and will not be done at a facility.
Procedure:	An official statement of the steps to take to do something at a facility.
Psychosocial:	Individual's mental or emotional processes combined with ability to interact with others.

THE HEALTHCARE TEAM

In a long-term care facility, many different people come together to provide care and supervision for the residents. Each member of this team has a specific function. These functions are explained in the **policies**, **procedures**, and job descriptions of each individual facility. It is important for you to know where the Policy and Procedure Manual is kept in your facility and for you to understand the portions which apply to your job. All of the team members must cooperate and work together to provide the best care possible for each resident. As a **nursing assistant**, you may work with some of these people occasionally, or once a week, or daily.

The healthcare team may include:

• Activity Coordinator	• Medication Nurse
• Nursing Assistant	• Occupational Therapist
• Chaplain	• Physical Therapist
• Charge Nurse	• Physician
• Dietitian	• Psychologist/ Psychiatrist
• Director of Nursing	• Social Service Coordinator
• Family	• Speech Therapist

Chapter 1: The Role of the Nursing Assistant

As a nursing assistant, you will work most closely with the nursing team. These are the members of the healthcare team who provide daily hands-on care to the residents. The nursing team includes:

- ▶ Registered Nurse

- ▶ Licensed Practical/Vocational Nurse

- ▶ Certified Nursing Assistant

A certified nursing assistant **(CNA)** has completed an approved precertification program and passed and examination. The certified nursing assistant is a member of this team and is often the one who provides the most hands-on care to the resident. Because of this, the nursing assistant has great influence on the resident's sense of well being as well as the resident's physical health. The nursing assistant is the most important link between the resident and the facility. The facility's successful operation depends on the care given by the nursing assistant.

The role of the nursing assistant can be broken down into four specific areas:

1. Providing a safe environment for the resident.
2. Meeting the resident's physical needs.
3. Meeting the resident's **psychosocial** needs.
4. Fulfilling responsibilities to employer.

As a nursing assistant, you will probably be supervised by a registered nurse. However you may accept direction from a licensed practical nurse, licensed vocational nurse, nurse practitioner or some other licensed healthcare professional. In some rare circumstances, such as a working in an assisted living facility, you may not have direct supervision present at all times. In that case you should know your precise responsibilities well, know who your supervisor is, and know who to call if you need advice or direction.

Providing A Safe Environment

The nursing assistant is responsible for knowing and following the facility's policies and procedures regarding emergency evacuation. It is also the nursing assistant's responsibility to:

1. Use all facility equipment in a safe manner. Report any hazardous conditions immediately to your supervisor.

2. Know and follow the proper use of protective devices (such as restraints and side rails).

3. Know and follow facility emergency procedures (evacuation plans for fire or other disasters).

4. Know and practice other fire safety procedures such as: knowing the location and operation of fire extinguishers and fire alarms; knowing how to use oxygen and electrical equipment safely; limiting smoking to specifically designated areas.

5. Be aware of potential hazards (such as liquid spills and obstructions). Either remove them or report them to the proper person.

6. Know how to dispose of dangerous chemicals such as cleaning solvents or acids. These should not be simply flushed down the drain or discarded in ordinary waste containers. You should wear gloves if you have to handle hazardous wastes and dispose of them carefully according to your facility's procedures.

7. Practice personal hygiene, cleanliness, and infection control.

Meeting the Resident's Personal Care Needs

The heart of the nursing assistant's job is fulfilling these needs. This includes assisting with all the **activities of daily (ADL)** living, such as bathing, oral hygiene, grooming, dressing, toileting, and feeding. It also includes healthcare and rehabilitative activities, such as taking vital signs, positioning, collecting specimens, and assisting with exercises and **ambulation**.

The amount of assistance required in activities of daily living will depend upon each individual resident's abilities. It is important for the nursing assistant to know what the resident can do without assistance, and to encourage the resident to be as independent as possible. Of course, the nursing assistant will help the resident with those things the resident is unable to do.

The psychosocial needs of the resident are often not as obvious as physical needs. Therefore, it requires skill and sensitivity to understand these needs in individual residents and to meet them.

Residents in a long-term care facility have many of the same needs we all do:

1. To be recognized as individuals.

2. To love and be loved.

3. To feel a sense of accomplishment.

4. To be treated with dignity and respect.

5. To feel secure.

6. To feel good about themselves.

The nursing assistant can fill these needs by providing individualized care, listening, treating each resident with respect, trying to understand what the resident is feeling, and showing genuine concern and interest. In other words, treating the resident just like you would like to be treated.

Fulfilling Responsibilities To Employer

Your responsibilities to your employer include:

1. Reporting to work on time.

2. Reliably fulfilling your assigned schedule.

3. Meeting the needs of the residents and their families.

4. Notifying your supervisor when you are ill.

5. Getting along with the rest of the staff.

6 Doing your job to the best of your ability.

7. Conserving supplies and equipment.

PERSONAL QUALITIES OF A NURSING ASSISTANT

It takes special qualities to be a nursing assistant. The following are some of the traits and attitudes important in being a successful nursing assistant. You should:

1. Be dependable, reliable, and honest.

2. Enjoy working with people and have a positive attitude.

3. Relate easily and get along with others.

4. Be tactful, patient and courteous.

5. Enjoy helping people and be flexible when needs change.

6. Show **compassion**.

7. Have **empathy**.

8. Understand and respect differences in people.

9. Be sensitive to the feelings of others.

10. Treat others the way you want to be treated.

Service to others can be one of the most fulfilling vocations. It can make your life meaningful and build your own self-esteem. The choice to remain in this field should be made after reflecting on the qualities needed to be successful in this career. It takes dedication and a sincere desire to help others.

It is important for you to look closely at yourself to see if you are this type of person. If you are, you will find being a nursing assistant a rewarding and satisfying career.

Now that you know what the role of a nursing assistant is, you are ready to learn how to become a Certified Nursing Assistant. The following lessons are designed to guide you in learning the skills required for certification. These skills are needed to fulfill your duties as a CNA. In addition, these lessons will help you understand yourself and your residents. There are many things to learn, and you will have to work hard, but when you finish and become a certified nursing assistant, you will be proud of your accomplishment.

*Circle the correct answer. There is only **one** correct answer.*

1. **The nursing assistant should remove or report potential hazards, such as liquid spills and obstructions, to the proper person.**

    a. True   b. False

2. **What are some activities of daily living in a long-term care facility?**

    a. Bathing.

    b. Oral hygiene.

    c. Grooming.

    d. Feeding.

    -e. All of the above.

3. **Residents in a long-term care facility have different needs than other people.**

    a. True   b. False

4. **Which of the following is NOT a responsibility of the nursing assistant as an employee?**

    a. Reporting to work on time.

    b. Getting along with coworkers.

    c. Supervising other workers.

    d. Notifying his or her supervisor when ill.

5. **A nursing assistant has special qualities.**

    a. True   b. False

6. **In describing the qualities of a good nursing assistant, which of the following would not apply?**

   a. Enjoys working with people.

   b. Honest.

   c. Compassionate.

   d. Uncooperative.

7. **There are no personal advantages to being a nursing assistant.**

   a. True   b. False

8. **Of all the members of a long-term care team, the nursing assistant provides the most hands-on care to the resident.**

   a. True   b. False

9. **Recognizing a resident as an individual is an example of recognizing what kind of need?**

   a. Psychosocial.

   b. Physical.

   c. Sexual.

   d. Social.

10. **Which of the following statements is true about meeting the resident's physical needs?**

   a. The resident should be encouraged to be as dependent as possible.

   b. The nursing assistant won't spend much time fulfilling the needs.

   c. The amount of assistance required will depend on each resident's abilities.

   d. Very few of the resident's physical needs can be met.

Chapter 2

WHAT IS LONG-TERM CARE?

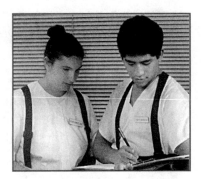

In this chapter... you will learn about:

▶ The care provided in a long-term care facility.

▶ The types of long-term care facilities.

▶ Some recent changes in the healthcare system.

DEFINITIONS

Nutrition:	The science of foods and how they affect health.
OBRA: (Omnibus Budget Reconciliation Act.)	A federal act that focuses on giving quality care to older people in long-term care facilities.
Outpatient:	Care given to a patient who visits a facility for the care rather than staying at the facility.

The resident in a long-term care facility has many needs. These needs include special medical care, special diets, personal care, specific therapies, nursing care, and recreational and social activities over a long period of time.

▶ Medical Care

The team members who are responsible for the resident's medical care are the physician, the pharmacist, the director of nursing, the charge nurse, and the medication nurse.

▶ Nutrition

The dietitian is responsible for the resident's **nutrition.**

▶ Personal Care

Personal care of the resident is the responsibility of the nurse and nursing assistants.

▶ Therapy

The physical and occupational therapists are responsible for the resident's rehabilitative therapies.

▶ Recreation

Recreational and social needs are the responsibility of the activity coordinator and the resident's family and friends, as well as the nursing staff.

▶ The Whole Team

All of these people together make up the healthcare team. The nursing assistant is an important member of this team and is the one who provides the most direct care for the resident. You may be asked to assist the other team members in providing some of these services.

Teamwork is very important. The team members must all cooperate in gathering information, planning, and performing what needs to be done for each individual resident. After care is given, team members must also cooperate to evaluate the services to be sure the resident's needs were met.

TYPES OF LONG-TERM CARE FACILITIES

There are many types of long-term care facilities to meet different needs. You should be aware of these different facilities. Some of the residents of your facility may need to move to a different type of care as their needs change.

Most long-term care facilities are often referred to as **nursing homes**. Long-term care is not just for older people, however. Many younger adults who need special care and assistance because of injury or disability also live in long-term care facilities.

The goals of long-term care are to provide the necessary physical care, medical care, rehabilitation and social activities that promote the health and well-being of each individual resident.

The following list includes most types of medical facilities:

Hospital — A facility that provides all types of medical care. It may also provide long-term care in a **transitional care unit**.

Subacute care unit — Sometimes called an **intermediate care facility**. It provides nursing care for patients who are recovering from surgery or illness, with some supervision by a registered nurse.

Long-term care facility — Sometimes called an **extended care facility**. An institution that provides nursing care 24-hours a day.

Board and care facility — An institution that offers some care and supervision for residents who need it. The residents are usually ambulatory. Often, some nursing care is provided, but not 24-hours a day.

Assisted living facility — A facility that provides meals, laundry, and transportation services for persons who cannot live independently. It does not usually offer nursing care.

Adult day care — A facility that provides meals and activities but not living facilities for adults who attend during the day only.

Mental health facility — A facility that provides care for mentally ill. Recently, mental illness is being treated more and more on an **outpatient** basis and in the home.

Hospice facility – A facility that provides 24-hour care for the terminally ill.

Home care — Healthcare provided for a person's needs in his or her own home. This is becoming more common because it is less costly and allows the person to recover at home.

HOW IS HEALTHCARE CHANGING?

Over the last 20 years there have been tremendous changes in the healthcare system in America. Some of these changes have come about because of rising medical costs, and some because state and federal governments have passed laws to try to protect patients and ensure quality of care. You should be aware of some of these changes.

What is OBRA?

One federal law that directly affects long-term care was passed in 1987 and took affect in 1990. You will hear it referred to as **OBRA**, which stands for the Omnibus Budget Reconciliation Act. OBRA focuses on the care of the older people in long-term care facilities. It defines the rights residents have (you will learn about these in the next chapter).

OBRA also sets standards for quality of care and for the training of nursing personnel. For example, under OBRA, to become a nursing assistant you must complete a nursing assistant course of at least 75 hours, and you must pass a competency exam that tests both written and manual skills. Some states have laws that set even stronger standards.

Medicare and Medicaid

Medicare is the federal program that pays for some of the healthcare of those over 65 and the permanently disabled. It covers only limited long-term care expenses.

Medicaid is a federal program that offers money to the states to pay for some of the healthcare of people who cannot afford it. Benefits vary from state to state. In some states Medicaid funds help pay long-term care costs.

Managed Care Systems

In the past, people who needed medical care simply went to a doctor or a hospital and paid them directly for their services. As costs went up, many employers offered health insurance that paid for a large part of these costs. Today, with costs still rising, a number of organizations have been developed to try to make medical care more efficient. Some terms used in this changing system are:

HMO (Health Maintenance Organization) — This is an institution that agrees to provide all of a person's health care for a single agreed amount. Some HMOs hire physicians and other staff and run their own hospitals.

PPO (Preferred Provider Organization) — This plan offers to pay a person's healthcare costs as long as they select physicians from a list of physicians who are part of the plan.

Disease Management — A plan that covers a specific chronic disease, such as asthma. It emphasizes patient education and following a definite set of procedures.

DRGs (Diagnosis Related Groupings) — Plans, introduced by the government, that cover specific conditions or diseases. The government pays a set amount for each condition or disease and the institution decides how to spend it.

*Circle the correct answer. There is only **one** correct answer.*

1. **A long-term care facility provides medical care, but not recreation or other therapies.**

    a. True   (b). False

2. **The word nutrition relates to what?**

    a. Bathing.
    b. Toileting.
    (c). Foods.
    d. Recreation.

3. **A board and care facility provides 24-hour nursing.**

    a. True   (b). False

4. **Which of the following is usually NOT a long-term care facility?**

    a. Subacute care facility.
    (b.) Hospital.
    c. Board and care facility.
    d. Assisted Living facility.

5. **A hospice treats people who are dying.**

    (a.) True   b. False

6. **OBRA is a government act that relates to setting standards for what?**

    a. Drug therapy.

    b. Long-term care.

    c. Emergency rooms.

    d. Outpatient care.

7. **Medicare covers all long-term care costs.**

    a. True   b. False

8. **Under OBRA, a nursing assistant must have at least how many hours of training?**

    a. 25.

    b. 50.

    c. 75.

    d. 100.

9. **Which institution usually hires its own physicians?**

    a. HMO.

    b. PPO.

    c. DRG.

    d. Medicaid.

10. **Which of the following statements is true about DRGs?**

    a. The government pays a set amount for each medical condition.

    b. The government pays whatever it costs to cure the condition.

    c. The government will not pay for them.

    d. The government pays 50% of the costs.

▶ The resident has the right to personal privacy and the confidentiality of his or her personal and clinical records. Personal privacy includes the residence area, medical treatment, written and telephone communications, personal care visits, and meetings of family and resident groups, but this does not require the facility to provide a private room.

▶ The resident has the right to voice grievances with respect to treatment or care that is, or fails to be furnished, without discrimination or reprisal for voicing the grievances.

▶ The resident has the right to privacy in written communications, including the right to send and receive mail promptly that is unopened, and have access to stationery, postage, and writing implements at the resident's own expense.

▶ The resident has the right to have regular access to the private use of a telephone.

▶ The resident has the right to retain and use personal possessions, including some furnishings and appropriate clothing, as space permits, unless to do so would infringe upon the rights or health and safety of other residents.

▶ The resident has the right to share a room with his or her spouse when married residents live in the same facility and both spouses consent to the arrangement.

▶ The resident has the right to be free from any physical restraints imposed or psychoactive drug administered for purposes of discipline or convenience, and not required to treat the resident's medical symptoms.

▶ The resident has the right to be free from verbal, sexual, physical or mental abuse, corporal punishment, and involuntary seclusion.

▶ The resident has the right to interact with members of the community both inside and outside the facility.

▶ The resident has the right to participate in social, religious, and community activities that do not interfere with the rights of other residents in the facility.

▶ The resident has the right to be treated with consideration, respect and full recognition of his or her dignity and individuality, including privacy in treatment and in care for his or her personal needs. (Never use nicknames such as "Honey," "Sweetie," "Gramps," or "Cutie." These nicknames show disrespect.)

Additional Rights of the Long-Term Care Resident Are As Follows:

▶ The resident has the right to inspect and purchase photocopies of all records pertaining to the resident, upon written request and 48 hours notice to the facility.

▶ The resident has the right to be fully informed in language that he or she can understand of his or her total health status, including but not limited to, his or her medical condition.

▶ The resident has the right to manage his or her financial affairs and the facility may not require residents to deposit their personal funds with the facility.

▶ The resident has the right to choose a personal attending physician.

▶ The resident has the right to be fully informed in advance about the care and treatment and of any changes in the care or treatment that may affect the resident's well-being.

▶ The resident has the right to, unless adjudged incompetent or otherwise found to be incapacitated under the laws of the State, participate in planning care and treatment or changes in care and treatment.

▶ The resident has the right to prompt efforts by the facility to resolve grievances the resident may have, including those with respect to the behavior of other residents.

▶ The resident has the right to examine the results of the most recent survey of the facility conducted by federal or state surveyors and any plan of correction in effect with respect to the facility. The results must be posted by the facility in a place readily accessible to residents.

▶ The resident has the right to receive information from agencies acting as client advocates, and be afforded the opportunity to contact these agencies.

▶ The resident has the right to refuse to perform services for the facility.

▶ The resident has the right to perform services for the facility, if he or she chooses.

▶ The resident has the right to choose activities, schedules, and healthcare consistent with his or her interests, assessments, and plans of care.

▶ The resident has the right to make choices about aspects of his or her life in the facility that are significant to the resident.

▶ The resident has the right to organize and participate in resident groups in the facility.

▶ The resident has the right to reside and receive services in the facility with reasonable accommodation of individual needs and preferences, except where the health or safety of the individual or other residents would be endangered.

▶ The resident has the right to receive notice before the resident's room or roommate in the facility is changed.

▶ The resident has the right to make choices about aspects of his or her life in the facility that are significant to the resident.

Advance Directives

In the last few years it has become more common for residents to state their wishes about what steps should be taken, or not taken, to keep them alive as they approach death. This is called an **advance directive**, or a **living will**. Some advance directives call for taking no special measures at all to keep the resident alive. Some call for no intravenous feedings. And some may insist on not having CPR in the case of a heart attack.

Any advance directives will be filed with the resident's chart. You should learn about them for each resident and work with the rest of the staff to follow them. In most states, advance directives are **legal** and you must obey them.

If a resident appears to be near death, you should check to see if there are any advance directives. And if a resident appears to change his or her mind at any time, even with a few words or a nod, you must honor that new wish and report it immediately to the person in charge.

Other Legal Terms

As a member of a healthcare team, there are a few other legal terms you should be familiar with. These will help you understand and meet your legal obligations.

▶ *Assault.* **Assault** is using physical violence against someone or even threatening to use violence. There is no excuse for the use of violence or threatening violence against any of your residents, and you are subject to arrest and prosecution for assault if you do.

▶ *Battery.* In the law, **battery** is the actual use of violence. Sometimes both terms are included in a single expression: "assault and battery."

▶ *Elder abuse.* **Elder abuse** is mistreatment of older people. Some older people become confused, argumentative, and uncooperative. There is a tendency for some caregivers to become impatient and strike out at these "troublesome" older people.

You cannot ever allow yourself to do this. It is illegal and it is wrong. In Chapter 6 you will learn some ways to deal with the frustrations and stress of the job to help prevent any acts of violence or abuse.

▶ *Informed consent.* **Informed consent** is obtaining permission to perform a procedure on a resident only after explaining all the risks. You must be certain you have informed consent before beginning any procedure, even something as simple as trimming the resident's fingernails.

▶ *Malpractice.* **Malpractice** is neglect or wrong treatment of a resident by a licensed professional person. You will learn about negligence in the next chapter.

▶ *Ombudsman.* **Ombudsman** is a guardian who is assigned to look out for the rights of others. Some facilities have a designated ombudsman who watches over the facility and tries to prevent any illegal, unethical, or unfair acts.

*Circle the correct answer. There is only **one** correct answer.*

1. **All residents have the right to be free from discrimination on the basis of age, sex, race, religion, ethnic origin, or physical handicap.**

    a. True   b. False

2. **The rules in the Resident's Bill of Rights are based on kindness and good sense but they are not legally required.**

    a. True   b. False

3. **Residents give up the right to have personal possessions when they enter a long-term care facility.**

    a. True   b. False

4. **Residents have the right to make telephone calls without the staff listening in.**

    a. True   b. False

5. **According to The Resident's Bill of Rights, which of the following statements is false?**

    a. Residents have the right to refuse treatment to the extent permitted by law.

    b. Abusing a resident is against the law.

    c. Critically ill residents are never allowed visitors.

    d. Information on a resident's chart is confidential.

6. **A resident has the right to complain about the facility, its care, and its staff members.**

    a. True   b. False

7. **It is okay to use nicknames, such as "Honey" or "Pops," when addressing residents.**

    a. True   b. False

8. **Advance directives define what steps to take or not to take to extend life as someone approaches death.**

    a. True   b. False

9. **Threatening to use physical violence against a resident is an example of:**

    a. Battery.

    b. Reprisal.

    c. Assault.

    d. Discrimination.

10. **Informed consent means the resident must:**

    a. Undergo a procedure whether the resident wants to or not.

    b. Undergo a procedure only when he or she *doesn't* want it.

    c. Understand and give consent to a procedure before it is performed.

    d. Give consent after a procedure is performed.

Chapter 4

ETHICS AND CONFIDENTIALITY

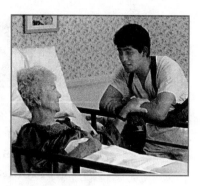

 See additional examples, descriptions and demonstrations of the concepts discussed in this chapter in the Medcom videotape "Confidentiality: Who Needs to Know" (M204).

In this chapter... you will learn about:

▶ The nursing care code of ethics.

▶ The importance of confidentiality.

▶ Avoiding negligence.

DEFINITIONS

Code of Ethics: An agreed upon set of moral principles or values.

Confidentiality: Not revealing information about residents except within the healthcare team.

Libel: A false and damaging written statement.

Negligence: Failure to give proper care, resulting in physical or emotional harm to a resident.

Slander: A false and damaging spoken statement.

THE NURSING CODE OF ETHICS

Nursing assistants have a great deal of responsibility. Not only must they take care of individual residents, but they must also obey certain rules in order to protect the residents' rights, the facility, and themselves.

In addition to legal regulations and facility rules, nursing assistants are expected to behave according to a **code of ethics**. Ethics refer to the honest, decent way to work with your residents and your employer.

Ethical Behavior Toward Your Residents

Ethical behavior toward your residents includes:

1. Treating all residents with respect and courtesy. By being considerate and courteous with your residents, you tell them you respect them as individuals and you are truly concerned about them.

2. Performing your duties to the best of your ability. It is the nursing assistant's responsibility to learn the skills necessary to fulfill his or her duties. It is important to always do your best. If you are unsure of any aspect of care, ask the charge nurse for assistance.

3. Responding to a resident's needs even though that particular resident is not assigned to you. Nursing assistants have many responsibilities and must work hard to carry them out for their assigned residents. However, it is unethical to ignore a resident's needs even though that resident may be assigned to someone else. Residents are not to be ignored.

4. Keeping yourself neat, clean, and professional looking at all times. This is another way of showing respect for your residents, your employer, and yourself.

5. Having a cheerful, positive attitude. Your attitude affects everyone around you and influences the care you give.

6. Remembering that the resident's well-being is your first concern. Your personal needs must be put aside when giving care to your residents.

Ethical behavior toward your employer includes:

1. Working your assigned shift, including being on time and working until your shift ends. Arriving late or not being ready to start work as soon as you arrive means more work for your coworkers and less help available for the residents.

2. Not being absent unless you are ill or there is an emergency. Absences cause extra work for your coworkers and less care for the residents.

3. Notifying your employer as soon as possible when it is necessary to be absent. Substitutes must be arranged when you are absent. The sooner you notify your employer, the easier it will be to find a substitute.

4. Following the instructions given by your supervisor and questioning any instruction that does not meet the resident's need. Individual care plans are developed to provide the best care for each resident, and you are responsible for following that plan of care.

5. Being helpful, friendly, and cooperative with other staff members. Nursing care is teamwork, and your attitude affects the team and the residents.

AVOIDING NEGLIGENCE

As a nursing assistant, you are required to provide the care ordered for every resident and to ensure their safety. Failure to respond to the duties assigned in a responsible and trustworthy manner is called **negligence**. Some examples of negligence are:

1. Serving the wrong diet to a resident.

2. Failure to put up bed rails when they have been ordered, resulting in the resident falling out of bed.

3. Failure to reposition a resident when ordered, resulting in the resident developing decubitus ulcers (pressure sores).

4. Administering medication or treatments. The nursing assistant is not trained or permitted by law to give any medication or treatments.

Negligence occurs when the nursing assistant does not follow the care plan. Negligence is judged by comparing your actions with those of someone else with the same experience and under similar circumstances. It is extremely important for the nursing assistant to follow orders and the care plan very carefully. In this way, you will be giving residents the best possible care.

CONFIDENTIALITY

Another important legal and ethical responsibility concerns **confidentiality** of information about residents. Residents have the right to privacy. This means that you may not share information about a resident's medical condition, personal or family problems, confidences, or any personal information. Unless private information is needed to provide care or treatment, it is unethical to repeat it. This would be considered an invasion of privacy and would violate the resident's right to privacy. Remember the golden rule and imagine how you would feel if people gossiped about your private medical information.

HIPAA

The legal rules regarding confidentiality have been strengthened through a federal law known as the Health Insurance Portability and Accountability Act, usually called HIPAA. HIPAA includes a large number of regulations for healthcare facilities and healthcare workers, but HIPAA's privacy requirements are what nursing assistants should be aware of most.

HIPAA rules prohibits the sharing of a resident's medical information in any form (orally, on paper, or in an electronic format) with anyone who is not directly providing care for that resident without the patient's written permission.

Your facility must have its privacy policies explained to the patient, and make a good faith effort to obtain the resident's written acknowledgement of this. HIPAA's privacy rules include serious criminal and civil penalties for privacy violations. So it is crucial that you know and follow the privacy policies of your facility and protect the privacy of your residents.

SLANDER AND LIBEL

It is also illegal and unethical to make damaging statements about residents. A false or damaging statement that is spoken is called *slander*. Those that are written are considered *libel*. Resist the temptation to gossip; it could be considered slander. Be careful not to discuss information about residents with others.

EXERCISES

*Circle the correct answer. There is only **one** correct answer.*

1. **Which of the following is an example of negligence?**

    a. Treating all residents with respect and courtesy.
    b. Gossiping about a resident.
    c. Serving a resident the wrong diet.
    d. Assaulting a resident.

2. **It is unethical to ignore a resident's needs.**

    a. True   b. False

3. **Two residents, Mrs. Jenkins and Mrs. Sloane, are overheard gossiping about another resident. What is the best action the nursing assistant can take?**

    a. Encourage the residents to talk about something they enjoy doing.
    b. Have them gossip about another resident instead.
    c. Yell at them.
    d. Tell them to be quiet.

4. **When is it ethical to share information about a resident?**

    a. Any time.

    b. Only when it is someone else's resident.

    c. When the information is needed to provide care or treatment.

    d. When you are with other staff members.

5. **Negligence occurs when you do not follow the care plan.**

    a. True   b. False

6. **When caring for a resident, it is okay to question your supervisor's instructions if you think they do not meet the resident's needs.**

    a. True   b. False

7. **Which of the following is NOT an ethical responsibility of the nursing assistant in his or her relationship with the resident?**

    a. Looking professional, neat and clean.

    b. Putting personal needs aside and taking care of your resident's needs first.

    c. Paying the resident's bills.

    d. Maintaining a cheerful, positive attitude.

8. **Which of the following is NOT an ethical responsibility of the nursing assistant as an employee?**

    a. Being on time for work.

    b. Being absent as little as possible.

    c. Being helpful, friendly, and cooperative.

    d. Working independently from your coworkers.

9. **It's okay to be absent from work if you do not wake up in time, and you miss your transportation.**

    a. True   b. False

10. **Teamwork among the staff and the residents is not particularly important in a long-term care facility.**

    a. True   b. False

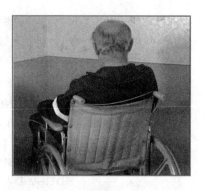

Chapter 5

ABUSE AND NEGLECT

 For additional examples and descriptions of the concepts discussed in this chapter, see the Medcom videotape, "Recognizing Elder Abuse: Working Together to Keep Residents Safe" (M217).

In this chapter... you will learn about:

▶ Signs of abuse or neglect.

▶ How to prevent abuse or neglect.

▶ Reporting abuse or neglect.

DEFINITIONS

Abuse:	Causing physical or emotional harm to someone in your care.
Active neglect:	Failing to provide needed care on purpose.
Financial abuse:	Taking money or possessions from those in your care.
Neglect:	Failing to provide needed care.
Passive neglect:	Failing to provide needed care, unintentionally.
Physical abuse:	Causing harm with a blow, a slap, or rough handling.
Psychological abuse:	Causing emotional harm by humiliating, insulting, or isolating someone.

WHAT ARE ABUSE AND NEGLECT

Federal laws says that all residents have the "right to be free from verbal, sexual, physical, and mental abuse, corporal punishment and involuntary seclusion." You must not abuse residents yourself, and you must remain alert for abuse by other caregivers, other residents, family members and visitors.

Abuse

Abuse is something you DO to harm a resident. It can be physical, such as a blow or a hard shaking, or it can be sexual or even psychological, such as yelling at a resident or humiliating him or her. Using restraints or isolation simply for your convenience, without a physician order, is a form of abuse. Financial abuse is stealing property or money from a resident.

Neglect

Neglect is something that you DON'T do that you should be doing. Since you are a caretaker and some residents are unable to do things for themselves, if you withhold needed care, it is called neglect. Active neglect is deliberately withholding care, such as leaving a bedridden person alone for long periods. Passive neglect is also withholding care, but not intentionally. Perhaps you don't know a resident's needs and don't try to find out.

You must also be alert for signs of self-abuse or self-neglect. Some residents, out of anger or confusion or loss of abilities, may perform acts of abuse or neglect on themselves.

WHO IS THE MOST VULNERABLE?

Obviously, everyone in a long-term care facility is vulnerable to some forms of abuse or neglect. Those who are particularly vulnerable are the elderly, those residents over 75 or 80 years old. In addition pay particular attention to:

> ▶ Those who are physically ill, disabled, or just very weak.
>
> ▶ Those who are developmentally disabled.
>
> ▶ Those who are mentally ill or mentally disabled.
>
> ▶ Those who are suffering from Alzheimer's or other forms of dementia.
>
> ▶ Those with communication problems, such as hearing, speech or vision loss.

These are the residents who most need your help to help prevent abuse and neglect. They may not be able to speak for themselves or protect themselves. They need the caregiver to assist them in this area.

SIGNS OF ABUSE

There are some signs you must watch for. These signs may not mean abuse, but if you see them you should report them to your supervisor.

Injuries

Some injuries are "suspicious" and should be reported to your charge nurse or your supervisor.

▶ Broken bones or other major injuries, such as puncture wounds

▶ Bite marks or scratches

▶ Strap marks

▶ Bruises

▶ Burn marks, or scalding burns, which occur when the water is far too hot

Other Signs of Abuse

Some other signs that might indicate abuse are not as obvious as injuries. You should be alert if a resident:

▶ Yells obscenities or shows anger or poor self-control

▶ Is afraid to be alone or afraid of certain caregivers

▶ Has constant pain

▶ Threatens to hurt others

▶ Hides or withdraws suddenly

SIGNS OF NEGLECT

Neglect can be more difficult to detect. Here are some signs you should watch for:

▶ Pressure sores

▶ A body that is not clean or is obviously uncared for

▶ Body lice

▶ Weight loss or dehydration

▶ Poor appetite

▶ Resident refuses care or refuses to use money for himself or herself

PREVENTING ABUSE OR NEGLECT

Working with residents can sometimes be frustrating and very difficult. One important way you can help prevent abuse is to take care of your own stress level so you do not snap and cause abuse yourself. We will discuss handling stress in the next chapter.

There are also ways you can be "proactive" in preventing abuse and neglect. This means taking steps ahead of time to prevent situations that might lead to abuse. Encourage residents, as much as possible, to maintain a normal life, connected to a circle of friends and family. Try to get residents to:

▶ Keep a group of friends

▶ Participate in community activities

▶ Go to personal care appointments, such as hairdresser and dentist, if possible

▶ Have one good friend outside the family and correspond regularly

▶ Invite guests to visit

▶ Remain neat and organized

▶ Protect their valuables and don't scatter them around

▶ Keep financial control, if possible

You should also post an abuse hotline telephone number and make sure the residents know where it is and have access to a telephone.

REPORTING ABUSE AND NEGLECT

If you remain alert for signs of abuse or neglect, you may eventually see them. Then you must act. In most states, you are required by law to report your suspicion. But you are not a detective or a police officer. It is not your responsibility to investigate or to confront anyone you suspect.

The correct action, if you suspect abuse, is to report it to your supervisor, and then keep it confidential. Do not go around the facility telling everyone about your suspicions.

Your facility will probably have a form for you to fill out and list the signs you have observed. You should learn the policies and procedures in your facility. Your supervisor will take any action necessary to stop the abuse or neglect, to relocate the victim if necessary, and contact any outside authorities.

Many residents in a long-term care facility are especially vulnerable to abuse or neglect. As a caretaker you must remain alert for the signs of these things and report them to your supervisor. Abuse and neglect are crimes and must not be allowed to continue.

*Circle the correct answer. There is only **one** correct answer.*

1. **Abuse only refers to harm caused by a caregiver.**

    a. True   b. False

2. **All of the actions below could be physical abuse EXCEPT _____.**

    a. Slapping a resident

    b. Locking a resident in a room for your convenience

    c. Calling a resident names

    d. Shaking a resident hard

3. **Neglect is always intentionally withholding needed care to a resident.**

    a. True   b. False

4. **Which resident below is most vulnerable to abuse?**

    a. A new resident

    b. A healthy resident with many friends

    c. A male resident

    d. A resident with dementia and speech difficulty

5. **All of the injuries or conditions below can suggest physical abuse except _____.**

    a. Bruises

    b. A runny nose

    c. A broken bone

    d. Burns

6. **All of the signs below can suggest abuse except _____.**

   a. Hiding
   b. Fear of a particular caregiver
   c. Yelling obscenities
   d. Having a large circle of friends

7. **All of the signs below suggest neglect except _____.**

   a. Tidy hair
   b. Pressure sores
   c. Lice
   d. Weight loss

8. **To help prevent abuse you should suggest the resident _____.**

   a. Avoid all friends
   b. Participate in group activities
   c. Avoid outside appointments, such as hairdressers
   d. Never invite guests

9. **If you suspect abuse, you should _____.**

   a. Investigate
   b. Confront the person you suspect
   c. Report it to your supervisor
   d. Immediately isolate the resident

10. **Once you have reported abuse, you should warn everyone in the facility about the caretaker involved.**

   a. True   b. False

Chapter 6

CARING FOR OTHERS AND DEALING WITH STRESS

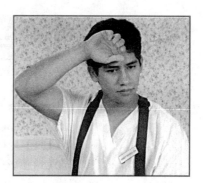

In this chapter... you will learn about:

▶ How your feelings can affect your ability to do your job.
▶ How to deal with stress.

DEFINITIONS

Prejudice: Preconceived, unreasonable judgement or opinion.

Stress: Tension and nervousness that build up in a
                     person.

All of us have much of the same basic needs. We need air, water, food, and shelter. But we also have emotional needs to feel loved, understood, important, worthwhile, and safe. You have these needs and so do your residents.

We also have differences. We do not look alike, our values differ, we sound different, and we react in distinctive ways. These differences make our world more interesting. If everyone were the same, it would be a dull world.

Sometimes differences cause us not to like someone. We may have developed **prejudices** against certain groups of people when we see them as being different from us. These feelings and attitudes affect our behavior. All of us have prejudices and we must find ways to deal with them.

Dealing with Prejudices

You will probably find that many of your residents are different from you. Many of them are probably older than you are, and they certainly are sicker or more handicapped than you are. They also may be a different race or from a different culture.

If you only see these differences as "something wrong" with the residents, you may end up becoming annoyed by their needs. You may think they are making unnecessary demands on you. Try to see the differences as a natural part of life. Older people naturally have more needs in some ways. People raised in other cultures naturally expect different things of people.

You have chosen a profession of caring about people. You should let your own life be enriched by these differences you will see every day. Talk to your residents whenever you can. Learn more about other peoples. Learn about the lives your residents have led, and the things they have learned. Learn about different foods, customs, beliefs, and different stages of life.

Most cultures honor the wisdom that comes with age. Your residents are not just helpless invalids to be moved and fed as quickly as possible so you can get on to the next task. They are experienced human beings you can learn from. The more you consider your residents as equals and talk with them, the more you will enjoy your job and grow in the job.

STRESS

Accepting and caring for your residents doesn't mean you will never feel frustrated, angry, or impatient. In fact, because you give so much of yourself as a nursing assistant, it can be a very difficult profession. Everyone has impatient feelings from time to time. When these negative feelings do occur, it is important for you to understand why you feel this way and not let the feelings be directed against your residents.

First, you should examine your home life for any causes that may be making your job **stress** worse. Here are some possible causes:

▶ *Working "two jobs."* Caring for the demands of a family by yourself can be overwhelming when you also work outside the home.

▶ *Lack of enough sleep.* This can make anyone irritable.

▶ *Dieting.* Hunger can make you tired and irritable.

▶ *A personal crisis.* A relationship breaking up or the loss of a loved one.

▶ *Lack of exercise.* Being out of shape can tire you out quickly.

▶ *Feeling unliked or misunderstood.* Everyone needs a sense of self-esteem.

Then examine your job for causes of stress on the job.

• Feeling overworked.

• Feeling isolated from your coworkers.

• Feeling unappreciated.

- Resentment because you feel you are expected to do more than other coworkers.

Dealing with the Causes

If possible, you should try to deal with the causes of your stress. Some of the things to do are obvious. If you aren't getting enough sleep, you can work on scheduling your life so that you have time to sleep. Balance the major activities of your life and cut back on some of the less important things. If you are dieting, you must eat at least three small but well-balanced meals a day. You can start to exercise. Even walking briskly twenty minutes a day can be a big help. This can be surprisingly effective in dealing with stress.

Talk to your supervisor, or at a team meeting about your feelings. Just talking about your concerns may help. And your coworkers may be able to suggest other ways to help.

Some causes of stress you may not be able to change. For many people, especially working mothers, there is simply no way around working "two jobs." In this case, you should investigate stress reduction techniques to help yourself. Some of these techniques can be learned by yourself and some may need professional help. If you feel that stress is seriously interfering with your life or affecting your job, you should seek professional counseling.

Stress Reduction Techniques

Here are a few things you can do by yourself:

- Regular exercise helps relax the body and the mind.

- Just sitting with your feet up for a few minutes can calm you down. Try picturing a peaceful place that you enjoy.

- Talking regularly about your problems with a friend can help.

- Take a few minutes of quiet to do nothing but drink a glass of juice or water.

- Listen to relaxing music for a few minutes.

- Take up a new relaxing hobby (as long as it doesn't eat up even more time that you need).

There are also several stress reduction disciplines. These you will probably have to learn from a class or from a videotape.

- Meditation.

- Yoga.

- Formal relaxation classes.

Don't let your stress build up until you reach burnout in your job or explode at your residents. Your feelings affect the way you relate to others. You owe it to the residents to take care of yourself so you can give them the best possible care.

EXERCISES

Circle the correct answer. There is only **one** correct answer.

1. **All people look alike.**

    a. True   b. False

2. **Only a few people have prejudices.**

    a. True   b. False

3. **Feelings of prejudice do not affect our behavior.**

    a. True   b. False

4. **Learning about different cultures can enrich our lives.**

    a. True   b. False

5. **If you are a caring person, you will never be affected by stress.**

    a. True   b. False

6. **Which is probably NOT a cause of stress at home?**

    a. Working "two jobs."
    b. The loss of a loved one.
    c. A caring friend.
    d. Lack of sleep.

7. **Exercise will usually increase your stress level.**

    a. True   b. False

8. **Talking to your supervisor and coworkers can be one way of dealing with stress.**

    a. True   b. False

9. **Your own stress will NOT affect your behavior toward your residents feelings.**

    a. True   b. False

10. **If all else fails you should seek professional counseling.**

    a. True   b. False

Chapter 7

DOCUMENTATION

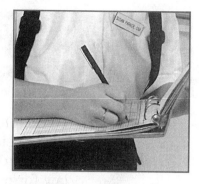

 Watch step-by-step demonstrations of the procedures discussed in this chapter in the Medcom videotape "Documenting Care:The Charting Process" (M207).

In this chapter... you will learn about:

▶ The resident care plan.

▶ The resident's chart.

▶ How to keep proper records.

DEFINITIONS

Chart:	The chart contains the healthcare plan, the physician's orders, and all the health information on one particular resident. It is a legal document and must be maintained properly.
Chronological:	Written in the order in which the events occurred.
Documentation:	Written information in the medical record.
Flow Sheet:	A graphic chart that is commonly used in long-term care to record resident information over time.
Kardex:	A card file kept at a convenient place that summarizes the nursing care plan for each resident.
Nursing Care Plan (Or Resident Care Plan):	The complete plan of care for each resident.
Objective Observation:	Observation based on facts you can see.
Subjective Observation:	Observation based on what you think.

DEVELOPING THE NURSING CARE PLAN

To enable everyone on the healthcare team to know what each resident needs, a *nursing care plan* (or resident care plan) is developed. The individual care plan is required by law for every resident of a healthcare facility. Each plan is different because each resident has different needs and goals.

All the health team members involved, the resident, the resident's family, the physician, and the nursing staff provide information for the development of the resident's care plan. The nursing assistant spends a great deal of time with individual residents and can contribute important information in developing and updating care plans.

Each member of the team identifies problems and goals for individual residents. Team members also develop a plan for achieving these goals in small identifiable steps. Goals are both short term and long term. Short term goals are easily attainable in a short period of time (e.g., "get out of bed within 1 week"). Long-term goals will probably take longer (e.g., "walk length of hall within 2 months").

The physician's orders are also included in the healthcare plan.

Examples of Nursing Care Plan Entries

Problem:	Resident is 15 pounds underweight.
Short-term Goal:	Resident will gain 2 pounds within 1 month.
Long-term Goal:	Resident will be at ideal body weight within 8 months.
Nursing Approach:	Encourage resident to eat. Provide dietary supplement prescribed. Monitor food intake.

All of these orders, plans, and goals are entered in the resident's **chart**. In this way, each member of the health care team knows exactly how to take care of each individual resident. This plan is the blueprint for resident care. You don't have to wonder how you are going to take care of your residents. The care plan will be your guide.

The daily entries on residents' charts help the healthcare team to continually review and update the individual care plans.

Everyone on the healthcare team will be working toward the same goals. As these goals are achieved, new ones are set. Helping a resident achieve a goal makes you feel good and helps to build your resident's self-esteem.

Remember, you can have an excellent care plan, but it is worthless unless it is followed carefully. It is the nursing assistant's responsibility to faithfully follow the care plan for each individual resident.

A summary of the nursing care plan is kept in the **Kardex.** This contains a card for each resident and is kept in a convenient place, usually the nursing station.

THE RESIDENT CHART

The nursing assistant has the legal and ethical responsibility to write accurate entries in every resident's chart. The chart is a legal **document**. The chart entries prove that something either has or has not been done. This protects the resident, the nursing assistant, the nurse, the healthcare team, and the facility. Information must be charted daily. Exact and timely records are extremely important.

The chart contains the nursing care plan, the physician's orders, and all the health information on that particular resident. It provides an accurate and continuing picture of the resident, the care and procedures ordered and provided, and the resident's response and progress. This information is used by the physician to review the resident's condition, to set new goals, and to order new treatment. It is used by the nursing staff as a guide to resident care, and as a record of the care.

The chart also contains information on safety precautions taken, observed changes in condition and behavior, potentially dangerous incidents (such as falls), and family and social background.

CHARTING

Depending upon the policies of the particular facility you work in, the nursing assistant may make daily entries and monthly summaries in the charts for each assigned resident. Or, you may be required to use a *flow sheet* to record the resident's activities of daily living. These entries are required to cover:

1. Nursing care and treatment provided to each resident.

2. The resident's response or lack of response to this care and treatment.

3. How the resident looks, reacts, and interacts.

4. The measures taken to protect the safety of the resident.

5. Changes in the resident's condition.

The entries are to be *objective observations*. This means that they are to be based on facts and not on your feelings or impressions. An example of an objective observation is: "The resident drank 2 oz. of water." When you include your own conclusions and impressions, the information becomes subjective. An example of a *subjective observation* is: "The resident didn't drink enough water." Subjective information is not appropriate for entries in the resident's chart. Remember, the resident's chart is a legal document. This means you are to chart only what actually occurred, and you are responsible for the accuracy of the entries you make.

▶ All entries must be written legibly in ink with a ballpoint pen, never with a felt tip pen.

▶ Every entry must be signed with your first initial, your last name, and your title.

▶ All entries must be in ***chronological*** order and contain the month, day, year, and time.

▶ Entries are to be exact, brief, and complete.

▶ Erasing and "white-out" are not allowed. If an error is made, draw one line through the incorrect words and write the word "error" above it. Initial and date it. Then make the correct entry.

▶ There should be no empty space left on a line or between entries. Draw a line through the center of the empty space and do not leave any empty lines between entries. This prevents anyone from adding information to your signed entry.

▶ Entries are to be made in the present tense. Example: "The resident ambulates without assistance."

▶ Use only approved medical abbreviations. Ditto marks are not to be used.

▶ Every sheet of paper in the chart must be properly identified with the resident's name and identifying information.

ABBREVIATIONS

You can use the commonly accepted abbreviations found in Appendix A to help you write brief, concise, but complete chart entries. As you study and use these abbreviations, you will become comfortable with using them.

Circle the correct answer. There is only **one** *correct answer.*

1. **A resident's nursing care plan is locked away and seen only by the physician.**

    a. True   b. False

2. **A nurse's entries in a resident's chart should be**

    a. Objective.

    b. Subjective.

    c. Written in felt pen.

    d. Written in pencil.

3. **Which of the following statements is subjective?**

    a. The resident gained six pounds.

    b. The resident ambulates without assistance.

    c. The resident is uncooperative.

    d. The resident cannot state his or her name.

4. **Which of the following statements is objective?**

    a. The resident looks thin.

    b. The resident is depressed.

    c. The resident's dress is inappropriate.

    d. The resident weighs 105 pounds.

5. **It is okay to erase errors in a resident's chart.**

    a. True   b. False

6. **All entries in the chart must be signed with your first initial, last name, and your title.**

    a. True   b. False

7. **The Kardex**

    a. Is a telephone list kept at the nursing station.

    b. Is a brief form of the nursing care plan.

    c. Is a device for erasing cards.

    d. Is given to the resident.

8. **A flow sheet**

    a. Is a way of measuring urine output.

    b. Is a way of tracking nursing assistant attendance.

    c. Is part of a nursing care plan.

    d. Is a chart used to record resident information.

    e. None of the above items.

9. **Only certain approved abbreviations may be used in chart entries.**

    a. True   b. False

10. **An objective statement is**

    a. "Temperature is 98.6 F"

    b. "Resident feels hot."

    c. "Resident looks hot."

    d. "Resident is very hot."

Chapter 8

ADMISSIONS

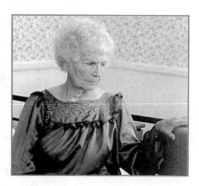

In this chapter... you will learn about:

▸ Welcoming a new resident to your facility.
▸ Preparing a resident unit.
▸ Welcoming a new resident into the unit.
▸ Assisting with the first observations of a new resident.

DEFINITIONS

Admission:	Steps followed when a resident is first brought to the facility.
Baseline Assessment:	First observations made on a new resident.

Coming to a long-term care facility for the first time can be very frightening and upsetting. In addition to being ill or weak, new residents may be leaving behind loved ones and familiar homes. They may also be leaving behind many activities that gave their lives meaning.

Some new residents may see this step as the "beginning of the end" of their life. Even if they hope the stay is temporary, it is in a very unfamiliar place. You should keep this in mind and treat every new resident just the way you would like to be treated in the same situation. Here are a few helpful hints for greeting a new resident:

- Be warm and friendly and try to make the new resident feel at home.

- Introduce yourself and always explain what you will be doing.

- Greet family and friends if they are present.

- Learn the resident's name and use it a lot. Do not use the resident's first name unless he or she asks you to.

- Introduce the new resident to other residents and to the facility.

- Answer any questions in a friendly and dignified manner.

- Remain confident and efficient.

PREPARING THE RESIDENT UNIT

Remember that the resident unit is about to become a new home for someone. The new resident was probably in a familiar and comfortable home only recently, and probably living with loved ones. You should do whatever you can to help in this change and make the resident unit seem comfortable and welcoming.

1. If the room is shared, inform the current resident that there will be a new roommate.

2. Make sure all the furniture is present and working properly.

3. Test all the lights to make sure they work. Test the TV, radio and telephone, if they are present.

4. Assemble the room kit that is used in your facility. This might include:

   • Water pitcher and glass. (Make sure the resident is allowed to drink water before filling the pitcher.)

   • Soap and washcloth.

   • Towel.

   • Basin.

   • Lotion and mouthwash.

5. Find out if any special medical equipment, such as an IV stand, is needed.

6. Make the bed, and fold the sheets and blankets neatly downward to open the bed and make it welcoming.

WELCOMING THE RESIDENT INTO THE UNIT

When the resident unit is prepared, you can bring the new resident to the unit.

1. Calmly conduct the resident and family to the room. Don't rush them.

2. Introduce the new resident and family to any roommates.

3. Show the new resident around and explain where things are kept. Explain how things like lights, the TV, and the nursing call signal work.

4. Help the resident make a list of his or her personal possessions.

5. Help the new resident into bed or into a chair if he or she is allowed to sit up.

6. Explain the other areas of the facility. Explain what services are available.

7. Explain facility rules and meal times.

8. Answer any further questions the resident or family may have.

One final note: You should always remember how frightened the new resident may feel in the first hours or days in your facility. He or she must not feel you are rushing through the **admission** to get on to something "more important." Take the time to explain things and be pleasant. Establish yourself as a new friend that the resident can trust.

ASSISTING WITH A BASELINE ASSESSMENT

Most facilities perform a series of observations when the resident is first admitted. This is called a **baseline assessment**. This can be checked against later observations to see if the resident is getting better or getting worse in any area. This procedure is generally the responsibility of the nurse, but you will probably assist and you may perform some of the routine observations.

Procedures in your facility may vary, but they will probably be similar to the following:

1. Wash your hands.

2. Assemble the equipment that will be needed in the resident unit.

    *   Admission checklist, worksheet, or chart.

    *   Thermometer.

    *   Stethoscope.

    *   Blood pressure gauge.

    *   A watch with a second hand.

    *   Scale.

    *   Urine specimen cup and rubber gloves (if required).

    *   Gown or pajamas (if used in your facility).

3. Identify the resident and double check the name against any paperwork.

4. Explain to the resident what is going to happen.

5. Ask family and friends to wait in the lobby or waiting area.

6. Provide privacy.

7. Assist the nurse as required.

*Circle the correct answer. There is only **one** correct answer.*

1. **Being admitted to a long-term care facility for the first time can be very frightening.**

   a. True   b. False

2. **You should not call the new resident by name.**

   a. True   b. False

3. **You should refer all questions from the new resident to your supervisor.**

   a. True   b. False

4. **You should hurry the new resident into the resident unit.**

   a. True   b. False

5. **In preparing the resident unit for a new resident, how should the bed be left?**

   a. Stripped.

   b. Stripped with new sheets folded and ready to put on.

   c. Made up with the blanket tucked under the pillow at the head of the bed.

   d. Made up with sheets and blankets folded neatly downward to the foot of the bed.

6. **You should test the lights when you are preparing the resident unit.**

   a. True   b. False

7. **Which item listed below is probably NOT in the room kit in the resident unit?**

   a. Water jug.

   b. Basin.

   c. Ashtray.

   d. Washcloth.

8. **You should introduce the new resident to any roommates in the unit.**

   a. True   b. False

9. **Which statement describes a baseline assessment?**

   a. Weighing the new resident.

   b. Performing a series of observations on the new resident.

   c. Observing the resident's height.

   d. Preparing the resident unit.

10. **Which item is probably NOT part of the equipment needed to perform an initial observation on a new resident?**

    a. Thermometer.

    b. Stethoscope.

    c. Hypodermic syringe.

    d. Watch with second hand.

Chapter 9

DISASTERS AND EVACUATION

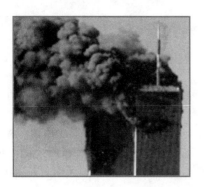

In this chapter... you will learn about:

▶ The importance of knowing what to do in a disaster

▶ Reporting emergencies

▶ Evacuating residents

DEFINITIONS

Centers for Disease Control (CDC): The government agency responsible for preventing or fighting the outbreak of epidemic diseases.

Disaster: Any event that disrupts the normal activities of a community and causes casualties.

Triage: Screening a number of disaster victims to determine who has the most severe injuries and needs to be treated first.

INTRODUCTION

The events of September 11, 2001 made it clear how important it is for every healthcare worker to think ahead and know what to do in emergencies. By a tragic coincidence, the disaster response center for all of New York City happened to be in the World Trade Center itself and was entirely destroyed by the collapse of the buildings.

Yet, within an hour a new center was up and running in the nearest healthcare facility--a long-term care center! This demonstrated how much of the community's ability to respond lay, not in the physical facilities themselves, but in the skills and training of people.

If your facility has a disaster plan, you should study it so you will know what to do in an emergency. If not, some of the simple actions listed below will help you be much better prepared if a disaster should strike near your facility.

TYPES OF DISASTERS

A disaster can be any event that disrupts the normal activities of your institution or community. There are many types, and they call for different types of responses.

Community Disasters

▶ Natural disasters such as fires, floods, tornadoes and earthquakes

▶ Other disasters such as terrorist incidents, bombs, airplane or train accidents with large numbers of casualties, and epidemics

In community disasters, or what are sometimes called mass-casualty disasters, you may expect that your facility will receive emergency patients from outside. Even a long-term care center may become a triage center or temporary hospital, and your supervisor may have you work with state or federal officials to help them use your facility for disaster management or recovery. Residents may need to be moved temporarily, and your facility's supplies may be needed for emergency relief.

To prepare yourself for this possibility, you should learn your facility's disaster plan, if it has one. Learn where all supplies are kept. Learn the location of fire extinguishers and any other relief equipment that might be available, such as respirators or first-aid supplies.

Institutional Disasters

These are disasters that may occur within your institution, and they are of two types.

▶ **Internal medical emergencies**, such as epidemics, poisonings, and the sudden death of key personnel.

You should report any suspected outbreaks of disease or poisoning immediately to your supervisor.

▶ **Internal non-medical emergencies**, such as loss of power, criminal activities, and computer failure.

Report any suspected non-medical emergencies immediately to your supervisor. If your supervisor is unavailable, you should know who to contact outside the facility.

For fire emergencies, refer to the chapter on fire safety.

THE DISASTER PLAN

The Joint Commission on Accreditation of Health Care Organizations (JCAHO) requires many healthcare institutions to have a disaster plan. Even if your facility is not required to have one, understanding what goes into a disaster plan can help you think ahead. The JCAHO plan contains four principles:

▶ **Easing the Disaster** – Make plans ahead of time to lessen the severity and impact of an emergency.

► *Preparation* – Build up needed organizational capacities, including supplies and equipment, staff orientation and training, planning processes, and organization-wide drills.

► *Response* – Define actions staff would take when confronted by an emergency, such as reporting to prearranged locations. Plan for a warning and notification process, priority-setting and becoming partners with other organizations.

► *Recovery* – Take steps to restore essential services and resume normal operations; plan for staff support and community response.

REPORTING EMERGENCIES

You should always report any suspected emergency first to your supervisor. But in some disasters your supervisor may not be available. You may be the only trained person present to take action. You should know where your facility keeps the home numbers of other staff in case you need to contact them, and you should know where each member of the staff resides. This may come in handy in a situation such as an earthquake or flood. Some personnel who live in the affected portions of the community may not be able to make it into work.

It is crucial that you also know where emergency telephone numbers are posted in your facility. You should have numbers for local police and fire, state health agencies, and other healthcare institutions in your area that may be able to lend you assistance.

Decide what sort of emergency you are facing. Is it medical? Is it internal or external? Is it criminal? Then decide the appropriate persons to contact for assistance.

WORKING WITH OUTSIDE OFFICIALS

In the event of any large-scale emergency with multiple casualties in your community, you may be asked to work with outside doctors, emergency personnel, investigators from the Centers for Disease Control (CDC) or many others. You should do your best to help make the supplies and the space of your facility available to respond to the emergency.

You are also responsible for all the residents in the facility. It is important to keep them calm in any emergency and to explain why any moves may be necessary, or why there are many other personnel suddenly using the building, for triage or other emergency procedures.

TRANSFER OR EVACUATION

Your supervisor will decide whether residents can be safely transferred within the facility in cases of internal disaster or evacuated to another facility in cases of external disaster.

Following is a general guideline regarding patient transfer during and after a disaster such as an earthquake:

Within Your Facility

1. Move all patients to a central area.

2. Issue extra blankets to all patients and keep them warm.

3. Close all drapes in the central area to protect against exposure to broken glass.

4. Close all doors to the central area including fire and smoke barrier doors.

5. Avoid using open flame devices.

6. Check for flashlights and extra batteries.

7. Reassure patients that all is well.

To Other Facilities

Should transfers of patients to other facilities be necessary, follow the guidelines set forth in your institution's policies and procedures.

Evacuation Procedures

If evacuation is necessary following an internal disaster, patients shall be evacuated until a search team has secured a place designated within the facility. Patients and personnel shall remain in the secured area until an "All Clear" has been given.

The use of elevators should be avoided. Supervisors should assign one staff member in each of their areas to remove patient charts. All such records shall be taken to an area designated by the person in charge.

No one shall be allowed to return to the building until an "All Clear" signal has been announced.

Assisting Evacuation

You should know how to assist those who cannot ambulate by themselves. The chapter on assisting ambulation explains how to assist those who can be evacuated with your assistance. In some cases, it may be preferable to use a wheelchair to help evacuate a resident more quickly, even if he or she is able to walk.

If wheelchairs are not available or are all in use, you should also know a few simple techniques for evacuating residents who are bedridden. You can use a blanket and work with two persons on each side of the blanket to carry a person into a safe area. In some emergencies, if you do not have assistance, you may have the person lie on a blanket and drag the resident to safety along the floor. The resident's safety is your first concern and if the resident must be evacuated rapidly, you must remain flexible and use whatever techniques you have available.

CONCLUSION

The keys to disaster planning are advance planning, preparedness and flexibility. It is important to minimize the disruptions of an emergency and handle a crisis in a calm and professional manner. The Disaster Plan in your facility must tell you how to address a wide variety of mass casualty events and you must be able to act quickly to address a specific event.

*Circle the correct answer. There is only **one** correct answer.*

1. **One lesson of the September 11, 2001 disaster was that _____.**

    a. Equipment is more important than trained personnel.

    b. Trained personnel are more important than equipment.

    c. Trained personnel and equipment are equally important.

    d. In a mass disaster no amount of planning will help.

2. **The following are all examples of natural disasters except _____.**

    a. Terrorism.

    b. Flood.

    c. Earthquake.

    d. Tornadoes.

3. **The following may all be examples of internal medical emergencies except _____.**

    a. Poisonings.

    b. Epidemics.

    c. Sudden death of key personnel.

    d. Loss of power.

4. **Which organization requires that many healthcare institutions have a disaster plan?**

    a. The police.

    b. CDC.

    c. The AMA.

    d. JCAHO.

5. **The "Easing the Disaster" portion of the disaster plan is meant to _____.**

   a. Restore essential services.

   b. Plan ahead of time to lessen the severity.

   c. Define who to contact.

   d. Set up disaster drills.

6. **The "Recovery" portion of the disaster plan is meant to _____.**

   a. Define who to contact in an emergency.

   b. Take steps to resume normal operations.

   c. Set up disaster drills.

   d. Plan ahead to lessen the severity.

7. **A long-term care institution must never be used for emergency care, even in a disaster.**

   a. True   b. False

8. **In the event of a disaster all medical supplies should be locked away to protect them.**

   a. True   b. False

9. **In the event of a disaster the use of elevators should be avoided.**

   a. True   b. False

10. **One technique you may need to use in an emergency evacuation is _____.**

    a. Dragging residents directly on the floor.

    b. Dragging residents on a blanket.

    c. Forcing bedridden residents to walk.

    d. Pushing wheelchairs down stairs.

Chapter 10

TRANSFERS, DISCHARGES AND HOMECARE

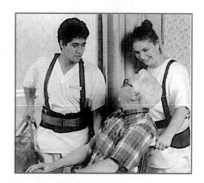

 Watch step-by-step demonstrations of the procedures discussed in this chapter in the Medcom videotape "The New Nursing Assistant 2000: Transfer and Ambulation" (CNA504).

In this chapter... you will learn about:

▶ Why a resident may need to be transferred.

▶ Preparing for a transfer.

▶ Assisting with a transfer.

▶ Assisting with the arrival.

▶ Discharges.

▶ Home Care.

DEFINITIONS

Client: A person receiving nursing assistant care in his or her own home instead of a long-term care facility.

Discharge: Steps followed when a resident is released from the facility.

Home Care: Care provided in a person's home.

Home Health Assistant (Home Healthcare Aide): A nursing assistant who goes to the patient's home to provide care.

Transfer: Steps followed when a resident is moved to another unit. The move may be to another room inside your facility or to another building.

WHY A RESIDENT MAY NEED TO BE TRANSFERRED OR DISCHARGED

Here are some possible reasons for a **transfer** or **discharge**:

▶ The resident's condition has changed. The resident may no longer need a room with oxygen, for example. Or the resident may now need a higher level of care that can only be given in another wing of your facility.

▶ The change may have been ordered by a physician.

▶ The resident may have asked for a new room.

▶ The resident's condition may have improved, and may be discharged to go home.

Any change, even a simple room change, can be frightening and upsetting. You should keep this in mind and try to reassure the resident. Find out the reasons for the transfer or discharge, and also find out what the resident has already been told about the reasons. Answer any questions in a friendly manner, keeping to the same reasons the resident has already been told.

PREPARING FOR A TRANSFER

There are a few things you can do ahead of a transfer to make the changes easier for everyone:

1. Make sure you have the permission of the resident or family for the transfer.

2. Make sure the resident knows the reasons for the transfer. Explain when and how the transfer will happen.

3. You may wish to speak to the nurse and nursing assistant in the new area. Share with them any information you have that would help them care for the resident.

4. You may wish to have the nurse or nursing assistant from the new area come over and meet the resident before the transfer.

ASSISTING WITH THE TRANSFER

The nurse is mainly responsible for the transfer, but you will probably assist. Your facility may even have a transfer team to take care of the transfer. Here are the steps to follow:

1. Make sure the new room is prepared before you begin.

2. Obtain the wheelchair, bed or cart to be used for the transfer.

3. Obtain any portable medical equipment that must move with the patient, such as an IV stand.

4. Wash your hands and check the resident's identification bracelet. Make very sure you are moving the right resident.

5. Explain to the resident what you will be doing.

6. Collect the resident's valuables from the unit and list them, if necessary. Have the resident place them all into a clearly marked bag or envelope, or do it with the resident watching.

7. Provide privacy. Help the patient into a robe and slippers if this is allowed.

8. Collect any medication, plus the chart and nursing plan to take with you.

9. Assist the nurse or transfer team with the transfer. Remain cheerful and reassure the resident.

It is very important to remember that you should never leave the resident alone during the transfer. And never leave the medications or records alone.

ASSISTING WITH THE ARRIVAL

Remember that the new room is about to become the resident's new home. Don't just leave the resident in the room and hurry away. You should do whatever you can to ease the transition and make the resident comfortable.

1. Help the resident into bed or into a chair, if he or she is allowed to sit up.

2. Make sure any roommates and the local nursing staff are introduced to the resident.

3. Transfer the valuables, chart, and medications to the local nursing staff. Help put these away if necessary.

4. Help explain to the resident anything that is different from the old room, and any different procedures.

5. Answer any questions the resident may have or make sure there is someone there who can answer them. Make sure the resident feels as comfortable as possible.

6. Wash your hands and complete any documentation necessary to describe the transfer.

You should bear in mind that a transfer is a little like an admission. The resident is moving into a new and unfamiliar home. You were a familiar part of the old home, and your presence can help the resident become comfortable in the new home. You may even want to offer to come back and visit from time to time.

There can be many reasons for a discharge. The resident may have improved enough to go to another facility or go home. The resident may wish to move to a facility that is closer to the family. Or the resident may not like your facility for some reason. In any case, the discharge must be approved by a physician.

Remember that a discharge can be an emotional time, just like any change. Remain calm and friendly, just as you would with a transfer.

Here are steps to follow for a discharge:

1. Make sure the physician has approved the discharge.

2. Obtain a wheelchair or other vehicle.

3. Wash your hands and help the resident dress, if possible. Explain what is happening.

4. Help the resident gather his or her belongings, if necessary. Check in all the drawers and closets. Help the family or resident gather any valuables placed in safe keeping in the facility.

5. Check with the nurse for any medications or medical equipment that must go with the resident.

6. When the appropriate vehicle arrives, assist in moving the resident to the discharge exit of the facility and into the vehicle.

7. Bid the resident and any family farewell.

8. Return to the unit and strip the bed and prepare it for another resident.

9. Wash your hands and complete any necessary paperwork to record the discharge.

Recently there has been a trend in medicine toward providing more nursing assistant care directly in a patient's home rather than in a facility. Not only is this often less expensive, but it also keeps the patient in a familiar place. A patient in a home is often called a **client**.

Nursing assistants who work in home care are often called **Home Health Assistants** or **Home Healthcare Aides**. They may work for an agency or they may be employed directly by a large company. Home Health Assistants work as part of a team with a nurse and physician, just as they would in a long-term care facility. They do many of the same tasks, but some of the tasks are very different. For example, tasks like infection control and safety are very different in a home than in a long-term care facility. Home Health Assistants may also help with many ordinary housekeeping tasks, such as cleaning up the kitchen or preparing a small meal.

If you wish to work as a Home Health Assistant, you should take special training in this work after you complete your nursing assistant training.

*Circle the correct answer. There is only **one** correct answer.*

1. **One reason for a transfer might be a change in a resident's condition.**

    a. True   b. False

2. **Simply changing from one room to another in the facility should NOT be frightening or upsetting to a resident.**

    a. True   b. False

3. **What might you tell the nurse and nursing assistant in the resident's new area?**

    a. Your own name.

    b. Anything that would help them care for the resident.

    c. How to do these duties.

    d. How to prepare the resident unit.

4. **You will not need to prepare the new room until after the transfer.**

    a. True   b. False

5. **What should you do with the resident's valuables during the transfer?**

    a. Leave them behind in the old room.

    b. Give them to the resident's roommate to hold.

    c. List them, put them in a bag and carry them along.

    d. Move them into the new room first.

6. **You must not leave the resident, the chart or any medications alone during the transfer.**

   a. True   b. False

7. **Once the resident reaches the new room, you should leave immediately.**

   a. True   b. False

8. **The only reason for a discharge is an improvement in the resident's condition.**

   a. True   b. False

9. **Before a discharge, check with the nurse for any medications the resident is taking so you can do what?**

   a. Discard them.

   b. Reuse them with another resident.

   c. Send them with the resident.

   d. Give them back to the nurse.

10. **Recently there has been a trend in medicine toward using more home care.**

    a. True   b. False

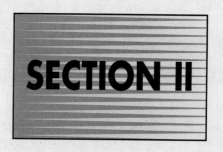

SECTION II

MEDICAL KNOWLEDGE

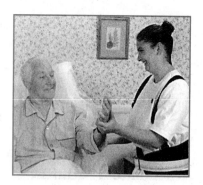

⚹ ANATOMY AND PHYSIOLOGY:
THE SKELETAL AND MUSCULAR SYSTEMS

In this chapter... you will learn about:

▶ The skeletal system.

▶ The muscular system.

▶ Some common problems of the skeletal and muscular systems.

DEFINITIONS

Abnormality:	Condition different from the normal.
Anatomy:	Parts of the body.
Anterior:	Front.
Atrophy:	The wasting away of unused muscle tissue.
Bursa:	A pad of cartilage that keeps bones from rubbing together.
Bursitis:	Inflammation of the bursa at a joint.
Contracture:	The permanent shortening of a muscle.
Disc:	Cushions of tissue between the bones of the spine.
Dislocation:	A change in the normal alignment of bones at a joint.
Fracture:	A broken bone.
Multiple Sclerosis:	A chronic degenerative disease of the nervous system resulting in the inability to move.

Definitions Continued...

Muscular Dystrophy:	A progressively crippling disease of the muscles.
Osteoarthritis:	Deterioration of cartilage in the joints with age, causing pain and stiffness.
Osteoporosis:	A condition that causes a decrease in the size and strength of the bones.
Paralysis:	Loss of voluntary control over a muscle.
Rheumatoid Arthritis:	Inflammation of the joints, causing limitation of movement.
Sprain:	A torn or stretched ligament or tendon.
Physiology:	How the body parts work.
Posterior:	Back.

SKELETAL SYSTEM

Bones

Our skeleton is made up of 4 different types of bones:

1. Long bones - such as leg bones.

2. Short bones - such as finger bones.

3. Irregular bones - Oddly shaped bones, such as the vertebrae of the spinal column.

4. Flat bones - such as the rib cage.

There are 206 bones in a skeleton. They are the framework of the body, giving it structure and support, and providing leverage for movement. Bones also protect some of the body's internal organs. The skull protects the brain; the rib cage protects the heart and lungs.

Bones also act as a storehouse for vital minerals, like calcium, needed by the body, and they produce red blood cells.

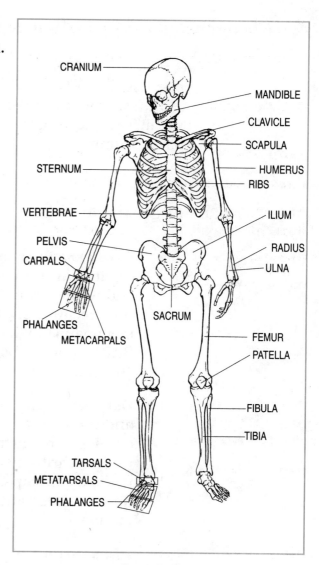

CRANIUM
MANDIBLE
CLAVICLE
SCAPULA
STERNUM
HUMERUS
RIBS
VERTEBRAE
ILIUM
PELVIS
RADIUS
CARPALS
ULNA
SACRUM
PHALANGES
METACARPALS
FEMUR
PATELLA
FIBULA
TIBIA
TARSALS
METATARSALS
PHALANGES

The skeleton

Joints

Joints are where bones are joined together. Joints form the hinges necessary for movement. Some joints, like the knees, work like a door hinge and allow the bones to flex. Some, like the hip, work like a ball and socket and allow the bones to rotate as well as flex. The joints in the spine both glide and pivot.

A fluid-filled capsule, called a **bursa** is a pad of cartilage that protects the joints and keeps the bones from rubbing together. The joints of the spine are protected by cushions called discs. These **discs** act as shock absorbers and help to protect the spinal cord.

Age Changes in the Skeletal System

As people get older, there is a natural and gradual loss of bone tissue. The bones tend to get weaker. This can also result from lack of movement. People tend to get shorter as they move into old age as a result of a shortening of the spinal column.

Abnormalities in the Skeletal System

▶ *Osteoporosis* is a condition in which the bones lose calcium and become porous and brittle. Both men and women can develop osteoporosis as they age, but, because of the hormone changes in menopause, older women are particularly at risk. Brittle, porous bones break easily. Even a strong sneeze may fracture a rib.

▶ *Osteoarthritis* is the deterioration of the cartilage and the resulting friction in the joints. Most people develop some arthritis as they become older. Osteoarthritis usually appears in the weight-bearing joints of the hips, knees, and vertebrae, and in the fingers. This causes pain, stiffness, and limited motion.

▶ *Rheumatoid arthritis* causes inflammation of the joints and may result in deformity. The joints become swollen, stiff, red, and warm to the touch. As the joints become more and more deformed, function decreases, which causes loss of movement in the joint.

▶ A *fracture* is a crack or break in the bone. The fracture must be immobilized while the bones manufacture new bone cells to seal and repair the fracture.

▶ *Dislocation* is a change in the normal alignment of the bones at the joint.

▶ *Sprains* are torn or stretched ligaments or tendons.

▶ *Bursitis* is an inflammation of the bursa at the joints.

MUSCULAR SYSTEM

The muscular system is made up of tendons, ligaments, and muscles. Tendons connect the muscle to the bone, and ligaments connect bones. Our muscular system is what enables us to move. Groups of muscle tissue flex (tighten) and extend to produce movement. The muscular system also provides our bodies with heat and protection and enables us to stand and sit straight.

There are three different types of muscle tissue, and each has a different function:

1. **Striated muscle** tissue, or skeletal muscle, is the muscle which makes it possible to walk, sit, lift, and bend. It is called voluntary muscle because we can control the movement.

2. **Smooth muscle** tissues provide the movement that internal body organs need to perform their functions. These are called involuntary muscles because we do not control them. Smooth muscles. move food and waste products through the digestive system.

3. **Cardiac muscle** tissue controls the beating of the heart. It is also involuntary because it works on its own.

A movement such as moving your hand is a result of the coordinated action of several muscles tightening and relaxing. If you bend your elbow, bringing your hand to your shoulder, the large muscle on the **anterior** portion of your arm contracts while the large muscle on the **posterior** relaxes. This is the muscle coordination that produces movement.

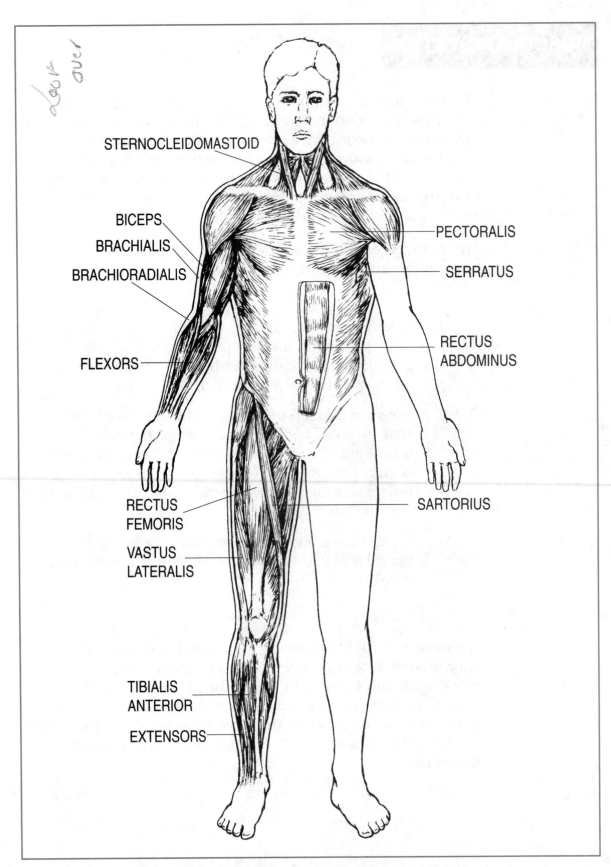

STERNOCLEIDOMASTOID

BICEPS

BRACHIALIS

BRACHIORADIALIS

FLEXORS

PECTORALIS

SERRATUS

RECTUS
ABDOMINUS

RECTUS
FEMORIS

VASTUS
LATERALIS

SARTORIUS

TIBIALIS
ANTERIOR

EXTENSORS

Muscular System - front view or anterior view

Chapter 11: Anatomy and Physiology:
The Skeletal and Muscular Systems

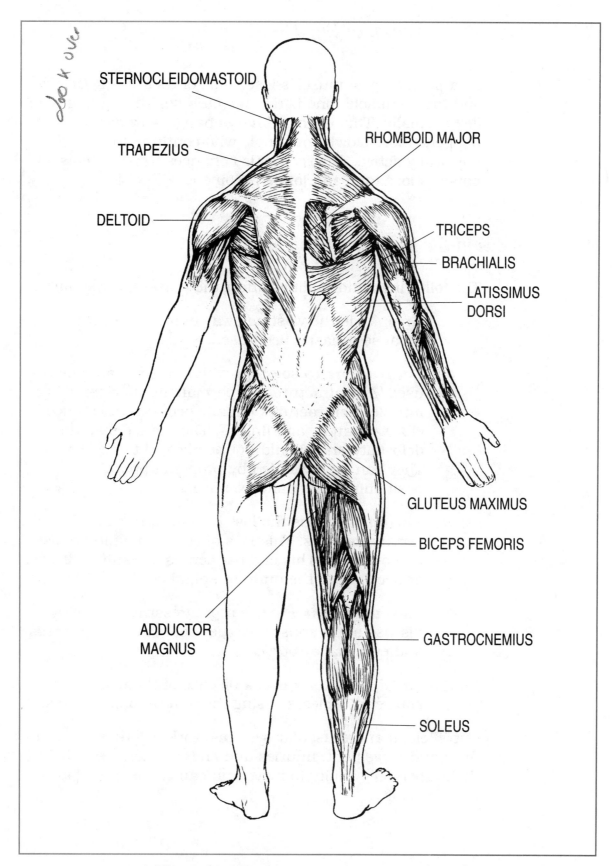

STERNOCLEIDOMASTOID

TRAPEZIUS

DELTOID

RHOMBOID MAJOR

TRICEPS

BRACHIALIS

LATISSIMUS DORSI

GLUTEUS MAXIMUS

BICEPS FEMORIS

ADDUCTOR MAGNUS

GASTROCNEMIUS

SOLEUS

Muscular System - rear or posterior view

Age Changes in the Muscular System

As a person ages, muscles lose some of their strength, size and tone. Muscle tone is the muscle's health and ability to flex normally. This is an ordinary change with age. It happens more slowly for people who continue to be physically active. There are also changes in posture as muscles lose tone and joints become less flexible.

Abnormalities in the Muscular System

The following abnormalities affect the muscular system:

▶ *Atrophy* is the wasting away of muscle tissue because it hasn't been used.

▶ *Contractures* also occur when muscles are not used. A contracture is a permanent shortening of a muscle. Contractures usually occur in hips, knees, elbows, hands, and fingers. They cause pain and deformity and should not be allowed to develop. They can be prevented by proper support, positioning, and daily exercise.

▶ *Paralysis* means the loss of voluntary control over certain muscles. This loss of control results in loss of movement. This can happen as a result of disease or accident to the brain or spinal cord.

▶ *Muscular Dystrophy* is a progressively crippling disease of the muscle tissues that causes weakness and eventual atrophy.

▶ *Multiple Sclerosis* is a disease of the nerves that control muscles, causing them to become useless.

The skeletal and muscular systems work together to give us form and movement. Injuries and changes can severely limit a person's ability to move and can cause great pain and deformity.

*Circle the correct answer. There is only **one** correct answer.*

1. **Our skeleton is made up of three different types of bones.**

    a. True   b. False

2. **The skeletal structure or bones**

    a. Act as shock absorbers.

    b. Prevent other bones from rubbing together.

    c. Provide heat and protection.

    d. Give the body structure and support.

3. **Osteoporosis is a condition where bones lose calcium and become porous and brittle.**

    a. True   b. False

4. **A fracture is**

    a. A change in alignment of bones at the joint.

    b. Similar to a sprain.

    c. A crack or break in a bone.

    d. An inflammation of the bursa.

5. **What body part works like a hinge, a ball and socket, or a pivot?**

    a. Ligament.

    b. Tendon.

    c. Joint.

    d. Bone.

6. **People tend to get taller as they move into old age.**

   a. True   b. False

7. **Involuntary muscles move food through the digestive tract.**

   a. True   b. False

8. **A person has conscious control of cardiac muscle tissue.**

   a. True   b. False

9. **Which of the following conditions results from a muscle's inactivity?**

   a. Paralysis.

   b. Multiple Sclerosis.

   c. Atrophy.

   d. Muscular Dystrophy.

10. **Older women tend to have osteoporosis more often than older men.**

    a. True   b. False

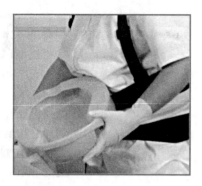

Chapter 12

ANATOMY AND PHYSIOLOGY: THE URINARY SYSTEM

In this chapter... you will learn about:

▶ The urinary system.

▶ Some common problems of the urinary system.

DEFINITIONS

Bladder:	Urinary organ which retains urine until it is excreted.
Cystitis:	Infection of the bladder.
Excrete:	To eliminate or expel from the body, such as waste or harmful materials.
Feces (fecal matter):	Solid or semi-solid body waste.
Immobile:	Unable to move.
Incontinent:	Unable to control functions of bowel or bladder.
Indwelling:	Staying inside the body.
Indwelling Catheter:	Tube inserted into the bladder to drain the urine.
Kidneys:	Two organs in the lower back which filter the blood.
Nephron:	A microscopic filtering unit in the kidneys.
Nephritis:	Infection of the kidney,
Nutrients:	Substances in food that the body uses to provide energy and build tissue.
Prostate:	A small gland that surrounds the urethra in men.
Trauma:	A wound or injury.
Ureters:	Tubes that carry urine from the kidneys to the bladder.
Urethra:	Tube that carries urine from the bladder out of the body.
Urine:	Fluid waste formed by the kidneys and excreted from the body.

The body is an efficient system. It takes in **nutrients**, uses what it needs to function, and then removes what it doesn't need in the form of waste products. The urinary system is this waste removal system.

The urinary system also adjusts the contents of the blood to maintain a chemical balance. The organs which make up this system include:

➤   Kidneys

➤   Ureter

➤   Bladder

➤   Urethra

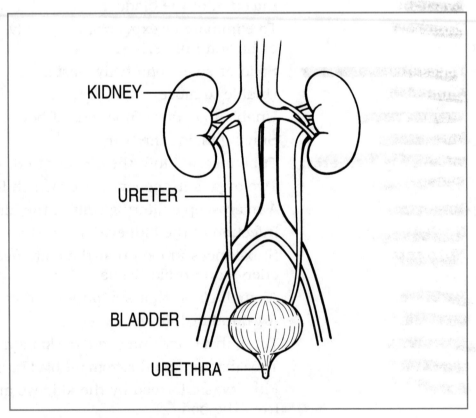

The Urinary System

KIDNEYS

People are born with two **kidneys**. Each kidney is about the size of a fist and weighs about 4 to 6 ounces. The kidneys lie on either side of the spine in the small of the back at the lower edge of the rib cage. Even though we are born with two kidneys, we can still live and function with only one.

In each of these small organs, there are more than a million **nephrons**. Nephrons are microscopic filtering units. Blood enters the kidney and passes through the nephrons where substances needed by the body are put back into the bloodstream. The substances which the body does not need are filtered out and create **urine**.

URETERS

The **ureters** are tiny tubes which connect the kidneys to the urinary **bladder**. The urine passes from each kidney through a ureter to the bladder.

BLADDER

The bladder is the organ in which the urine collects before it is **excreted** from the body. The bladder is capable of gently stretching to hold the incoming urine. The muscular walls of the bladder contain receptors which are stimulated when the bladder gets full. These receptors then signal the brain, and the person has the urge to void or urinate. This usually occurs when the bladder contains about 1/2 pint or 250 to 300 cc of urine.

Normal urine is clear and straw colored. If the urine is dark, bloody, or unusual in any way, the nursing assistant must report these conditions to the charge nurse.

The tube which carries the urine from the bladder to the outside of the body is the *urethra*. In the female, this tube is about 1-1/2 inches long; in the male, it is about 8 inches long because it runs through the penis. Since this tube opens outside the body, it is a potential entry for an infection.

Bacteria can travel up the urethra to the bladder and the kidneys, causing an infection. *Cystitis* is a bladder infection. *Nephritis* is an infection in the kidney. These infections can be very painful and dangerous, especially to an older resident. To help prevent urinary tract infections and bladder and kidney infections, it is important to keep the area of urination clean. It is particularly important to keep *fecal* material from coming in contact with the area of urination by wiping the urinary and anal areas from front to back. This avoids spreading fecal material to the area of urination.

Another important way to prevent urinary tract infections is by seeing that the resident drinks at least 8 glasses of water every day. Providing adequate fluids is important in the care of all residents, but it is even more important for residents with *catheters* and residents who are *incontinent*. The fluids help to keep the bladder "flushed out" and to prevent infection. Before encouraging fluid intake, the nursing assistant needs to check the physician's orders to be sure there is no fluid restriction on the particular resident.

In men, the **prostate** surrounds the urethra. In older men, the prostate gland tends to swell up and harden, pressing on the urethra. This makes urination slower and more difficult. You shouldn't hurry someone who has difficulty starting his urine flow.

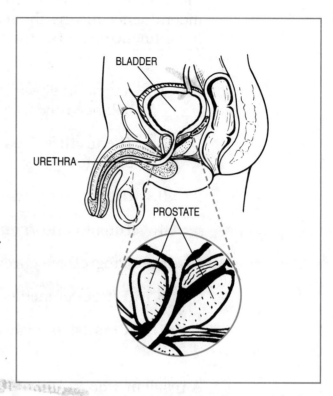

Location of the Prostate

AGE CHANGES

As a person ages, the kidneys function less efficiently. Many of the nephrons in the kidneys are lost. The kidneys' ability to filter waste materials from the blood decreases. It will take longer for a medication to be filtered through the kidneys of an older person than it would for a younger person. This means a drug stays in the bloodstream longer and could cause problems. It is the nursing assistant's responsibility to observe a resident for drug reactions and report these to the charge nurse.

The muscle tone of the bladder decreases with aging. This decreases the amount of urine it can hold. The older resident may not be aware of the need to urinate until the bladder is almost full. There may be a frequent need to urinate with a feeling of urgency--being unable to wait. The resident may experience this urgency at night also, and may wake up often to urinate.

Incontinence is a problem for many older people. Bladder incontinence means the inability to control urination. Incontinence may be due to several problems:

1. A general slowing down of the body's ability to balance fluids.

2. The urethra's loss of ability to expand and contract.

3. Urinary tract infections.

4. Tumors and *trauma.*

5. Progressive chronic disease processes.

6. Effects of medication,

7. Confusion, disorientation.

A resident who is *immobile* may have urinary tract problems. Urinating while lying flat results in an incomplete emptying of the bladder and kidneys. Bacteria may grow in the remaining urine, causing urinary tract infection, bladder stones, and kidney stones. These can be extremely painful.

A resident with urinary problems may have an *indwelling catheter*. A catheter is a tube inserted manually into the bladder for the purpose of draining the urine by gravity into a collection bag. The potential for developing a urinary tract infection is greater for residents with catheters. It is the nursing assistant's responsibility to keep the catheter and surrounding body areas clean and free from contamination.

Residents who are incontinent cannot help it. They do not wet or soil themselves on purpose. They must never be punished or ridiculed for these accidents. Residents are usually embarrassed by this lack of control. The nursing assistant should handle the situation with tact and understanding.

*Circle the correct answer. There is only **one** correct answer.*

1. **Even though we are born with two kidneys, we can still live and function with only one.**

    (a.) True   b. False

2. **On average, how much urine has to collect to create an urge to urinate?**

    a. 1/2 pint.

    b. 1 pint.

    c. 2 pints.

    d. 1/10 pint.

3. **Mr. Bowman was unable to get to the bathroom in time to relieve himself and urinated on his trousers. How should the nursing assistant react?**

    a. Scold him.

    b. Tell him he can't have dessert for a week.

    c. Tell the other residents what he did.

    d. Assure him that you understand and, if he requires assistance, help him clean his clothing.

4. **How can urinary tract infections be prevented?**

    a. Wipe the urinary and anal areas from front to back.

    b. Reduce the amount of fluids the residents drink every day.

    c. Have the residents take long walks on a regular basis.

    d. There is no way you can prevent urinary tract infections.

5. **It takes longer for medication to be filtered through the kidneys of an older person than it would for a younger person.**

    (a.) True   b. False

6. **Age changes exhibited by older men include:**

    a. Increase in muscular tone of the bladder.

    (b.) Decrease in the kidneys' ability to filter waste from the blood.

    c. Shrinking of the prostate.

    d. Hardening of the urethra.

7. **The organs that make up the urinary system are the**

    a. Bladder, bowels, kidneys, urethra.

    (b.) Kidneys, ureter, bladder, urethra.

    c. Liver, kidneys, ureter, bladder.

    d. Liver, kidneys, bladder, bowels.

8. **An indwelling catheter is inserted into the:**

    a. Kidney.

    b. Ureter.

    (c.) Bladder.

    d. Liver.

9. **Incontinence can be caused by a urinary tract infection.**

    (a.) True   b. False

10. **The potential for developing a urinary tract infection is less for residents with catheters.**

    a. True   (b.) False

Chapter 13

ANATOMY AND PHYSIOLOGY: THE INTEGUMENTARY SYSTEM

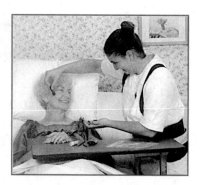

In this chapter... you will learn about:

▶ The integumentary system (the skin).

▶ Some common problems of the integumentary system.

DEFINITIONS

Cyanosis:	Bluish color of skin due to lack of oxygen.
Dermis:	Inner layer of skin.
Eczema:	Dry, reddish, scaly patches on the skin.
Elasticity:	Ability to expand and contract.
Epidermis:	Outer layer of skin.
Erythema:	Redness of skin.
Evaporate:	Give off moisture.
Follicle:	Tube holding hair root.
Integumentary:	Outer covering; skin, hair, nails.
Lubricate:	To oil or grease.
Perspiration:	Sweat.
Podiatrist:	Foot doctor.
Pressure Sores (Decubitus Ulcers):	Areas of the skin that break open due to constant pressure.
Psoriasis:	Reddish scaly patches, usually on elbows and knees.
Shingles:	Scaly painful patches on the sides, caused by a virus.

The ***integumentary*** system includes the skin, hair, nails, sweat glands, and oil glands. This is the most visible body system, and it has many functions. The integumentary system:

▶ Protects the body from dirt and germs.

▶ Regulates body temperature.

▶ Eliminates waste materials through perspiration.

▶ Produces vitamin D from sunlight.

▶ Detects pain through nerves contained in the skin.

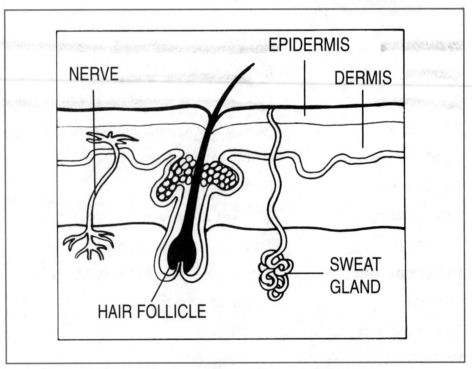

Magnified cross-section of the skin

SKIN

Skin is our largest organ, and it completely covers the body. Our skin has two layers. The outer layer is called the **epidermis**. This layer is very thin over all the body except on the palms of the hands and the soles of the feet. The palms and the soles receive a great deal of hard use and the epidermis on these areas needs to be thicker. The cells of the epidermis are constantly dying and being shed. This dead skin is normal.

Beneath the epidermis is the inner layer of skin called the **dermis**. The dermis is thicker than the epidermis. New skin cells are produced in the dermis to replace those dying in the epidermis. Blood vessels, nerves and sweat glands are found in the dermis.

GLANDS

Sweat glands in the skin eliminate waste products through perspiration. **Perspiration** also helps regulate body temperature. When the perspiration **evaporates** in the air, it carries away heat and cools the body.

Oil glands function to **lubricate** the skin. They keep the skin soft and flexible. These glands also supply the hair follicles with oil.

HAIR AND NAILS

Hair and nails are considered appendages or attachments to the skin. Hair grows in **follicles**, which are tubes that extend from the dermis to the epidermis and hold the hair root. The health and growth of hair and nails reflects the general health of the resident.

Skin

Skin is our largest and most visible organ. The aging changes in the skin are also very evident. As the person ages, the skin becomes thin and dry. It may become as fragile as tissue paper and tear very easily. Particular care must be taken when caring for a resident with fragile skin to avoid injury.

The older residents may have lost some of their fat stores under the skin. This may make sitting and lying on hard surfaces uncomfortable. Since fat acts as an insulator, the older residents may feel the changes in temperature more acutely. The nursing assistant can make residents more comfortable by padding hard surfaces and keeping the older resident warmly dressed and adequately covered.

The skin wrinkles and sags as the person ages due to the loss of muscle and *elasticity*. Brown spots may appear on those areas of the skin which are usually exposed to sunlight (hands, arms, face). These brown spots may not be considered attractive, but they do not harm the resident.

Hair

Hair often loses its color, turning gray or white as the person ages. It also may become dry and sparse. Facial hair, especially around the mouth and chin, may increase on women. Shaving or tweezing the face may become a choice for some aging women.

Nails

Both fingernails and toenails tend to thicken and become abnormal in shape as the person ages. The nails may become too thick for the resident to be able to perform adequate nail care. Often an appointment with a *podiatrist* is necessary to safely provide toenail care.

Changes Which Should be Reported

Changes in a resident's skin can be a signal that something else is wrong. Any change must be reported to the charge nurse. Here are some examples:

1. Pale, white skin color could indicate shock.

2. Blue or gray skin color indicates a lack of oxygen. This condition is called **cyanosis** and is extremely serious.

3. Redness of the skin may indicate infection, injury, pressure, or elevated temperature. This is called **erythema**.

4. Skin diseases. There are a number of skin diseases that are common in the older resident. You should report any signs of abnormal skin to the charge nurse:

    - *Psoriasis.* Reddish patches with scales, often on the elbows and knees.

    - *Eczema.* Dry, reddish, scaly, itchy patches on the skin.

    - *Shingles.* Scaly, very painful patches, often on the sides, caused by a virus.

    - *Pressure sores (Decubitus ulcers).* Areas of the skin that break open, due to constant pressure, often on knees, elbows, or buttocks. These can become very serious, and later in this course you will learn about the need to reposition residents who are immobile to prevent pressure sores from occurring.

It is the nursing assistant's responsibility to observe the resident's skin, hair, and nails while giving daily personal care. If any abnormalities are seen, the nursing assistant must report them to the charge nurse and note the changes in the resident's medical record.

*Circle the correct answer. There is only **one** correct answer.*

1. **Where are new skin cells produced?**

    a. Beneath the skin.

    b. In the pores.

    c. In the epidermis.

    d. In the dermis.

2. **The health and growth of hair and nails reflects the general health of the resident.**

    a. True   b. False

3. **Older residents do not often have skin problems.**

    a. True   b. False

4. **The integumentary system is the most visible body system.**

    a. True   b. False

5. **The integumentary system**

    a. Includes skin, hair, and nails.

    b. Includes sweat glands and kidneys.

    c. Includes skin, hair, and the bladder.

    d. Includes skin and hair only.

6. **Why might older residents find it uncomfortable to sit and lie on hard surfaces?**

    a. They are too used to standing or walking.

    b. They do not have good posture.

    c. They may have lost some of the fat under their skin.

    d. Their skin may have lost its elasticity.

7. **What do sweat glands do?**

    a. Lubricate the skin.

    (b.) Eliminate waste products.

    c. Warn you about pain.

    d. Kill bacteria.

8. **As part of the aging process, fingernails and toenails.**

    a. Become thinner.

    b. Stop growing.

    c. Become brittle.

    (d.) Thicken and become abnormally shaped.

9. **The nursing assistant finds Mrs. Jamison lying in bed and notices that her skin is reddish in color and she has a temperature. What should the nursing assistant do?**

    a. Continue with her other duties.

    (b.) Report Mrs. Jamison's condition and note it in her medical record.

    c. Open a window.

    d. Nothing.

10. **A podiatrist usually treats.**

    a. Hands.

    (b.) Feet.

    c. Hair.

    d. Nerves.

Chapter 14

ANATOMY AND PHYSIOLOGY: THE CARDIOVASCULAR SYSTEM

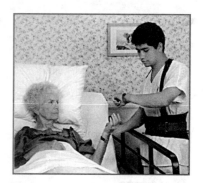

In this chapter... you will learn about:

▶ The cardiovascular system.

▶ Some common problems of the cardiovascular system.

DEFINITIONS

Angina	Acute pain in the chest from low blood supply to the heart.
Arrhythmia:	An abnormal rhythm in the heartbeat.
Arteries:	Blood vessels which carry oxygenated blood away from the heart.
Arterioles:	Tiny arteries which carry blood from large arteries to capillaries.
Arteriosclerosis:	Hardening of the arteries.
Atrium:	Upper chamber of the heart.
Blood Pressure:	The force of the blood pressing against artery walls.
Capillaries:	Small blood vessels which carry nutrients to individual cells.
Congestive Heart Failure	Gradual loss of the heart's ability to pump blood.
Heart attack (Myocardial Infarction):	Death of tissue in the heart due to a lack of blood supply.

Definitions Continued...

Hypertension:	High blood pressure.
Lymph Vessels:	Structures which collect body fluid.
Lymph Nodes:	Small glands which filter body fluid.
Pacemaker:	Initiates and transmits electrical impulse to cause heart to contract.
Plasma:	The fluid portion of the blood.
Platelets:	Elements of blood which form clots.
Red blood Cells:	The red-colored cells in the blood that carry oxygen.
Septum:	Tissue dividing heart in half.
Stroke (Cerebral Vascular Accident or CVA):	Sudden stoppage of the blood supply to an area of the brain.
Varicose Vein:	Weakened swollen vein, usually seen in the legs.
Veins:	Blood vessels which carry unoxygenated blood back to the heart.
Ventricle:	Lower chamber of heart.
Venules:	Tiny veins which carry blood from capillaries to large veins.
White Blood Cells:	The white-colored cells in the blood that fight infection.

THE CARDIOVASCULAR SYSTEM

The *cardiovascular* system is the system that pumps and carries blood through the body. It is made up of the:

▶ Heart

▶ Blood vessels

▶ Blood

▶ Lymph vessels

This system has the important job of carrying oxygen and nutrients to all the body's cells and then removing the waste products.

The heart is the pump of this system. It is about the size of a fist and located to the left of the center of the chest behind the breastbone.

The heart has four chambers or compartments. The top compartments are called atria. There is a left **atrium** and a right atrium. The lower chambers are called **ventricles**, of which there is also a right and a left ventricle.

The heart beats about 100,000 times a day to keep this system working. An electrical impulse is generated by a specialized area in the right atrium called the **pacemaker**. This impulse causes the ventricles to contract and force the blood through the vessels.

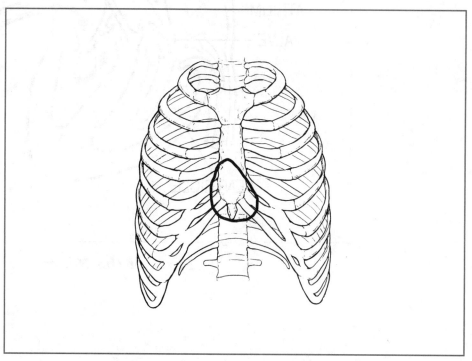

Position of the Heart in the body

Blood bringing waste products from the cells enters the right atrium, flows through a valve into the right ventricle. The heart, or pump, contracts and forces the blood to the lungs.

In the lungs, the blood delivers carbon dioxide (a waste product) and exchanges it for oxygen. It is then returned to the heart by way of the left atrium and ventricle. From there it is pumped through the aorta and out through the blood vessels to feed all the cells of the body.

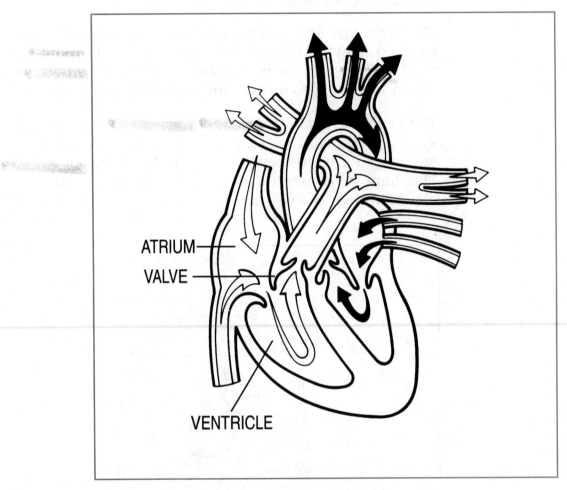

Parts of the Heart

BLOOD VESSELS

There are three main types of blood vessels in the body:

- ▶ Arteries.

- ▶ Capillaries.

- ▶ Veins.

These three types of blood vessels carry blood, oxygen, and nutrients to all parts of the body and carry waste products back to the lungs, kidneys, and sweat glands to be eliminated.

Arteries

Arteries are large blood vessels that carry the oxygen-rich blood from the heart to all parts of the body. The arteries are elastic, which enables them to constrict and relax. This motion helps move the blood along the system. The blood moves from the arteries to the capillaries by way of **arterioles**. Arterioles are tiny arteries which are not elastic. The color of arterial blood is bright red.

Veins

Veins are the blood vessels which carry oxygen-poor blood and waste products back to the heart, lungs, and kidneys. The blood reaches the large veins by way of **venules** which are tiny veins that bring the blood from the capillaries to the large veins. The color of venous blood is dark red.

The measurement of the force of the blood circulating through the vessels is called **blood pressure**.

Capillaries

Capillaries are the smallest blood vessels. The walls are only one cell thick so oxygen and nutrients can pass through their walls to nourish the body cells and carbon dioxide can be removed from the cell as a waste product.

BLOOD

The average adult has about five quarts of blood circulating through the cardiovascular system. Blood serves many functions in the body:

1. Blood delivers oxygen to all the body cells. It also removes carbon dioxide and other waste products from the cells.

2. Blood distributes nutrients to all body cells.

3. Blood helps regulate body temperature by expanding and contracting blood vessels.

4. Blood helps protect the body by fighting infection.

5. Blood helps maintain the fluid balance of the body.

Blood is composed of:

▶ Plasma.

▶ Red blood cells.

▶ White blood cells.

▶ Platelets.

Plasma

Plasma is the fluid portion of the blood. It is light colored and clear. It contains chemicals, proteins, and sugars.

Red Blood Cells

Red blood cells far outnumber white blood cells. Their main function is to carry oxygen from the lungs throughout the body. These cells give blood its red color.

White Blood Cells

The main function of the **white blood cells** is to fight infection. They block germs and bacteria from causing disease in the body.

Platelets

Platelets are formed in bone marrow. Their main function is to cause clotting and stop bleeding.

LYMPH VESSELS

Lymph vessels collect excess lymph fluid which surrounds all body cells. This fluid passes through the **lymph nodes** which filter out and destroy bacteria in the fluid. Eventually, the fluid is emptied into the large veins.

AGE-RELATED CHANGES

In the older person, blood vessels thicken and lose some of their elasticity, which increases the blood pressure, causing *hypertension*. This may cause the older resident's heart to enlarge. Blood vessels lose their elasticity causing the heart to work harder to pump the blood. This extra work causes the heart muscle to enlarge.

As a person ages, all body systems slow down. In the cardiovascular system, this means the heart rate slows, the heart contractions slow, and less blood is pumped. This means that less oxygen and nutrients are carried to body cells, resulting in a decrease in a person's strength and energy.

COMMON CARDIOVASCULAR DISEASES

The following are some common cardiovascular diseases in the older resident. You should report any signs of these conditions to the charge nurse.

Angina. Acute pain in the chest caused by lack of blood to the heart muscle tissue.

Arrhythmias. Abnormal rhythms in the heartbeat, sometimes evident when taking a pulse.

Arteriosclerosis. Hardening of the arteries, causing decreased blood flow to areas of the body. Often resulting in cold extremities (hands and feet).

Congestive heart failure. The gradual loss of the heart's ability to pump out all the blood that returns to it, often resulting in difficulty in breathing, edema, and general weakness.

Stroke (CVA, or cerebral vascular accident). Sudden stoppage of the blood supply to an area of the brain, sometimes by a blood clot getting caught in a blood vessel. This can result in permanent damage to the brain, loss of control of some part of the body, or slurring or loss of speech.

Heart Attack (Myocardial infarction). The death of tissue in the heart due to a lack of blood supply. This can cause death.

*Circle the correct answer. There is only **one** correct answer.*

1. **The cardiovascular system carries oxygen and nutrients to all body cells.**

    a. True   b. False

2. **The four chambers of the heart are the left and right atria, the left ventricle, and the**

    a. Aorta.

    b. Septum.

    c. Right ventricle.

    d. Lymph vessel.

3. **The fluid part of the blood is called:**

    a. Platelet.

    b. Plasma.

    c. Capillary.

    d. Aorta.

4. **There are two main types of blood vessels—arteries and veins.**

    a. True   b. False

5. **Arteries carry oxygen-rich blood from the heart to all parts of the body; veins carry what back to the heart, lungs, and kidneys?**

    a. Oxygen-poor blood and wastes.

    b. Waste only.

    c. Urine.

    d. Lymph.

6. **The main function of platelets is to**

    a. Move blood from arteries to capillaries.

    b. Collect excess fluid surrounding body cells.

    (c.) Cause clotting and stop bleeding.

    d. Fight infection.

7. **What does plasma contain?**

    a. Arterioles.

    b. Capillaries.

    c. Venules.

    (d.) Proteins.

8. **What do white blood cells do?**

    a. Carry oxygen from the lungs throughout the body.

    b. Cause clotting.

    (c.) Fight infection.

    d. Bring blood from capillaries to veins.

9. **Angina means what?**

    a. Uneven heart rhythms.

    b. Hardening of the arteries.

    c. Stroke.

    (d.) Acute heart pain.

10. **High blood pressure may cause an older resident's heart to enlarge.**

    (a.) True   b. False

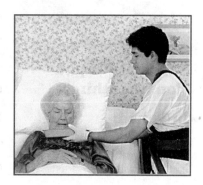

Chapter 15

ANATOMY AND PHYSIOLOGY: THE RESPIRATORY SYSTEM

In this chapter... you will learn about:

▶ The respiratory system.

▶ Some common problems of the respiratory system.

DEFINITIONS

Alveoli	Tiny air sacs in the lungs.
Aspiration:	Inhaling of food, liquid, mucus, or vomitus into air passages.
Asthma:	A disease of the bronchi, causing narrowing air passages and difficulty breathing.
Bronchi:	Tubes which connect trachea to lungs.
Bronchitis:	Inflammation of the bronchi.
Chronic Obstructive Pulmonary Disease (COPD):	A lung condition arising from repeated injury of the tissue, with tissues becoming less elastic and breathing becoming difficult.
Cilia:	Microscopic hair-like appendages that sweep foreign matter out of the trachea and bronchi.
Diaphragm:	Muscle which separates the chest cavity from the abdomen.
Emphysema:	A condition of the lungs in which bronchioles become plugged with mucus and breathing becomes difficult.

Definitions Continued...

Chapter 15: Anatomy and Physiology:
The Respiratory System

125

Epiglottis:	Tissue that closes during swallowing to cover the top of the trachea.
External Respiration (Breathing):	The exchange of gases between the body and the outside world.
Inflamed:	Red, swollen.
Internal Respiration:	The exchange of gases between the blood and the cells of the body.
Larynx:	Voice box.
Lungs:	Two organs in the chest cavity responsible for exchanging gases with the blood.
Metabolism	All the physical and chemical processes involved in sustaining life.
Pneumonia	A disease caused by a virus or bacteria in which the lung tissue is inflamed and the airways fill with fluid.
Pharynx:	Throat.
Pleura:	Lining of chest cavity.
Respiratory System	Organs involved in the transfer of gases between the body and the environment.
Respiration:	Breathing.
Trachea:	Windpipe.

THE HEALTHCARE TEAM

Respiration means breathing. Breathing in is called inspiration; breathing out is expiration. Every organ and every cell in the body needs oxygen to live. As body processes are carried on, waste products accumulate and must be removed. Therefore, the *respiratory system's* main function is to exchange oxygen for carbon dioxide and water from the bloodstream which then carries it to all the body cells.

The respiratory system is made up of many different parts:

- ▶ Lungs
- ▶ Bronchi
- ▶ Alveoli
- ▶ Diaphragm
- ▶ Trachea
- ▶ Nasal Cavity
- ▶ Oral Cavity
- ▶ Pharynx
- ▶ Larynx

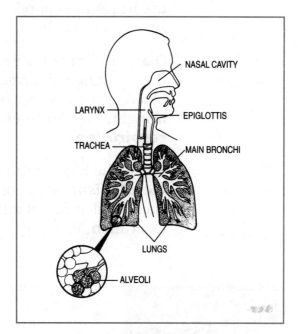

The Respiratory System

Breathing is regulated by the brain. We can control our breathing, but usually we breathe without thinking about it.

Breathing pulls air into the body through the nose or mouth *(external respiration)*. The air travels down the *pharynx*, past the *larynx*, into the *trachea*. At the top of the trachea, covering the opening, is a piece of cartilage called the epiglottis. When food or liquid is swallowed, the *epiglottis* closes off the trachea so nothing enters the windpipe.

Aspiration occurs when small pieces of food, liquid, mucus, or vomitus enter the air passages. This can cause choking, obstruction, or infection.

The air travels from the trachea through the *bronchi* to each of the *lungs*. *Cilia* sweep foreign matter out of the trachea and bronchi, helping to prevent infection. The lungs are the main organs of the respiratory system. When you breathe, the lungs expand and contract in the chest cavity. This movement is smooth because the chest cavity is lined with a moist membrane called the *pleura*.

Also helping the chest cavity to expand and contract is the *diaphragm*. This is a muscular organ which flattens when you breathe in. This makes the chest cavity bigger, allowing the lungs to expand. The lungs sit on the diaphragm and it separates the chest cavity from the abdomen.

Oxygen from the air enters the ***alveoli*** of the lungs where the exchange of oxygen for carbon dioxide takes place. The blood is then pumped through the cardiovascular system, bringing oxygen to all the cells of the body ***(internal respiration)***.

When the blood returns, it brings the waste products of cell ***metabolism***. Some of these wastes are carbon dioxide and water which are eliminated from the body through expiration, or breathing out.

AGE-RELATED CHANGES

As a person ages, changes occur in the respiratory system:

- The lungs lose some of their elasticity. They no longer expand and contract as easily. This reduces the amount of air exchanged and the amount of oxygen circulating in the blood.
- The rib cage becomes more rigid, preventing full expansion of the lungs during breathing.
- The posture becomes more stooped. This reduces the air capacity of the chest cavity.
- Secretions, or mucus, thicken and become more difficult to expel.
- There is less resistance to diseases of the respiratory system.

These changes generally do not interfere with an older person in normal functioning. However, the older resident is more at risk for developing a respiratory problem due to these changes. Any changes observed by the nursing assistant in breathing patterns, respiratory difficulty, cough or chest pain should be reported to the charge nurse.

Those residents who continue to smoke or smoked earlier in their life are at greater risk for all respiratory diseases. Smoking weakens and destroys lung tissues.

COMMON RESPIRATORY DISEASES IN THE OLDER RESIDENT

Pneumonia

Pneumonia can be caused by either a bacteria or a virus. These microorganisms are always present in the upper respiratory tract and usually do not cause disease. However, if the person is weak, the body may not be able to fight off the effects of these organisms. Then the lungs may become infected or **inflamed.**

The resident who does not move around is at risk for developing pneumonia. In this condition, the lungs do not expand completely when the resident is in a reclining position. The body fluids and mucus are not eliminated and tend to collect in the lungs. This can encourage the growth of bacteria and cause pneumonia.

This is a serious disease for the weak and older resident. The nursing assistant can help the dependent resident by frequent position changes and encouraging deep breathing, coughing, and fluid intake to bring up the secretions and prevent complications leading to pneumonia.

Emphysema

Emphysema has been called the smokers' disease as it often affects people after years of smoking. Smoking destroys the cilia in the mucous membrane lining of the trachea, thereby allowing foreign matter into the lungs and minimizing the ability to cough up mucous. Other pollutants can also cause emphysema, as well as chronic **bronchitis**, **asthma**, and tuberculosis. With emphysema, the bronchioles, tiny branches of the bronchi, become plugged with mucus. Breathing is difficult because the lungs lose much of their elasticity. Air remains trapped in the lungs because it is difficult to exhale.

Residents with emphysema will be short of breath after even mild exertion and may cough and wheeze. The nursing assistant can help the residents with emphysema by helping them do activities at a slower pace.

Chronic Obstructive Pulmonary Disease (COPD)

Chronic Obstructive Pulmonary Disease (or COPD) is a condition in which many of the airways in the lungs are blocked, and the tissues of the lungs become less elastic and less able to exchange gases. It can develop from repeated injury to lung tissue caused by many other lung conditions, such as asthma, bronchitis or emphysema.

Asthma

Allergies to foods, animals, and environmental pollens and plants may cause asthma. Asthma is a disease of the bronchi. Muscle spasms narrow the air passages, causing the resident to wheeze and have difficulty breathing. Emotional stress can also produce an asthma reaction. By helping the resident to remain calm and away from irritants, the nursing assistant can help the resident avoid an asthma attack. There are medications to ease the symptoms.

*Circle the correct answer. There is only **one** correct answer.*

1. **Every organ and cell in the body needs oxygen to live.**

    a. True   b. False

2. **When small pieces of food, liquid, mucus, or vomitus enter the air passages, what occurs?**

    a. Respiration.

    b. Metabolism.

    c. Aspiration.

    d. Asthma.

3. **The exchange of gases between the body and the outside world is called:**

    a. External respiration.

    b. Internal respiration.

    c. Metabolism.

    d. Emphysema.

4. **How do cilia help prevent infection?**

    a. They break down food and oxygen in the cells.

    b. They sweep foreign matter out of the trachea and bronchi.

    c. They line the chest cavity.

    d. They remove waste products from the body.

5. **In addition to the lungs, what organ helps the chest cavity expand and contract?**

    a. Trachea.

    b. Pharynx.

    c. Epiglottis.

    d. Diaphragm.

6. **As a person ages,**

    a. The lungs become more elastic.

    b. The air capacity of the chest cavity increases.

    (c.) Secretions thicken and become difficult to expel.

    d. Resistance to diseases of the respiratory system increases.

7. **The exchange of oxygen and carbon dioxide takes place in the diaphragm.** Lung

    a. True   (b.) False

8. **Mrs. Riebers, who is 78 years old, has been diagnosed as having pneumonia. How can the nursing assistant help her recover?**

    a. Keep Mrs. Riebers from changing position.

    (b.) Encourage her to cough and drink fluids.

    c. Cut down her fluid intake.

    d. Keep her from coughing.

9. **Residents with emphysema will be short of breath even after mild exertion.**

    (a.) True   b. False

10. **What effect does smoking have on lung diseases?**

    a. It increases the risk for pneumonia only.

    (b.) It increases the risk for all lung diseases.

    c. It has no relation to lung diseases.

    d. It helps prevent lung diseases.

Chapter 16

ANATOMY AND PHYSIOLOGY: THE ENDOCRINE SYSTEM

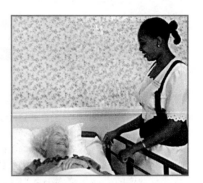

In this chapter... you will learn about:

▶ The endocrine system.

▶ Some common problems of the endocrine system.

DEFINITIONS

Carbohydrates:	Sugars and starches.
Diabetes (Diabetes Mellitus):	A condition in which the body cannot break down and use carbohydrates because there is insufficient insulin.
Electrolyte:	A fluid that conducts electricity.
Endocrine System:	System of glands which secrete hormones into the blood.
Exocrine Glands:	Glands which secrete hormones into a body cavity or directly outside the body.
Fallopian Tubes:	Tiny tubes connecting the ovaries with the uterus.
Hormones:	Fluid which starts a set of reactions within the body.
Immune:	Protected against infection.
Secrete:	Give off.

The endocrine system is made up of the following glands:

- Pituitary
- Thyroid
- Parathyroid
- Thymus

- Adrenal
- Pancreas
- Ovaries (female sex glands)
- Testes (male sex glands)

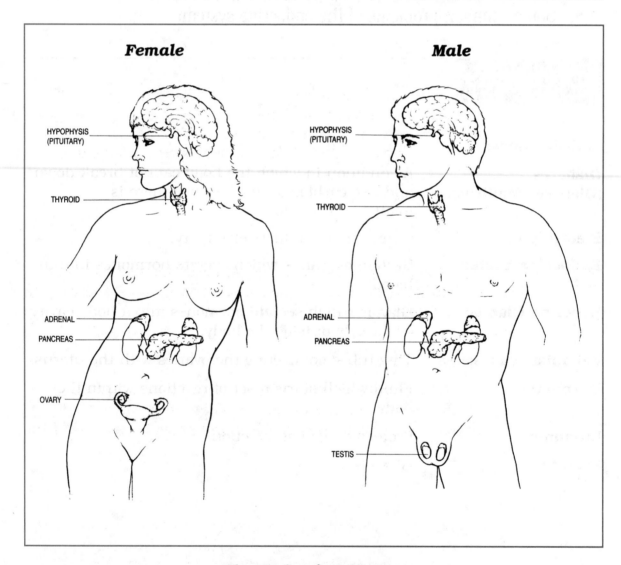

The Endocrine System

These glands **secrete** fluids called **hormones** directly into the bloodstream. These hormones are necessary to set in motion and regulate body functions involved with:

▶ Growth.

▶ Development.

▶ Metabolism.

▶ Reproduction.

GLANDS

Each gland secretes a particular hormone or group of hormones. Each hormone is responsible for a particular function.

Pituitary Gland

The pituitary gland is located at the base of the brain and is the smallest **endocrine** gland. It is called the master gland because its hormone regulates the work of all the cells, or metabolism, and stimulates other endocrine glands to **secrete** their hormones. The pituitary is the master regulator of the body.

Thyroid Gland

The thyroid gland is a large gland located at the base of the throat. Its hormones are responsible for growth, energy, sexual development, and skin texture.

Parathyroid Glands

The parathyroid glands are two pairs of very small glands located within the thyroid gland. Their hormone is necessary for regulating calcium and phosphorus within the body.

Thymus Gland

The thymus is located in the center of the chest, behind and above the heart. This gland is not fully understood. It is believed that it plays a part in the body's **immune** system.

Pancreas

The pancreas is located behind and underneath the stomach and liver. It secretes two hormones, insulin and glucagon, which regulate the level of sugar in the blood.

Adrenal Glands

The adrenals are two small glands which are located on top of each kidney. They are responsible for secreting hormones which regulate the use of nutrients in the body and regulate fluid and **electrolyte** balances. The adrenals also secrete hormones which help the body react to stress.

Sex Glands

Ovaries. In females, the ovaries are located at the end of the **fallopian tubes** in the lower pelvic area. These glands stimulate the regular release of an ovum, or egg. They also produce the female hormones needed for reproduction and physical female characteristics.

Testes. In males, the testes are located in the scrotum, or sac behind the penis. These glands produce sperm and the male hormone which stimulates sperm production and physical male characteristics.

Exocrine Glands

The **exocrine glands** differ from most of the endocrine glands by secreting their hormones directly to the outside of the body or into body cavities. Some of the exocrine glands are:

Lacrimal Glands. The lacrimal glands are located behind the eyes and are responsible for secreting the fluid, or tears, which keeps the eyes moist.

Sweat Glands. Sweat glands are located all over the surface of the skin. Their function is to release moisture to the surface where it will evaporate and produce cooling of the body. This process also eliminates some waste products.

Salivary Glands. The salivary glands are located inside the mouth. They produce saliva which keeps the mouth moist, makes food easier to chew and swallow, and begins the digestion of the food.

AGE-RELATED CHANGES

There is a gradual decrease in hormone secretion as a person ages. The ovaries stop producing the female hormone estrogen after menopause. The testes continue to produce the male hormone, testosterone, but the amount decreases with age.

DISEASES OF THE ENDOCRINE SYSTEM

The most common disease of the endocrine system in the older resident is diabetes mellitus. Diabetes affects people of all ages and puts them at risk for other complications and problems. It is a disorder of carbohydrate metabolism. The body cannot break down and use sugars and starches because there is insufficient insulin secreted by the pancreas.

> ▶ In *Type I* diabetes (insulin-dependent), the body completely lacks the hormone insulin and the person must take the hormone regularly by injection.
>
> ▶ In *Type II* diabetes (non-insulin dependent), the condition can sometimes be brought under control with exercise, careful diet, and medications. This condition becomes more common with aging.

It is important for the nursing assistant to monitor the diabetic resident carefully and report any eating problems to the charge nurse as these can affect the older diabetic. Good skin care and foot care can also be important in this group of residents.

*Circle the correct answer. There is only **one** correct answer.*

1. **Which one of the following glands is not part of the endocrine system?**

    a. Pituitary.

    b. Pancreas.

    c. Heart.

    d. Ovaries.

2. **All glands secrete the same hormone.**

    a. True   b. False

3. **What does the thyroid do?**

    a. It is the master regulator of the body.

    b. It regulates level of blood sugar.

    c. It regulates electrolyte balances.

    d. It is responsible for growth.

4. **The hormones of the pancreas are responsible for regulating:**

    a. Growth and development.

    b. Reproduction.

    c. Sugar in the blood.

    d. Respiration.

5. **Which gland secretes a hormone that helps the body react to stress?**

    a. Pituitary.

    b. Adrenal glands.

    c. Pancreas.

    d. Thyroid.

6. **What do the lacrimal glands do?**

   a. Produce saliva.

   b. Secrete enzymes.

   c. Secrete tears.

   d. Release moisture.

7. **As a person ages, his or her glands gradually secrete fewer hormones.**

   a. True   b. False

8. **What is the most common disease of the endocrine system?**

   a. Parkinson's disease.

   b. Alzheimer's disease.

   c. Cancer.

   d. Diabetes mellitus.

9. **Diabetes affects only older residents.**

   a. True   b. False

10. **Hormones from the parathyroid glands regulate calcium and phosphorus.**

   a. True   b. False

Chapter 17

ANATOMY AND PHYSIOLOGY: THE SENSORY SYSTEM

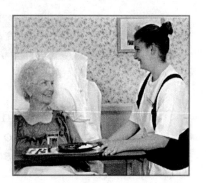

In this chapter... you will learn about:

▶ The sensory system.

▶ Some common problems of the sensory system.

DEFINITIONS

Bifocal:	Two different prescriptions in one eyeglass lens.
Cataract:	Clouding of the lens of the eye.
Environment:	The world around you.
Glaucoma:	Increased pressure in the eye, due to the inability of the fluid in the eye (vitreous humor) to circulate properly.
Myopia:	Difficulty seeing things that are far away.
Peripheral Vision:	Vision seen to the side while looking straight ahead.
Presbyopia:	Decrease in the ability of the eye to focus.
Presbycusis:	Hearing loss for high-pitched sounds.
Senses:	Sight, hearing, smell, taste, and touch.
Sensory System:	Eyes, ears, nose, tongue, and skin.
Stimulus:	Action that causes a response.
Tinnitus:	Constant ringing in the ear.

THE SENSORY SYSTEM

All the information we receive from the world around us comes to us through organs that are responsible for our five **senses**. These organs and senses are:

1. Eyes: **Sight**

2. Ears: **Hearing**

3. Nose: **Smell**

4. Tongue: **Taste**

5. Skin: **Touch**

The **sensory system** is made up of these five organs that bring information to our brains about changes in the world around us. Any change in our **environment** is called a **stimulus**. The sense organ reacts to a stimulus by sending a message about the change to the brain. This information can be used by the brain to start a response to the change. For example, if you step into a warm room, your skin picks up the stimulus of the heat. The information that the room is very warm travels from your skin to your brain. The brain then sends a message that may result in your removing your sweater.

If any one of these sense organs is impaired, some of the input from your environment will be missing.

The eye is the organ of sight. It works like a camera, giving the brain a picture of the environment. The parts of the eye are:

1. *Sclera.* The white part of the eyeball.

2. *Iris.* The circle of color in the center of the eye (blue, brown, green, violet, hazel).

3. *Pupil.* The dark opening in the center of the iris where light enters.

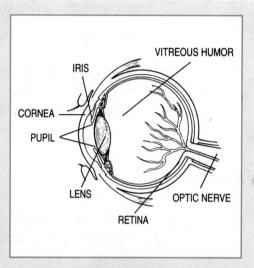

The Eye

4. *Cornea.* Clear circular area of the eyeball, called the "window" of the eye.

5. *Vitreous Humor.* Clear liquid which fills the eyeball.

6. *Aqueous Humor.* Fluid produced by the eye which fills the space between the cornea and the lens.

7. *Lens.* Lies directly behind the pupil and focuses the picture of what you see on the retina.

8. *Retina.* Back part of the eye which receives the picture and sends nerve impulses to the optic nerve.

9. *Optic Nerve.* Receives the nerve impulse from the retina and sends it to the brain so the brain can interpret what you see.

The most common change in the eye as the person ages is a condition called **presbyopia**. The lens loses some of its elasticity and ability to focus rapidly and clearly, particularly on an object close to the eye. The person must hold small print farther and farther away in order to read it. Reading glasses which slightly magnify the print are the usual way of correcting presbyopia.

With age there is also a loss of **peripheral vision**, or side vision.

Myopia is difficulty seeing things that are far from the eye. If the person has myopia and begins to develop presbyopia as well, **bifocals** are usually the answer.

Diseases of the Eye

There are two diseases of the eye often found in the older resident: **cataracts** and **glaucoma**.

► *Cataracts.* When a cataract occurs, the eye lens becomes cloudy. Since the lens is no longer transparent, vision is impaired. As the lens becomes yellow and cloudy, the perception of color changes. This change affects colors in the blue-green range. The ability to tolerate glare and bright light is also decreased. Eventually, blindness will result. Fortunately, surgery to remove the clouded lens is now a relatively safe and simple procedure.

► *Glaucoma.* This is a much more serious disease of the eye. Pressure from accumulated fluid builds up in the eye and can damage the optic nerve. The person who is developing glaucoma may complain of pain in the eye or see halos around lights. There may also be a loss of peripheral and central, or front, vision. If detected early, glaucoma can be treated to prevent damage to the optic nerve. The test for glaucoma is simple and painless, and it should be a routine part of any eye examination for persons past middle age. If untreated, glaucoma results in permanent blindness. Treatments include medication and surgery.

Hearing is the function of the ear. The ear is also involved in the sense of balance. Sounds enter the ear and are transmitted to the brain. There are 4 main parts to the ear:

1. **Outer Ear.** This is the body part which we can see.

2. **Eardrum.** The membrane which separates the outer ear from the middle ear.

3. **Middle Ear.** This contains three tiny bones which are set into vibration by the eardrum. These bones are the hammer, anvil, and stirrup.

4. **Inner Ear.** This contains two parts. One is the cochlea, a snail shell-shaped tube, which contains the fluid necessary for us to maintain our sense of balance. The other part of the inner ear contains tiny hairlike nerve cells which receive the signals from the middle ear and transfer them to the brain.

OUTER EAR

MIDDLE EAR

INNER EAR

EAR DRUM

The Ear

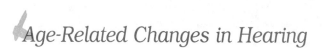

Age-Related Changes in Hearing

Most older people will have some hearing loss. The most common hearing deficit in aging is called **presbycusis**. This results in a reduction in the ability to hear higher-pitched sounds. The person with presbycusis may hear the sound of a conversation, but be unable to understand some of the words, especially with speakers who have high-pitched voices. Increasing the volume of speech often helps the person hear more clearly.

Another hearing problem among the older residents is **tinnitus**, a continual ringing, roaring, or hissing sound in the ears. It is not known what causes tinnitus or how to correct it. This can be very frustrating, and the only remedy is to learn to ignore the noise.

Severe loss of hearing may seriously interfere with a resident's ability to interact and communicate with others.

Hearing aids amplify all sounds but do not correct or cure the hearing problem. Hearing aids help the resident hear better. This is because the hearing aid makes the sounds louder, though it does not make them clearer. Hearing aids are expensive and must be handled carefully and cared for properly by the nursing assistant.

SMELL

The special lining of the upper part of the nose enables us to smell and detect differences in odors. This sense is the least understood, and it is not known how this information is transmitted to the brain.

Age-Related Changes in Smell

The sense of smell declines with age. Many older people have difficulty identifying common odors. Since the sense of smell is important to taste, this can contribute to a loss of appetite.

The tongue is the organ for the sense of taste. Tiny taste buds on the tongue allow us to tell the difference among sweet, sour, bitter, and salty tastes. The taste buds for sweet and salty are located near the tip of the tongue. The buds for sour are in the middle, and those for bitter are located at the base of the tongue. In more complicated tastes, the brain combines these four tongue sensations, plus information from the sense of smell.

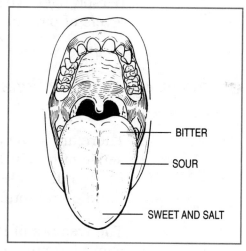

Areas of Taste

Age-Related Changes in Taste

The number of taste buds decrease as a person ages. The tastes for sweet and salty seem to decline first, causing the older person to increase the use of sugar and salt. The loss of taste often causes a loss of appetite.

TOUCH

The skin is the organ for the sense of touch. Special sensory nerve cells send different messages about touch to the brain. These nerve cells can identify pressure, pain, heat, and cold.

Age-Related Changes in Touch

The special nerve cells lose some of their sensitivity as a person ages. The older person may not experience normal levels of pain or accurately perceive hot and cold.

Diseases Affecting the Sense of Touch

There are some diseases which can affect the older person's sense of touch. Rheumatoid arthritis causes deformities in the hands, making it difficult and painful for the person to handle and touch things.

The tremors of Parkinson's disease may cause the person to avoid touching things for fear of dropping or damaging them.

SENSORY INPUT

We all require varied sensory input to function normally. Age and disease affect all five of the senses. This results in less information being sent to the brain about the environment. If the loss is severe, the person can become confused and angry, as well as have difficulty with the activities of daily living.

*Circle the correct answer. There is only **one** correct answer.*

1. **Which part of the eye receives the picture and sends nerve impulses to the optic nerve?**

    a. Pupil.

    b. Iris.

    c. Lens.

    d. Retina.

2. **What is the most common change in the eye as a person ages?**

    a. Peripheral vision.

    b. Glaucoma.

    c. Presbyopia.

    d. Cataract.

3. **Which part of the ear contains the fluid necessary to maintain our sense of balance?**

    a. Outer ear.

    b. Inner ear.

    c. Eardrum.

    d. Middle ear.

4. **Presbycusis involves an inability to hear what?**

    a. Low-pitched sounds.

    b. High-pitched sounds.

    c. Mid-range sounds.

    d. All sounds.

5. **The sense that we know least about is**

  a. Taste.

  b. Hearing.

  c. Smell.

  d. Touch.

6. **With age, the sense of smell**

  a. Improves.

  b. Declines.

  c. Remains the same.

7. **Which taste buds are located near the tip of the tongue?**

  a. Sweet and sour.

  b. Salty and bitter.

  c. Bitter and sour.

  d. Sweet and salty.

8. **Loss of taste often causes a loss of appetite.**

  a. True   b. False

9. **The older resident may not accurately perceive hot and cold.**

  a. True   b. False

10. **What disease can affect the older person's sense of touch?**

  a. Rheumatoid arthritis.

  b. Pneumonia.

  c. Glaucoma.

  d. Tinnitus.

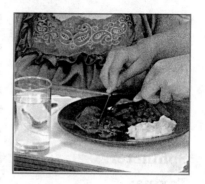

ANATOMY AND PHYSIOLOGY:
THE DIGESTIVE SYSTEM

In this chapter... you will learn about:

▶ The digestive system.

▶ Some common problems of the digestive system.

DEFINITIONS

Anus:	The opening of the rectum located between the buttocks.
Bile:	Substance manufactured by liver, stored by gallbladder; aids in the digestion of fats.
Bowel:	The intestines.
Colon:	The large intestine.
Defecation:	Eliminating fecal matter through the anus.
Digest:	To break down food substances.
Duodenum:	First loop of small intestine where most of digestion occurs.
Enema:	Insertion of fluid into the rectum and colon.
Feces (Fecal Matter):	Solid or semi-solid body waste.
Gastric Juices:	Digestive fluids secreted by the stomach.
Gastrointestinal (GI):	Referring to the stomach and intestines.
Glucose:	Simple sugar to which food is converted.

Definitions Continued...

Insulin:	Hormone secreted by pancreas.
Laxative:	A substance that aids defecation.
Peristalsis:	Rhythmic contractions of the intestine that help move food along.
Rectum:	The lowest part of the large intestine that connects to the anus.
Sphincter:	Muscles that contracts to close a body opening.
Toxins:	Waste products released by disease-producing organisms.
Villi:	Tiny fingerlike projections in the duodenum which absorb digested food particles and release them into the bloodstream.

THE DIGESTIVE SYSTEM

The digestive system is a tube running from the mouth to the rectum and is about 30 feet long. It is also referred to as the **gastrointestinal tract**, or **GI** tract. The functions of this system are to take in food, **digest** it so that the body cells can use it, and eliminate body wastes. The breakdown of food is done both mechanically by chewing and chemically by **gastric juices** and saliva.

The parts of the digestive system are:

1. Tongue
2. Teeth
3. Salivary glands
4. Esophagus
5. Stomach
6. Small intestine
7. Pancreas
8. Liver
9. Gallbladder
10. Large intestine
11. Rectum

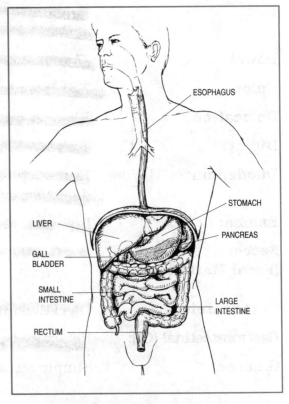

The Digestive System

Tongue, Teeth, and Salivary Glands

Food is taken into the mouth where the teeth grind it into pieces small enough to swallow. During this grinding process, it is mixed with saliva, the fluid produced by the salivary glands. Saliva contains enzymes that initiate the breakdown of food and moistens the food so that it is easily swallowed. The tongue aids in moving the food around in the mouth and moving it down the throat into the esophagus.

Esophagus

The esophagus is a tube approximately 10 inches long which connects the throat with the stomach. The food moves down the esophagus and enters the stomach.

Stomach

The stomach is a pear-shaped muscular sac. It can expand to accommodate food. The muscles of the stomach contract and churn and mix the food with gastric juices and digestive enzymes which break the food down into a thick, soupy substance. This can take from three to five hours. The churning action then passes this substance into the small intestine.

Small Intestine

The small intestine is a coiled, muscular tube about 26 feet long. The first loop of the coil, just below the stomach, is called the **duodenum**. This is the most important area for digestion. The partially digested food from the stomach is mixed with more digestive juices from the duodenum, pancreas, and gallbladder. Water is also essential to this process. Within the lining of the small intestine are thousand of **villi** which absorb the digested food particles and release them into the bloodstream to be carried to the body cells. The food mass moves through the 26 feet of small intestine by a process called **peristalsis**. Here the process of digestion is completed.

Pancreas

The pancreas is part of the endocrine system. It is a long, thin gland which lies just behind and slightly below the stomach. The pancreas plays a part in digestion because it secretes **insulin** into the small intestine, which helps break down starch and sugar in the food mass.

Liver

The liver is a large organ lying to the right of the stomach. **Bile**, which breaks down fats, is manufactured and secreted by the liver. The liver is also a storage area for **glucose**. And it serves as a filtering system which removes **toxins** from the blood and produces and stores blood proteins.

Gallbladder

The gallbladder lies directly under the liver and functions as a storage bag for the bile produced by the liver. Bile is released by the gallbladder into the duodenum to break down fats in the food being digested.

Large Intestine

The large intestine, or **colon**, is a continuation of the small intestine. It is bigger in diameter, but is only about five feet long. The parts of the food which have not been absorbed by the villi pass into the large intestine. Here most of the water remaining in the food is reabsorbed through the walls of the large intestine. The remaining solid mass is waste material called **feces**. This is moved by peristalsis through the large intestine to the **rectum**, where it is removed from the body by **defecation**.

Rectum

The rectum is a small canal about six inches long which connects the large intestine with the **anus**, the opening to the outside of the body. This canal is surrounded by **sphincter** muscles which keep the anus closed until voluntary elimination, or **bowel** movement, occurs.

AGE-RELATED CHANGES

There are a number of changes which occur in the digestive tract as a person ages. There is a general slowing down of these systems:

1. Movement of the esophagus decreases.

2. Movement of the colon decreases.

3. There is a decrease in the active ingredients in saliva from the salivary glands.

4. Less gastric juice is secreted by the stomach.

5. Food is absorbed more slowly in the small intestine.

COMMON DISORDERS OF THE DIGESTIVE SYSTEM

Many older people complain of digestive and elimination problems. Some of the most common are:

> ▶   *Ulcer.* An ulcer is a loss of tissue or a hole in tissue. Ulcers can occur in the esophagus, stomach, or duodenum. They are caused by an excess of gastric juice, which destroys the mucous

membranes in these areas. Ulcers usually cause a burning pain in the stomach area an hour or more after eating. Ulcers are treated with medication and diet.

▶ **Gallstones.** Gallstones are cholesterol crystals which settle out of the bile in the gallbladder and form gallstones. These stones may block the secretions of bile. This produces pain and nausea. The treatment involves removing or crushing the stones or removing the gallbladder.

▶ **Diverticulitis.** Diverticula are small, sac-like extensions of the intestinal wall that form and become inflamed. This disease can cause extreme pain. The treatment is a modification of diet, usually to a diet low in fat and very high in roughage.

▶ **Hemorrhoids.** Hemorrhoids are blood vessels surrounding the rectum that become enlarged and are particularly painful when having a bowel movement. They are usually treated with medication but may have to be surgically removed if they become very bad.

▶ **Constipation.** Constipation is the buildup of fecal material in the large intestine, which is not easily eliminated. Treatment is usually with *laxatives*, stool softeners, or *enema*. Prevention is preferable to treatment, and it consists of diet change, increased fluids and increased exercise. You should immediately report any pain, liquid stool or an absence of bowel movements to the charge nurse.

▶ **Fecal Impaction.** Fecal impaction is a serious complication of constipation. Feces stay in the colon and rectum where water is absorbed, which causes the feces to become dry and very hard. The intestinal passage may be totally blocked and the abdomen becomes distended and is very painful. This needs the attention of the licensed nurse.

It is the nursing assistant's responsibility to report promptly any GI symptoms to the charge nurse if there are signs or complaints of nausea, vomiting, constipation, diarrhea, or abdominal pain.

Chapter 18: Anatomy and Physiology:
The Digestive System

*Circle the correct answer. There is only **one** correct answer.*

1. **About how long is the normal human digestive system?**

    a. 3 inches.

    b. 3 feet.

    c. 30 feet.

    d. 300 feet.

2. **Saliva contains enzymes that initiate the breakdown of food.**

    a. True   b. False

3. **Which organ of the body filters toxins?**

    a. Esophagus.

    b. Small intestine.

    c. Pancreas.

    d. Liver.

4. **Where are villi located?**

    a. Stomach.

    b. Small intestine.

    c. Large intestine.

    d. Gallbladder.

5. **Another name for the large intestine is**

    a. Duodenum.

    b. Bile.

    c. Colon.

    d. Peristalsis.

6. **Where is glucose stored?**

   a. Gallbladder.

   b. Small intestine.

   c. Large intestine.

   (d.) Liver.

7. **As a person ages, what changes occur in the digestive tract?**

   (a.) Movement of the colon is decreased.

   b. More gastric juice is secreted.

   c. Food is absorbed more quickly.

   d. The active ingredients in saliva increase.

8. **Ulcers can be caused by an excess of:**

   (a.) Gastric juice.

   b. Food.

   c. Saliva.

   d. Roughage.

9. **Gallstones are formed by cholesterol crystals which settle out of the bile in the gallbladder.**

   (a.) True   b. False

10. **Hemorrhoids are:**

    (a.) Enlarged blood vessels.

    b. Holes in tissue.

    c. Impacted feces.

    d. Abnormal secretions.

Chapter 19

ANATOMY AND PHYSIOLOGY: THE NERVOUS SYSTEM

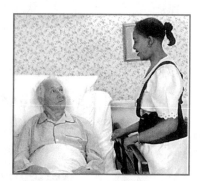

In this chapter... you will learn about:

▶ The nervous system.

▶ Some common problems of the nervous system.

DEFINITIONS

Aphasia:	Loss of language or verbal communication.
Chronic Brain Syndrome (Alzheimer's Type Dementia)	Large areas of the brain stop functioning, causing memory loss, fear and poor judgment.
Dementia:	Mental deterioration, loss of ability to think clearly.
Equilibrium:	Balance.
Hemiplegia:	Paralysis on one side of the body.
Hemisphere:	Half of a round mass of tissue.
Linear:	Following in order along a line.
Neurons:	Specialized cells of the nervous system.
Parkinson's Disease:	Disorder of the nervous system resulting in body stiffness and shakiness.
Peripheral:	Away from the center of something.

Definitions continued...

^x**Reflex:**	An automatic response to stimulation.
^x**Spatial:**	Oriented in space.
Stroke (Cerebral Vascular Accident or CVA)	Sudden stoppage of the blood supply to an area of the brain.
^x**Vertebrae:**	Bones of the spine.

THE NERVOUS SYSTEM

The nervous system is the control and communication center for the body. It causes all the other body systems to function. It enables you to see, hear, feel, talk, smell, taste, move, think, and remember.

The nervous system is made of:

1. The brain, which has three main parts.

2. The spinal cord, which extends from the brain down your spinal column.

3. *Peripheral* nerves, that extend outward from the brain and spinal column and carry messages to and from all parts of the body.

These three parts work together to control and coordinate all body activities.

Brain

The brain fits inside our skull and weighs about three pounds in an adult. The soft, wavy material we associate with the word brain is called the cerebrum or cerebral cortex. This is the largest part of the brain, and it controls all the functions associated with thinking and voluntary activity. Deciding to walk across the room is a voluntary activity.

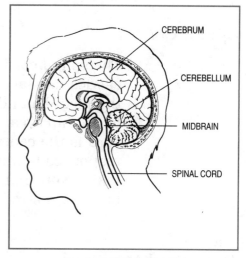

Parts of the Brain

Sitting beneath the cerebrum, or top part of the brain, in the back of the skull is the cerebellum. The cerebellum is involved in coordinating voluntary movements and helps maintain **equilibrium**.

Beneath the cerebrum is the midbrain. This section connects the cerebrum with the spinal cord and carries messages to and from the cerebral cortex. It also controls all the involuntary functions of the body, such as breathing, peristalsis in your intestine, and heartbeat. You don't have to think about these activities; they happen automatically.

Scientists have learned that the cerebrum contains specific areas which control specific functions. The main division is into right and left **hemispheres**. The right hemisphere controls the left side of the body and is usually the site of the centers for **spatial** and creative functions. The left hemisphere controls the right side of the body and, for most people, it is the site of speech and **linear** thought. These hemispheres look basically the same. Each is divided into lobes which are the sites of specific functions:

1. Frontal lobes - area of speech, reason, and thought.

2. Parietal lobes - sensations of touch, pain, pressure, and temperature change.

3. Occipital lobes - sight.

4. Temporal lobes - hearing.

Spinal Cord

The spinal cord is a long bundle of nerves, like a cable, that carries messages to and from the brain. It is connected to the medulla and runs down the spine inside the **vertebrae** to the hip area. In addition to relaying messages, the spinal cord is the center for **reflexes**. These are automatic responses to stimulation. You don't have to think about taking your hand off a hot stove; when your hand jerks back, it is a reflex action.

Peripheral Nerves

The information relayed by the spinal cord comes from and is sent to nerves running to all parts of the body. If you stub your toe, this information travels from your toe, up your leg to the spinal cord which tells your brain that your toe hurts.

The cells of the nervous system are called **neurons**. Neurons are different from other cells because it is believed that they do not reproduce themselves. Even if neurons are not replaced when they die, this should not seriously affect functions since we each have billions of neurons in our nervous system.

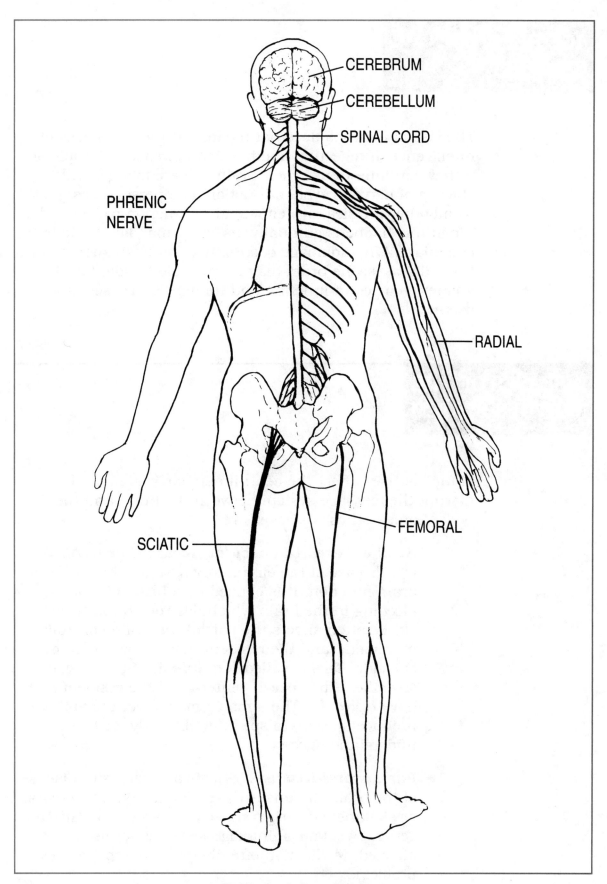

CEREBRUM

CEREBELLUM

SPINAL CORD

PHRENIC
NERVE

RADIAL

FEMORAL

SCIATIC

Some Peripheral Nerves

AGE-RELATED CHANGES

The loss of neurons does not mean that there is a loss of intelligence. Intellectual abilities can increase as people age if they continue to use their brains. There is a general slowing of nervous system function as a person ages, just as all other physical systems tend to function more slowly. When this happens gradually, as in normal aging, the brain can adapt. When damage occurs more quickly, such as in some diseases, the brain may not be able to adapt and greater changes in function and thought processes may occur.

DISEASES OF THE NERVOUS SYSTEM

Many diseases affect the central nervous system and can disrupt the message system between the brain and the body. Some of these diseases are:

▶ *Stroke (Cerebral vascular accident or CVA).* This is a disease of the circulatory system which affects brain function. It is caused by a blood clot or bleeding in the brain which destroys brain tissue. A stroke often affects the part of the brain controlling movement, and the resident may be paralyzed on one side. This is called *hemiplegia*. Strokes can also affect the speech centers and the resident may have *aphasia*. The aphasia may affect the ability to produce speech, to speak intelligently, or to understand speech.

▶ *Parkinson's Disease.* This is a progressive disease of the brain. It causes the resident to have tremors, or shaking; stiff, rigid muscles; a shuffling gait; and general weakness. Intelligence, however, is not affected. Medication often helps ease some of these problems.

▶ ***Chronic Brain Syndrome (also called Alzheimer's-Type Dementia).*** In this condition large areas of neurons cease to function and the resident cannot remember what just happened, has poor judgment, and has great fear and anxiety. Residents may forget who family and friends are, how to do simple tasks, and how to care for themselves. These residents need a safe, caring environment. Behavior will change due to diseases of the nervous system. It is important to remember that the disease causes the change. The behavior is not intentional. You will learn more about dealing with Alzheimer's and other dementias in a later chapter.

*Circle the correct answer. There is only **one** correct answer.*

1. **The nervous system is the control and communication center for the rest of the body.**

    a. True   b. False

2. **What body part is not part of the nervous system?**

    a. Brain.

    b. Spinal cord.

    c. Peripheral nerves.

    d. Pancreas.

3. **Which part of the brain controls the involuntary functions of the body, such as breathing and sleeping?**

    a. Cerebrum and cerebellum.

    b. Cerebellum and cortex.

    c. Midbrain.

    d. Neuron and vertebrae.

4. **In most people, the right side or hemisphere of the brain controls the left side of the body.**

    a. True   b. False

5. **Hemispheres are divided into neurons which are the sites of specific functions.**

    a. True   b. False

6. **The spinal cord controls reflex actions.**

    a. True   b. False

7. **What are the nerves called that run to all parts of the body?**

    a. Spinal nerves.

    b. Neurons.

    c. Peripheral nerves.

    d. Lobes.

8. **As a person ages, the nervous system functions more slowly.**

    a. True   b. False

9. **Mrs. Jarrett had a stroke which left her paralyzed on her right side. What is this condition called?**

    a. Aphasia.

    b. Hemiplegia.

    c. Parkinson's disease.

    d. Alzheimer's disease.

10. **The loss of the ability to think clearly is called:**

    a. Stroke.

    b. Parkinson's disease.

    c. Dementia.

    d. Hemiplegia.

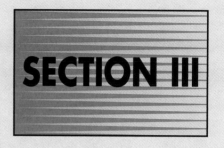

SECTION III

INFECTION CONTROL AND COMMON DISEASES

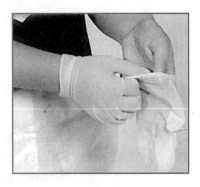

Chapter 20

INFECTION CONTROL

 Watch step-by-step demonstrations of the procedures discussed in this chapter in the Medcom videotapes "The New Nursing Assistant 2000: Infection Control" *(CNA501),* "Bloodborne Safety: Universal Precautions, Standard Precautions, and Needlestick Prevention in Long Term Care" *(UP200T), and* "Standards for Infection Control: An Update for Long Term Care" *(M167).*

In this chapter... you will learn about:

▶ What causes infections.

▶ What you can do to help prevent infections in the facility.

▶ What you can do to protect yourself from infections

DEFINITIONS

Asepsis:	Preventing the growth and spread of dangerous microorganisms.
Autoclave:	A machine used to kill all microorganisms on medical instruments or supplies.
CDC (Centers for Disease Control):	The government agency that investigates outbreaks of diseases and sets standards to try to prevent the spread of diseases.
Clean:	Considered to be free from pathogens.
Disinfection:	Process of killing microorganisms.
Highly Transmissible:	Easily spread through the air or by contact.
Immune System:	System of the body which protects from invasion of certain diseases.
Infection:	Invasion of the body by disease-producing organisms.

Definitions continued...

Inflammation:	Tissue reaction to disease or injury displayed by redness, heat, swelling, and pain.
Microorganism:	Tiny living objects seen only with a microscope
OSHA (Occupational Safety and Health Agency):	The government agency that investigates and promotes safety and health issues in the workplace.
Organism:	Any form of life (such as a germ).
Pathogen:	A microorganism that is harmful and can cause an infection (for example, a bacteria or virus).
Standard Precautions:	Standards set by CDC to decrease disease transmission through body fluids.
Sterile:	Free from all microorganisms.
Universal Precautions:	Standards set by OSHA to decrease disease transmission through contact with blood and body fluids containing blood.

INFECTION CONTROL

Infection control is a necessary part of keeping the residents safe. Every facility has policies and procedures to accomplish control and must constantly monitor the infection control program. It is important for the nursing assistant to be familiar with and follow these established procedures.

The purposes of the infection control program are:

▶ To provide an environment that is as germ-free as possible for residents, visitors, and staff (environmental control).

▶ To protect residents, visitors and staff from getting an infection from someone else (cross infection).

▶ To prevent residents from getting an infection a second or third time (re-infection).

Infections are caused by **microorganisms**. Microorganisms are on all outer surfaces and inside everything around us, including the human body. Fortunately, the body's natural **immune system** usually protects us from these **pathogens**. The skin and mucous lining in the mouth and nose act as barriers to these foreign substances. Two of the common microorganisms which cause the most disease in humans are bacteria and viruses.

Not all bacteria are harmful. Many bacteria normally live on your skin, in your nose, mouth, and intestinal tract. These "friendly" bacteria are necessary in body processes, such as breaking down waste products.

Two types of harmful bacteria which cause serious infections are:

▶ *Staphylococcus* which enters the body through natural openings or cuts and can cause severe local or entire body infections.

▶ *Streptococcus* which also enters through a natural opening or cut and causes sore throat, rheumatic fever, local or general infections.

Bacteria grow best in a warm, moist, dark environment. Bacteria grow well in food and in waste products. There are specific drugs, such as antibiotics, which kill specific bacteria.

Viruses are much smaller than bacteria, but they cause many human diseases, such as colds, influenza, polio, measles, and smallpox. Viruses can only survive in living cells. For this reason, they are more difficult to treat as the medication must kill the virus, and this often destroys the cell in which it lives. There is no one drug to kill all viruses. Vaccines have been developed which destroy or control specific viruses, such as polio, smallpox, and influenza.

When pathogenic microorganisms enter the body, they release toxins, or waste products, which poison the body's system. The immune system works to fight these toxins. The symptoms of this process which indicate an infection has occurred are:

- ▶ Elevated temperature or chills.

- ▶ ***Inflammation.***

- ▶ Swelling.

- ▶ Pain.

- ▶ Drainage from wound, nose, ears, or eyes.

- ▶ Disorientation, fatigue, or nausea.

Asepsis

Asepsis means preventing the conditions that allow pathogens to live and spread. These germs are destroyed or controlled with soap, water, disinfectant, and heat.

Sterilization is the process of killing all microorganisms. This requires the use of an ***autoclave***, a machine used to sterilize surgical instruments with high-temperature pressurized steam. Some autoclaves use chemical gases to sterilize objects that are vulnerable to heat, such as plastics.

- ▶ ***Sterile.*** An object is ***sterile*** when it is free from all microorganisms. An object which is not free of all microorganisms is contaminated. When a sterile object touches a nonsterile object, it becomes contaminated.

- ▶ ***Clean.*** This means an object is considered free from pathogens, but not necessarily free from all microorganisms (sterile). ***Disinfection*** with chemicals kills most microorganisms and slows the growth and activity of others. The object is considered clean, but not sterile.

> ▶ *Dirty.* This means an object can be presumed to be contaminated. It has been exposed to disease-producing organisms and can pass them on to other objects. If an object touches the floor, it may still look "clean," but it has been contaminated and cannot be used.

PROTECTING YOURSELF FROM INFECTION

There are several things you can do to protect yourself and others from infections.

Standard Precautions

To prevent the spread of infection, the Centers for Disease Control (CDC) has developed guidelines for hospitals called STANDARD PRECAUTIONS. In addition, the Occupational Safety and Health Administration (OSHA) enforces regulations called UNIVERSAL PRECAUTIONS, designed to protect workers from bloodborne pathogens, such as HIV (the human immunodeficiency virus that causes AIDS) and HBV and HCV (the hepatitis B and C viruses).

Standard Precautions are designed to reduce the transmission of pathogens from both recognized and unrecognized sources. They are to be used for the care of all residents, whether they have been diagnosed with infectious disease or not. Standard Precautions apply to:

1. All human blood.

2. All body fluids, secretions and excretions, except sweat, regardless of whether they contain visible blood.

3. Nonintact skin.

4. Mucous membranes.

Universal Precautions enforced by OSHA are aimed only at blood and body fluids that contain blood. Standard

Precautions are broader in that they apply to all body fluids, secretions, or excretions except sweat.

The primary modes of transmission of bloodborne pathogens, such as HIV (AIDS) and HBV (hepatitis B), on the job are:

▶ Puncture wounds from contaminated needles or other sharps.

▶ Broken skin contact with infectious fluids, such as blood.

▶ Contact with infectious fluids through the mucous membranes of the eyes, nose and mouth.

By observing the following rules, you can observe Standard Precautions and help protect yourself and others from transmission of potentially infectious materials:

Rule 1: Consider all residents potentially infectious, because you can never be sure who may be a carrier of infection.

Rule 2: Assume that all blood and other body fluids, secretions, or excretions, except sweat, are contaminated with pathogens that can infect you.

Rule 3: Assume that all used needles and other sharps are contaminated. Be on the alert for sharps hidden in beds or dirty linen. Never recap used needles by hand, and place all used sharps into approved disposal containers.

Rule 4: Wear protective gloves at all times when handling blood, body fluids, secretions, excretions, and any contaminated items. And wear gloves when performing procedures that involve possible contact with mucous membranes or nonintact skin. Remember to wash hands after wearing gloves.

Rule 5: Wear a mask and protective eyewear if risky material is likely to splash or spray into the eyes, nose, or mouth.

> Rule 6: Wear a gown to protect your clothing when there is possible contact with infectious materials, such as when handling fluid-soaked linens.
>
> Rule 7: Dispose of infectious waste according to the policies of your facility. For waste that is dripping or oozes fluids when pressure is applied, place it in a leak-proof container.

In addition, OSHA recommends that all workers who come into contact with blood or other potentially infectious body fluids be vaccinated against hepatitis B.

Hand Hygiene

As a nursing assistant, your hands are continually coming in contact with your residents and objects which can be contaminated. The best infection control you can practice is frequent, thorough hand hygiene.

Routine handwashing is an effective means of infection control. But often handwashing is not done due to the time it takes to wash hands with soap and water, and the availability of handwashing facilities. To address this, the CDC's most recent hand hygiene guideline, recommends the use of waterless antiseptic agents, such as alcohol-based handrubs, for the routine decontamination of hands that are not visibly soiled.

You reduce the chance of infection if you always use an antiseptic handrub:

- ▶ Before and after contact with each resident, even if gloves are worn.

- ▶ Before handling food or food trays.

- ▶ After contact with contaminated objects.

- ▶ After blowing your nose.

- ▶ After using the bathroom.

- ▶ After contact with soiled linen.

To use an antiseptic hand rub:

▶ Apply the manufacturer's recommended amount of the agent to the palm of one hand.

▶ Rub the hands together so the agent covers all surfaces of the hands and fingers.

▶ Continue to rub until the hands are dry. Do not rinse.

Hand washing with soap and water should still be done anytime hands are visibly soiled, and at the beginning of your shift. Following are guidelines for proper handwashing.

1. Keeping your fingertips down, completely wet your hands and wrists under warm running water.

2. Apply soap, spreading it over your entire hands, wrists, between fingers, and under nails. (Use an antimicrobial agent if there was contact with nfective material, such as fecal material or wound drainage).

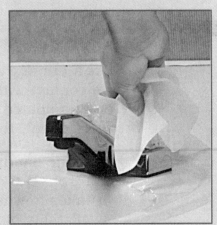

3. Vigorously rub hands together, between fingers, under nails, and two inches above wrists for one full minute.

4. Rinse under warm running water, holding fingers down.

5. Dry hands and wrists thoroughly with paper towels.

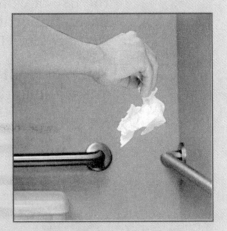

6. Turn off faucet with a paper towel between the faucet and your hand and immediately discard the towel. The faucet is considered dirty and will contaminate your hand.

Any body fluid, including saliva, wound drainage, urine, and feces which contain pathogens, and disposable items which come in contact with *any* body discharges are considered infectious waste. You must wear gloves when handling any of these substances, and these items must be carefully disposed of in accordance with the policies of the facility.

Linen Handling

The nursing assistant must also handle the residents' linen in a way that reduces the possibility of infection. Guidelines for proper linen handling are:

1. Wash hands before touching clean linen.

2. Hold clean linen away from your body. Your uniform can transfer microorganisms to the clean linen. Also hold soiled linen away from your body. It can transfer microorganisms TO your uniform.

3. Avoid shaking or fluffing linen as this spreads microorganisms.

4. Soiled linen must never be placed on bedside furniture or the floor. Soiled linen must be placed immediately in a soiled linen hamper and the lid must be tightly closed.

5. Wash your hands immediately after handling soiled linen.

Transmission-Based Precautions

Your facility will probably not have any residents with **highly transmissible** pathogens, such as those that cause tuberculosis or other infectious diseases. If one of your residents is diagnosed with one of these diseases, the charge nurse will inform you of further precautions to take. These precautions may include:

- *Airborne Precautions.* To prevent spread through microorganisms suspended in the air. You will probably be instructed to wear a special N-95 mask (respirator) to filter out contaminated air.

- *Droplet Precautions.* To prevent spread through pathogens contained in small droplets in a cough or sneeze. You will probably be instructed to wear a surgical mask in this case.

- *Contact Precautions.* To prevent skin-to-skin or object-to-skin spread of pathogens. You will wear gloves and you may be asked to wear other protective clothing such as a face shield or use protective covers on other surfaces to prevent direct contact. Patient care equipment may need to be dedicated to a single patient.

Personal Cleanliness

In addition to the above infection control measures, as a nursing assistant you must keep yourself clean. A clean uniform should be worn each day. Hair should be clean and well groomed. Fingernails should be kept short and clean. Do not wear unnecessary jewelry because it can harbor microorganisms.

If you have a cold or any type of infection, it is your responsibility to report this to the charge nurse who will determine whether or not you should provide resident care.

Infection control is one of the primary responsibilities of a nursing assistant. By practicing good infection control techniques, you will be safeguarding your residents, their families, other employees, yourself, and your family.

Circle the correct answer. There is only **one** *correct answer.*

1. **Infection control is necessary to keep the resident safe.**

    a. True   b. False

2. **In what type of environment do bacteria grow best?**

    a. Cool and dry.

    b. Light.

    c. Warm and moist.

3. **There is no one drug that kills all viruses.**

    a. True   b. False

4. **Chills or fever, inflammation and swelling are some signs of infection.**

    a. True   b. False

5. **It is only necessary to wash your hands once a day or when you can actually see dirt on your hands.**

    a. True   b. False

6. **If an object falls on the floor it is considered:**

    a. Clean.

    b. Disinfected.

    c. Dirty.

    d. Dirty only if you can see dirt on it.

7. **To avoid contamination, turn off the faucet.**

    a. After handling food.

    b. After touching a resident.

    c. With a paper towel between the faucet and your hand.

    d. With your bare hands.

8. **Disinfectants kill all organisms.**

    a. True   b. False

9. **Some examples of infectious waste are saliva, wound drainage, urine, and feces.**

    a. True   b. False

10. **Mrs. Morton falls asleep and urinates in bed. In changing her bed, it's okay to place the soiled linen on a chair for few minutes before putting it in a hamper.**

    a. True   b. False

Chapter 21

OPTIMUM LEVELS OF HEALTH

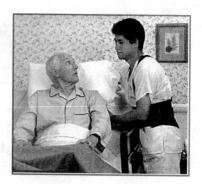

In this chapter... you will learn about:

▶ Optimum levels of health.

▶ How to help residents reach optimum levels of health.

DEFINITIONS

Optimum Level of Health:

The most favorable level of health and well-being possible.

OPTIMUM LEVELS OF HEALTH

The goal of **optimum level of health** is to be as independent as possible and to feel as good as possible. Optimum health is not simply a question of avoiding disease. It also includes physical, emotional and social well being. The resident has many needs which must be met in all these areas. When all these needs are met, the resident will be as healthy as possible.

Physical Needs

To reach and maintain optimum physical health, the resident must have:

> ▶ Proper food.
>
> ▶ Adequate rest.
>
> ▶ Proper medical care.
>
> ▶ Prescribed medication and treatments.
>
> ▶ Movement and exercise.
>
> ▶ Cleanliness.

The nursing assistant is responsible for fulfilling many of these daily physical needs. When the resident is encouraged to eat the diet provided, helped to relax and rest, encouraged and assisted in ambulation and exercise, and assisted in daily hygiene, he or she will have a good chance of reaching an optimum level of health. Helping to meet a resident's physical needs will be discussed in more detail in Chapter 30.

Psychosocial Needs

Everyone also has psychosocial and emotional needs. These include needing to feel:

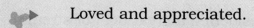

> Loved and appreciated.
>
> ▶ Approved of and respected.
>
> ▶ A sense of accomplishment.
>
> ▶ Recognized as an individual.
>
> ▶ Worthwhile and important.

How residents feel about themselves affects their physical health. Listening, encouraging, and reinforcing positive actions help the resident feel worthwhile and able to strive toward greater health.

Socialization Needs

We all have a need to interact with other people every day. This is called socialization. Socialization provides us with:

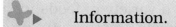

> Information.
>
> ▶ Ideas.
>
> ▶ Support.
>
> ▶ Affection.
>
> ▶ Stimulation.

Our needs for affection, affirmation, and feelings of worth are met by the response we receive from others. The nursing assistant interacts with residents every day and provides a great deal of emotional and socialization support. Helping residents interact with each other will also provide them with many opportunities to fill their emotional needs. Helping to meet a resident's socialization needs will be discussed in more detail in Chapter 51.

Spiritual Needs

For many residents, a great deal of strength, patience, and acceptance is gained through a belief in a being or force greater than themselves. The nursing assistant can help residents by accepting individual beliefs, whatever they are, and helping residents follow these beliefs. Cultural and religious beliefs will be discussed in more detail in Chapter 56.

SETTING AN EXAMPLE OF OPTIMUM HEALTH

You can help motivate residents by being an example of good physical and mental health yourself. There are things you can do for yourself at any age to promote optimum health and become an example to others of the habits of good health.

Be aware of what you eat and choose foods which help you to be strong and healthy. Good habits can start at any age. A healthy diet includes a variety of foods including fresh fruits and vegetables, whole grains, dairy products, and meat, poultry, and fish which are low in fat. Limiting sweets, salt, and foods high in fats can help you keep from gaining excess weight, increase your energy, and promote good health.

Avoid smoking. This habit damages your respiratory system and shortens your life. Smoking interferes with breathing, tasting food, and it smells bad. It can also harm those around you. Be smart, don't start. If you already have, stop.

Regular activity and movement is necessary for everyone to maintain optimum health. Regular participation in a sport, aerobics, or a brisk walk will increase your strength and endurance, burn calories, and make you feel great. Brisk walking as little as 20 minutes three times a week can make a tremendous improvement in your health.

Having a positive attitude about yourself and others is just as important as the positive physical things you do for yourself. Concentrate on the good things happening in your life. Enjoy the people you are with and they will enjoy being with you. It's just as easy to look on the bright side as it is to see only the gloom. Take pride in who you are and what you do.

Maintaining optimum levels of health for your residents is an important responsibility. But, an equally important responsibility is gaining and maintaining optimum levels of physical and emotional well being for yourself. You can hardly expect your residents to be very enthusiastic if you do not set a positive example yourself.

*Circle the correct answer. There is only **one** correct answer.*

1. **An optimum level of health is being as independent as possible and feeling as good as possible.**

    (a.) True   b. False

2. **To reach an optimum level of health you only need to worry about avoiding diseases.**

    a. True   (b.) False

3. **Exercise is not an important part of maintaining an optimal level of health.**

    a. True   (b.) False

4. **How residents feel about themselves has no effect on their physical health.**

    a. True   (b.) False

5. **Psychosocial needs refers to**

    a. Eating properly.

    (b.) Emotional health.

    c. Getting exercise.

    d. Avoiding disease.

6. **Which of the following foods does not promote good health?**

    a. Apple.

    (b.) Chocolate bar.

    c. Oat bran cereal.

    d. Chicken.

7. **Which of the following statements is not true about smoking?**

    a. It can add years to your life.

    b. It smells bad.

    c. It interferes with breathing.

    d. It affects the taste of food.

8. **How can you set a good example of optimum health.**

    a. Continue smoking.

    b. Explain to the residents what they must do.

    c. Maintain your own optimum health.

    d. Avoid exercise.

9. **Having a positive attitude about yourself and others is just as important as the positive physical things you do for yourself.**

    a. True   b. False

10. **Maintaining optimum levels of health for yourself is not nearly as important as it is for your residents.**

    a. True   b. False

Chapter 22

AGE-SPECIFIC ISSUES

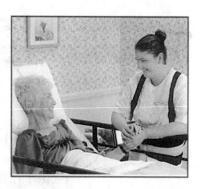

 See additional examples, descriptions and demonstrations of the concepts discussed in this chapter in the Medcom videotape "Aging: The Natural Process" (M203).

In this chapter... you will learn about:

▶ Issues of puberty.

▶ The process of aging.

▶ Wrong ideas about older people.

▶ Some common diseases and conditions of the older resident.

DEFINITIONS

Carbohydrates:	The chemicals in foods that supply quick energy, such as sugars and starches.
Dementia:	A mental state in which the mind no longer functions properly.
Insulin:	A hormone that the body needs to turn carbohydrates into energy.
Menstruation:	The monthly loss of blood and some tissue from a woman of sexual age who is not pregnant.
Osteoporosis:	A condition that causes a decrease in the size and strength of the bones.
Puberty:	The age when boys and girls become capable of sexual activity and reproduction, usually from age 11 to 13.
Secondary sexual characteristics:	Breasts, pubic hair, and other traits that develop during puberty.
Tremor:	A rapid shaking or trembling, often noticeable in the hands or face muscles.

Puberty is a time of great change and emotional worry in boys and girls. On average girls reach sexual maturity sooner than boys, as early as nine years old in some cases, though more often at 11 or later. Boys do not usually reach puberty until age 12 or later. At whatever age, the young people who enter puberty suddenly grow taller and heavier, and they experience a rush of new hormones in their blood. These sexual hormones make them more interested in romance and sexual activity.

The hormones also cause the growth of secondary sexual characteristics that may make young people self-conscious. Girls begin menstruation, develop breasts, and grow pubic hair. Boys grow pubic hair, beards and mustaches, and often their voices change and grow deeper. These powerful changes can lead to personal and social problems.

Problems of Puberty

If you work with young people who are entering puberty, there are a number of problems and issues to watch out for. Just being in an institution will not shield a young person from the problems of puberty.

Grow Distant from Parents

It is natural for many young people at this age to grow distant or even angry at their parents. You shouldn't agree with them if they complain about their parents, but listen with sympathy. Counsel the parents, if they are upset, that this is a natural stage of growing up that many young people experience and pass through.

Love Attachments

Young people in puberty tend to fall in and out of love, to develop strong attachments quickly, and become very sad when relationships end. You should remain sympathetic and listen to their concerns. Even if you know they will feel better in a few days, it doesn't help to tell them things like, "You'll get over it soon," or "We all felt this way when we were young." Take them seriously as people. If possible, provide activities to help give them a new focus.

Worry about their Body Image

Girls at this age are beginning to develop breasts, and boys experience sudden growth that makes them feel awkward or a change of voice. And some young people see their friends going through these changes before they do--or they go first and experience the changes while their friends are still unchanged. These new looks and sounds can make them very self-conscious, private, and nervous about being seen. It is best at this age for women to counsel girls and men to counsel boys. If you are the "wrong" sex to give advice, try to find someone of the same sex as the young person. Reassure them that these changes are a natural part of life. Express interest in the changes and share any experiences you have had.

Menstruation

Menstruation is a normal part of life for all young women, but it can be very frightening the first few times it happens without much warning. It is best to find a women to counsel a girl who is first experiencing menstruation. As with other changes of puberty, remain sympathetic, patiently explain the change matter-of factly as a normal part of life, and offer your own experiences.

Sexual Activities

Adults have the right to engage in sexual activities, even in an institution, but minors do not. They are children, in your care, and you are responsible for them. No matter how intense their feelings, this must be made clear to them. Discuss sex openly with them, and without embarrassment or shame, but make it clear that you cannot tolerate any sexual contact in the institution.

And some young people may try to express their sexual feeling by reaching out to you or even touching you where you don't want to be touched. Handle the situation calmly but firmly, and insist that you don't want them to do that.

Masturbation

Masturbation, or sexual self-stimulation, is a normal part of adolescence, and it does no harm. Discuss it calmly and without trying to shame anyone. If you observe anyone masturbating, do not call attention to it. Try to provide privacy discreetly by closing the door.

Young people going through puberty are in a difficult time of their lives. This can be made worse for them if some accident or medical condition has put them in nursing care. Try to understand, talk to them sympathetically, and treat them as young adults. Try to involve them in their own health care decisions. You shouldn't belittle their fears and worries, but discuss them openly and calmly. Use sympathy and praise, and compliment them on any positive responses to their fears.

As a nursing assistant in a long-term care facility, it is likely that you will work with a number of older adult residents. It is important that you understand the processes of aging, how they affect your residents and what common conditions and diseases the residents are more likely to have as they grow older.

The Process of Aging

Aging happens at a different rate for everyone. The rate is influenced by heredity, general health and lifestyle. Some people remain active and alert into their nineties and beyond, while others begin to slow down and lose mental alertness much sooner. There is no specific date at which someone is "old."

Despite this, there is no way to escape the processes of aging entirely. Sooner or later, everyone loses some coordination, bones become more brittle, joints get stiffer, and vision and hearing may become weaker. These are normal processes.

Wrong Ideas about the Older Person

There are a few common ideas about older people that it will be important for you to put aside. These are not true, or certainly not true of everyone.

"Old people think of themselves as old." Since aging is a continuous process, many old people think of themselves as the same as they were ten or twenty or more years ago. In fact, many can still do the same things. Many old people are quite proud of how well they have aged and the things they can still do.

"Old people are all confused." Confusion is usually the result of a specific condition such as Alzheimer's or another form of dementia. Some loss of the ability to memorize new information is very common in older people, but many old people are just as alert and well oriented as they ever were.

"Old people are no longer interested in sex." Some older people experience a decline in sexuality, but many do not. Many simply have lost a loving partner and have no outlet for their sexual feelings.

"Old people are all bitter and unhappy." Some people who have lost loved ones, or have had to leave familiar homes, will go through a period of mourning. Others may become upset by their declining powers. But a state of permanent depression or unhappiness is NOT normal for the older resident. If one of your residents seems permanently unhappy, you should discuss it with the nurse. The resident may need psychological help.

The older residents you care for are just as varied and different as any group of people you will meet. There are very few general rules that apply to all of them.

COMMON DISEASES OF THE OLDER RESIDENT

There are some diseases and conditions that become more common with age. Of course, not all the elderly will get these. But it is important to watch out for signs and symptoms of these conditions as you carry out your daily caregiving.

Alzheimer's Disease

A progressive mental disorder that slowly takes away all mental functioning. There is no cure.

Arteriosclerosis

A hardening of the arteries, reducing blood flow to some parts of the body, causing poor circulation of blood, particularly to the extremities (especially hand and feet). Moderate exercise and a low-fat diet may help prevent it.

Broken Bones (fractures)

As people age, their bones become more brittle and break more easily. Fractures of the hip can be common from falls. Older women with **osteoporosis** are especially prone to breaking bones.

Cataracts

Clouding of the lens of the eye, causing decreased vision. Surgery can sometimes repair the damage.

Congestive Heart Failure

Inability of the heart to pump enough blood, which causes, difficulty breathing, and accumulation of fluid in the extremities.

Dementia

A term used to describe mental disorders caused by changes in the brain which affect a person's ability to think, reason, judge, understand and behave normally. This is commonly caused by Alzheimer's Disease, but it may be due to a curable condition. Speak to your nurse if you notice new signs of confusion or disorientation in a resident.

Diabetes Mellitus

Sometimes just called diabetes. A disease of the metabolism that makes it hard for the body to turn **carbohydrates** into energy.   In Type I diabetes, the body lacks the hormone called **insulin** and the person must take it regularly by injection. In Type II, which becomes more common with aging, the condition can sometimes be brought under control with exercise, careful diet, and oral medications.

Emphysema

The tiny airways in the lungs grow rigid and become blocked by fluids, making breathing very difficult. The person coughs a lot, coughs up thick secretions, and becomes very anxious about difficult breathing. It is more common in people who smoke or have smoked. Persons diagnosed with emphysema may have to take oxygen regularly because their lungs no longer work properly.

Gastritis (stomach upset)

An inflammation of the stomach that can be caused by infections, or poor nutrition, or excessive eating or drinking. Gastritis is more common in older people. If it persists, notify the nurse. A physician should try to determine the cause.

Heart Attack (myocardial infarction)

This happens when there is a sudden blockage of the arteries to the heart. This may kill some heart tissue, causing the heart to stop functioning. Death may result.

Hemorrhoids (piles)

Enlarged blood vessels around the rectum, which are more common as people become less active and sit a lot. They cause burning and itching around the rectum and blood can sometimes be seen on the stool or on toilet paper.

Hypertension (high blood pressure)

You should discover this condition when you take the resident's blood pressure. There are often no symptoms, but if it becomes very high there can be headaches and changes in vision. Treatments usually include exercise, diet (no salt) and medications. This is common in older people, due to changes in the blood vessels as a person ages.

Multiple Sclerosis (MS)

A slow progressive disease of the nervous system that causes loss of control of muscles and speech problems.

Parkinson's Disease

A slow progressive disease of the nervous system that causes **tremors**, a shuffling way of walking, and very slow movements. Mental function is usually unaffected. Treatment includes drugs, the but resident usually needs help with activities of daily living.

Pneumonia

Infection of the lungs. Some forms can be treated with antibiotics. Fluids building up in the lungs may have to be suctioned out by a respiratory therapist.

Pressure Sores (pressure ulcers, decubitus ulcers)

Areas of the skin that become reddened and then break open. Caused by continuous pressure in one area, usually where bones stick out such as the sacral area, ankles and hips. Bed-ridden patients are turned regularly to prevent pressure sores.

Prostate Disease (benign prostatic hypertrophy or BPH)

In most men, the prostate gland that surrounds the urethra swells and hardens with age. This makes it harder to urinate. If the resident has had surgery on the prostate, it can cause urinary incontinence.

Scabies

Tiny mites (insects) that infest the skin, particularly in folds or in the genital area. They cause itching and inflammation. Report any suspicious rash or itching to the nurse. Scabies infestations spread easily through some nursing homes and care should be taken when found on a resident.

Stroke (cerebral vascular accident or CVA)

The blood supply to an area of the brain is suddenly cut off, sometimes by a blood clot getting caught in a blood vessel. This can result in permanent damage to the brain, loss of control of some part of the body, and/or slurring or loss of speech.

Varicose Veins

Some blood veins become swollen and painful, particularly in the legs. They often show as swollen blue lines under the skin. This is due to poor circulation and makes the feet cold and discolored.

As you carry out your daily activities with the residents, you should watch for signs of any of these conditions. Report anything new immediately to the nurse.

*Circle the correct answer. There is only **one** correct answer.*

1. **If you exercise regularly and eat well, you will never show any signs of aging.**

    a. True   (b.) False

2. **The word "cataract" means**

    a. A broken bone.

    b. Heart failure.

    (c.) Clouding of the lens of the eye.

    d. Forgetfulness.

3. **Which of the following is NOT characteristic of puberty:**

    a. Menstruation

    b. Breast development

    (c.) Dementia

    d. Voice changes

4. **Arteriosclerosis means**

    a. Hardening of a vein.

    b. Dementia.

    c. Confusion.

    (d.) Hardening of the arteries.

5. **Dementia means confusion and the inability to think properly.**

    (a.) True   b. False

6. **Diabetes mellitus can usually be cured with surgery.**

    a. True   (b.) False

7. **Hemorrhoids are swollen blood vessels around the rectum.**

   (a.) True   b. False

8. **Tremor might be caused by**

   a. Diabetes mellitus.

   b. Varicose veins.

   (c.) Parkinson's disease.

   d. Heart attack.

9. **Slurred speech might be caused by**

   (a.) Stroke.

   b. Hemorrhoids.

   c. Scabies.

   d. Pneumonia.

10. **A reddened itchy patch in the genital area might be caused by**

    a. Parkinson's disease.

    b. Emphysema.

    c. Dementia.

    (d.) Scabies.

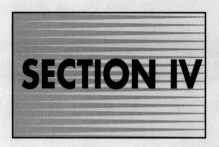

SECTION IV

OBSERVING THE RESIDENT

Chapter 23

COMMUNICATING WITH THE RESIDENTS

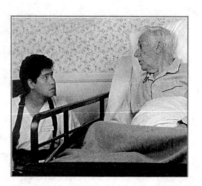

In this chapter... you will learn about:

▶ The importance of effective communication.

▶ Types of communication.

▶ The barriers to communication.

▶ Courtesy in use of a language other than English.

DEFINITIONS

Aphasia: Loss of the ability to use language effectively.

Body Language: Communicating through posture or facial expression or actions.

Communicate: To exchange information or opinions.

THE IMPORTANCE OF EFFECTIVE COMMUNICATION

Before you can provide care, or even make observations, you must be able to **communicate** effectively with your residents. You have to learn what they are thinking and feeling and you have to tell them what you are going to be doing.

Communication occurs whenever two or more people are together. Even if no one speaks, information is communicated through actions, **body language**, posture, facial expression, or even lack of action. We are always communicating.

SPEAKING AND LISTENING

When you talk, meaning is conveyed not only by the words you choose, but also by *how* you say them. Your attitude and how you feel affect how and what you say. People can often "hear" your attitude even if you don't think you are revealing it.

Talking is only part of verbal communicating — listening is also an important part. Too often we become so involved in talking that we forget to listen. Listening carefully will help you learn things about the residents, and it will also tell the residents that you care and are interested in them.

Good communication practices also include telling the resident what you are going to do before you do it. A simple explanation can decrease fear and suspicion in a resident and increase trust and cooperation.

The nursing assistant should speak in a pleasant voice that is neither too loud nor too soft. Speaking slowly and clearly will help the resident understand what you are saying. The use of slang or vulgar words or phrases by the nursing assistant is never appropriate.

The nursing assistant should always assume that the resident can hear and understand what is being said. Even if the resident appears to be confused or unconscious, the nursing assistant should never speak as though the resident cannot understand. Hearing is the last of the five senses to leave the body and is present even in a deep comatose state. You have no way of knowing what is heard or understood at this time.

WRITTEN COMMUNICATION

You will communicate every day with other staff members by writing in the chart. It is important that you keep this communication accurate and complete. If you forget to record a procedure or observation, or if you record it in a way that others cannot understand it, you may be risking harm to a resident.

You may even have to communicate in writing with a resident. A resident who has trouble speaking may pass you a note, or a resident who cannot hear may ask you to write what you are going to do. It is important that you practice your writing skills so your written communications will not be misunderstood.

NONVERBAL COMMUNICATION

Body Language

Your posture, facial expressions, and actions often reveal your true attitudes and feelings better than your words do. This is called body language. Moving slowly and having a slumped posture tells people that you are tired or bored. Clenched teeth, a frown, and a rigid posture could tell people you are angry. These are not the messages a nursing assistant will want to give to the residents. Moving briskly, standing erect, and smiling reassures the residents that you are skilled, alert, and interested.

It is important that your body language agrees with what you are saying. Telling a resident not to hurry while you are tapping your foot, or hurrying yourself, is sending two different messages. The resident will get the message that you are impatient. Remember, actions often speak louder than words.

Eye Contact

Maintaining eye contact is also important. This shows your residents that they have your complete attention.

Touch

A good way to communicate feelings is often through touch. Holding a hand, touching an arm or shoulder conveys tenderness, caring, concern, and warmth. We all have a need to be touched by another human being. Many older people are touched only when it is necessary to carry out a function such as bathing or positioning, yet the need for a warm, caring touch does not disappear with age.

BARRIERS TO COMMUNICATION

The Hearing Impaired Resident

It is important to know the degree of hearing loss for all your residents. Determine on which side the resident hears better and always speak to that side. Since older residents often lose the capacity to hear the higher-pitched sounds, it is best to keep your voice lower so it will be easier to hear you. Speaking in a clear, moderate voice is preferable to yelling. It will also help to stand in front of the resident so he or she can see you.

If the resident cannot hear at all, you may have to use written messages in order to communicate. Carrying a small tablet and pen in your pocket may be helpful.

The Blind Resident

Your words and tone of voice will be even more important when you are communicating with a blind or near-blind resident. Blind people often become very sensitive to tone of voice.

The Difficult Resident

Being ill and dependent is very stressful, and a resident may be very demanding and irritable. This behavior is often directed at you as the nursing assistant because you are the person most involved in the resident's care. It is important for you to remember this and not take negative comments and behavior personally.

Often the resident will be more cooperative and pleasant after he or she has had the opportunity to let the anger and frustration out. Reacting to the anger with disapproval, scolding, or your own anger will only make the problem worse.

It is important for the nursing assistant to listen to what the resident has to say and then respond appropriately without becoming defensive. Complaints should be taken seriously and checked out to see if they are valid.

The Confused Resident

Some residents have trouble understanding language. **Aphasia**, for example, is a condition that makes it difficult for the impaired resident to understand even simple speech. Speak as slowly and simply as you can. Use non-verbal cues, such as displaying the food you are bringing. Gently guide the resident's actions, but do not let yourself become frustrated and use force.

Some residents may have grown up speaking a language other than English. They may never have learned English well, or they may have forgotten a lot of it. Try to speak simply and slowly. Using single words will help. Use non-verbal cues. You might even learn a few words or a few phrases of the resident's language to help make yourself understood. If there is someone else at the facility who speaks the second language, you might ask for assistance translating what the resident is saying. Be patient. Imagine what it would be like to be in an unfamiliar place where most of the people don't speak your language.

COURTESY WHEN YOU SPEAK OTHER LANGUAGES

In some facilities there may be several nursing assistants who know and speak a second language. They may even feel more comfortable in the second language. If you are in this position, you must remember that staff members should not speak a second language in front of the residents.

Imagine that you are a resident at a facility where the people caring for you whisper to each other in a language you don't understand. You are going to think they are gossiping about you even if they are only talking about the weather. Or you are going to think that they are saying something serious about your medical condition that they don't want you to hear. It can be very frightening or upsetting.

When residents can hear you, it is only common courtesy to speak in a language that they can understand.

COMMUNICATION HELPS EVERYONE

The nursing assistant interacts with the residents more than anyone else. You and the residents communicate for most of your eight-hour shift. Good communication techniques help to make your job easier and your residents' lives more enjoyable.

*Circle the correct answer. There is only **one** correct answer.*

1. **You can make effective observations without communicating.**

   a. True   b. False

2. **Even if no one speaks, communication occurs when two or more people are together.**

   a. True   b. False

3. **Telling a resident what you are going to do before you do it is not a good idea because it arouses fear.**

   a. True   b. False

4. **Body language means**

   a. Writing on your body.
   b. Communicating by sign language.
   c. Communication by posture and facial expression.
   d. Writing.

5. **The need for a warm, caring touch decreases with age.**

   a. True   b. False

6. **A resident can hear even when in a deep comatose state.**

   a. True   b. False

7. **Your body language should be consistent with what you are saying.**

   a. True   b. False

8. **Mr. Brown is hard of hearing. How should the nursing assistant communicate with him?**

    a. Speak in higher-pitched tones.

    b. Shout into Mr. Brown's ear.

    c. Stand directly in front of Mr. Brown so he can see you speak.

    d. Whisper.

9. **When a resident becomes demanding and irritable, you should**

    a. Express your anger.

    b. Scold the resident.

    c. Become defensive.

    d. Listen and respond appropriately.

10. **Complaints from residents should be taken seriously and investigated to determine if they're valid.**

    a. True   b. False

Chapter 24

PRINCIPLES OF OBSERVATION

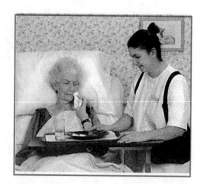

In this chapter... you will learn about:

▶ How to observe a resident.

▶ How to report what you observe.

DEFINITIONS

Observation:	Noticing a fact or event (activities, looks, speech, behavior).
Oriented:	Knowing the month, day, year, your name, and where you are.
Pertinent:	Important information related to the observation.

As a nursing assistant, you work closely with the residents and have the greatest opportunity for observing them. That is why it is extremely important for you to become a skillful observer. The changes that you see and report are vital information needed in managing the residents' care, and may prevent a serious condition from going untreated.

The nursing assistant gathers information about the resident in many different areas. These areas include:

- ▶ General appearance.

- ▶ If resident is *oriented*.

- ▶ Activities.

- ▶ Intake-Output.

- ▶ Responsiveness.

- ▶ Unusual signs or occurrences; changes in behavior or mood.

The nursing assistant observes, or gathers information, through the four senses of seeing, hearing, smelling, and touching. The more you practice observing, the better observer you will become.

Practice observing the resident every time you are with him or her. This means being alert to changes while bathing, dressing, toileting, and feeding the resident; making the bed; taking vital signs; and when listening to and talking with the resident. The more you interact with your residents, the easier it will be to notice changes.

What You See

The word **observation** makes us think first of looking. You can observe a great deal just by looking at your resident. The first thing you will observe is the resident's general appearance. Does the resident look different than usual?

Look at the resident carefully. Check the resident's skin for a change in color. Do you see any signs of rash, reddened areas, skin breaks, or swelling? Are the resident's eyes clear or cloudy?

Observe the resident's ability to move. Is the resident having more or less difficulty in movement. Does the resident appear to be in pain?

Does the resident appear restless or nervous? How does he or she interact with other residents, staff, and visitors?

Observing the resident's tray after meals will tell you how much is being eaten, fluids taken, what foods are being rejected, and if there is any change in eating habits.

If the resident has been independent in dressing and grooming, daily observations will alert you to changes in functions. Is the resident dressed appropriately? Is the resident's hair combed? Are the resident's teeth brushed?

What You Hear

Listening can also alert the nursing assistant to changes in the resident. Listen to what the resident has to say. Follow up on resident complaints. Residents will usually tell you when they are in pain. Listen for how the resident describes the pain, where it is, and how long it has been there.

The resident may also tell you of abnormal changes occurring in his or her body or functioning. Listen for this information.

Listen for the appropriateness of what the resident says. Is the resident oriented to time, place, and who he or she is?

Listening to the resident's breathing can alert you to changes, such as wheezing, coughing, or difficulty in breathing, which could mean a change in physical condition.

What You Smell

Your sense of smell can alert you to changes in a resident's condition. Does the urine or feces have a different odor? Is there a bad odor coming from sores on the resident's body? A peculiar odor to the resident's breath also can mean a change in the resident's physical condition. Is there a strange odor coming from a cast that the resident is wearing?

What You Touch

As you touch your resident during caregiving, you should be alert to changes. Is the resident's skin hot or cool? Damp or dry? Do you feel any puffiness, bumps, or swellings? How does the resident react to your touch?

REPORTING CHANGES

All changes in a resident's condition, appearance, and behavior are to be reported promptly to the charge nurse and recorded in the resident's chart. When reporting, it is important to include all the **pertinent** information:

1. Resident's name, room, and bed number.

2. Exactly what you observed.

3. Time of observation.

Observing your residents and reporting all changes in condition or behavior are two of your most important duties as a nursing assistant. Learn to observe all the time you are working. Try to be as objective as possible in your observations by reporting exactly what you observe. Instead of "the resident seems hot," you should report "the resident is sweating and her forehead felt hot to the touch."

The better you know your residents, the quicker you will notice any change in condition or behavior. There is a good feeling when a potentially harmful situation is avoided because you were observant and reported significant changes.

*Circle the correct answer. There is only **one** correct answer.*

1. **You never use the sense of touch in observing a resident.**

    a. True   b. False

2. **An advantage of being a skillful observer is that you may prevent a serious condition from remaining untreated.**

    a. True   b.False

3. **Inappropriate dress is one example of an unusual sign or occurrence.**

    a. True   b. False

4. **The less you interact with your residents, the easier it is to notice changes.**

    a. True   b. False

5. **Changes in a resident's condition, appearance, and behavior should be reported to the charge nurse and recorded.**

    a. True   b. False

6. **Pertinent information about a resident includes the**

    a. Nursing assistant's address and phone number.
    b. Number of residents in the facility.
    c. Resident's name, room, and bed number.
    d. Number of staff members in the facility.

7. **Orientation refers to:**

    a. Noticing a fact or occurrence.
    b. Observing and reporting.
    c. Knowing the month, day, year, your name, and your location.
    d. A rash or eruption on the skin.

8. **Mood changes are common among residents in a care facility and need not be reported.**

    a. True   b. False

9. **A nursing assistant's sense of smell can alert him or her to changes in a resident's condition.**

    a. True   b. False

10. **The nursing assistant should report:**

    a. Only normal behavior in a resident.

    b. Any changes in a resident's behavior.

    c. What other nursing assistants are doing.

    d. The clothing a resident is wearing.

MEASURING WEIGHT AND HEIGHT

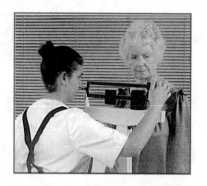

 Watch step-by-step demonstrations of the procedures discussed in this chapter in the Medcom videotape "Measuring Weight" (CNA206).

In this chapter... you will learn about:

▶ How to measure a resident's weight.

▶ How to measure a resident's height.

▶ How to measure weight and height of residents who cannot stand up.

DEFINITIONS

Aligned:	Formed into a straight line.
Centimeter:	Metric measurement of height; 1 cm = 1/100 of meter. About 0.39 inch.
Contracture:	Shortening of muscle due to inactivity.
Fluctuate:	To change continually from one condition or position to another.
Kilogram:	Metric measurement of weight; 1 kg = 1,000 grams. About 2.2 pounds.
Segment:	A part into which something naturally separates or is divided.

WEIGHT AND HEIGHT

Federal law requires that all residents be accurately weighed and measured on admission to a licensed healthcare facility.

MEASURING WEIGHT

After admissions, residents are routinely weighed according to facility policy and when ordered by the resident's physician. These weights can then be compared to the weight on admission. Changes in weight can indicate nutritional and/or medical problems, such as fluid retention, malnutrition, and disease. Therefore, a resident's weight is very important information and must be accurate.

There are three types of scales used in a healthcare facility:

▶ Standing Balance Scale - This is used for all residents who can stand unassisted.

▶ Wheelchair Scale - This is used for residents who cannot stand unassisted.

▶ Mechanical Lift Scale - This is used for residents who cannot sit in a wheelchair nor stand unassisted.

Scales may weigh in pounds and ounces (U.S. Customary Scale) or in *kilograms* and grams (metric). One kilogram equals 2.2 pounds.

Following are some general guidelines for obtaining accurate weight measurements:

- Weigh a resident at the same time each day. Weight *fluctuates* during the day. The best time to weigh a resident is the first thing in the morning, before the resident has anything to eat or drink.

Chapter 25: Measuring Weight and Height

- Have the resident empty his or her bladder before measuring weight.

- Weigh a resident on the same scale every time. There are inconsistencies in different scales.

- Have the resident wear the same clothing each time he or she is weighed. Some clothing is heavier than others. Use as little clothing as possible, always maintaining the resident's privacy.

- If the resident wears a brace, prosthesis, or cast when being weighed, record this with the weight measurement.

- If possible, do not move the scales. Moving may cause inaccurate measurements. Take the resident to the scales.

- Always check the scale for proper balance by pushing the weights to zero with no one on it and checking that the scale balances.

The Standing Balance Scale

For residents who are able to stand without assistance and without leaning on something, a standing balance scale is used. The procedure for weighing a resident on a standing balance scale is as follows:

1. If the resident is just being admitted, ask the resident what his or her normal weight is. If this is a scheduled weighing of a previously admitted resident, note the previous weight from resident's chart.

2. Explain to the resident what you are going to do. wash your hands and put a gait belt on the resident for support.

3. Take the resident to the scale.

4. Check the scale for proper balance prior to having the resident stand on it.

5. Assist the resident onto the scale. Be sure the resident stands on the center of the scale with arms at the sides. Hold onto the resident's gait belt for support and to prevent the resident from losing balance. Let go only for a moment while you actually take the measurement. Be prepared to hold the belt again immediately if the resident needs support.

6. Adjust the weights until the scale is balanced.

7. Read the weight and write it down immediately.

8. Place the weights back to zero.

9. Assist the resident off the scale and back to the room. Remove the gait belt from the resident's waist and wash your hands.

10. Notify the charge nurse if there is an increase or a decrease in the resident's weight from the last weighing.

11. Record the weight in the resident's medical chart.

Wheelchair Scale

Residents who cannot stand on a regular scale but can sit in a wheelchair can be weighed on a wheelchair scale. A wheelchair scale is a standing balance scale with a special wheelchair unit attached. The procedure for using a wheelchair scale is as follows:

1. If the resident is being admitted, ask the resident what his or her normal weight is. If a resident is being re-weighed, check the resident's chart and note the previous weight.

2. Explain to the resident what you are going to do and wash your hands.

3. Take the resident's wheelchair to the scale.

4. Check the scale for balance prior to putting the resident on the scale.

5. Push the empty wheelchair onto the scale, and adjust the weights until the scale is balanced Read the weight, and write it down immediately.

6. Place the resident in the same wheelchair, reverse the wheelchair, and push it onto the scale so the resident is facing away from the scale. Lock the wheelchair brakes.

7. Adjust the weights until the scale is balanced.

8. Read the weight and write it down immediately

9. Put the weights back to zero.

10. Unlock the brakes and roll the wheelchair off the scale.

11. Subtract the weight of the empty wheelchair from the weight of the resident in the wheelchair. The remainder is the resident's weight.

12. Wash your hands.

13. If there is a weight loss or gain, notify the charge nurse.

14. Record the resident's weight in the chart.

Mechanical Lift Scale

The mechanical lift scale can be used to weigh residents who cannot be transferred safely to a wheelchair. A mechanical lift scale has a cloth sling to hold the resident and a hydraulic lift to raise and lower the resident. The proper procedures for using a mechanical lift scale are as follows:

1. Move the mechanical lift scale next to the resident's bed.

2. Explain to the resident what you are going to do, provide privacy and wash your hands.

3. If the resident is being admitted, ask the resident what his or her normal weight is. If a resident is

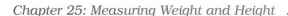

being re-weighed, check the resident's chart and note the previous weight.

4. Have the resident flat on his or her back. Roll the resident onto one side. Place half the sling between the resident's shoulders and knees. Roll the resident to the opposite side, pulling the other half of the sling under the resident.

5. Place the lift scale over the resident with the base under the bed.

6. Attach the sling to the scale using the hooks provided. The open part of the hook should be away from the resident.

7. Use the hand crank or pump handle to raise the resident. The buttocks should be clear of the bed, and the resident should be **aligned** comfortably in the sling. If the resident's body is not touching the bed, the weight can be taken at this point. If the body is touching the bed, proceed with steps 8 and 9.

8. Swing the resident's feet and legs over the edge of the bed.

9. Move the lift away from the bed so that the resident's body is not touching the bed.

10. Adjust the weights until the scale is balanced.

11. Read the weight and write it down immediately.

12. Move the resident back over the bed.

13. SLOWLY release the knob which will lower the resident onto the bed.

14. Unhook the sling and gently remove it from under the resident.

15. Return the mechanical lift scale to its proper storage area and wash your hands.

16. If any weight loss or gain is noted, inform the charge nurse.

17. Record the weight in the resident's chart.

Ideal weight are calculated in relation to the resident's height. Height is measured in either feet and inches or **centimeters**. A centimeter is about 0.39 inch.

$$1 = 0.39.$$

Measuring Residents Who Can Stand

Residents who can stand unassisted can be measured while standing on a regular standing scale. Use a gait belt on the resident if there are any balance problems when ambulating to the scale.

1. Explain to the resident what you are going to do and wash your hands.

2. Have the resident stand facing away from the scale.

3. Raise the measuring rod above the resident's head.

4. Lower the rod until it rests gently on top of the resident's head.

5. Read the measurement and assist the resident off the scale.

6. Return the resident to the room and record the measurement in the resident's chart.

7. Wash your hands.

Measuring Stooped Residents

Some residents' posture is stooped and they cannot stand straight. These residents must be measured differently.

1. Explain to the resident what you are going to do and wash your hands.

2. Have the resident stand up.

3. With a tape measure, measure the resident from the top of the head to the shoulder. Write this measurement down.

4. Measure from the shoulder to the heel and write this measurement down.

5. Add these two measurements together. This is the resident's height.

6. Record this height measurement in the resident's medical chart.

7. Wash your hands.

Measuring Residents in Bed

Residents who cannot stand must be measured in bed.

1. Explain to the resident what you are going to do, provide privacy, and wash your hands.

2. Position the resident so that he or she is lying flat and straight on the bed.

3. Using a pen or pencil, mark the sheet at the top of the resident's head and at the bottom of the resident's heels.

4. Roll the resident on to one side.

5. Using a tape measure, measure the distance between the two marks and write it down.

6. Roll the resident back.

7. Record the measurement in the resident's medical chart.

8. Wash your hands.

Chapter 25: Measuring Weight and Height

Residents who have **contractures** and cannot lie straight and flat must be measured in **segments**.

1. Explain to the resident what you are going to do, provide privacy, and wash your hands.

2. Position the resident on his or her back in the bed.

3. Using a tape measure, measure from the top of the head to the bottom of the buttocks. Write this measurement down.

4. Measure from the top of the leg to the knee. Write down this measurement.

5. Measure from the knee to the heel. Write down this measurement.

6. Add these three measurements together. The sum is the resident's height.

7. Record this height measurement in the resident's medical chart.

8. Wash your hands.

Height and weight measurements are an important part of the resident's medical record and provide necessary information for the resident's physician. Taking these measurements accurately and consistently is another important function of the nursing assistant.

*Circle the correct answer. There is only **one** correct answer.*

1. **It is important to measure the resident's weight accurately because weight changes can indicate nutritional or medical problems.**

    (a.) True   b. False

2. **You should weigh the resident at a different time of day each time.**

    a. True   (b.) False

3. **If a resident cannot stand unassisted, how can he or she be weighed?**

    a. With a standing balance scale.

    (b.) With a wheelchair scale.

    c. The resident should not be weighed.

    d. All of the above.

4. **What should you do with the weights when you are finished weighing a resident?**

    a. Put them up to the maximum weight.

    b. Leave them where they are.

    c. Add more weights to them.

    (d.) Put them back to zero.

5. **Any weight gain or loss must be reported to the charge nurse.**

    (a.) True   b. False

6. **When a resident cannot be transferred safely to a wheelchair, what type of scale is best for weighing?**

    a. Standing balance scale.

    b. Wheelchair scale.

    (c.) Mechanical lift scale.

    d. Sliding scale.

7. **How should you measure residents who are stooped or have contractures?**

   a. Only in centimeters.

   b. In segments.

   c. When they are asleep.

   d. First thing in the morning.

8. **Residents who cannot stand must be measured while sitting.**

   a. True   b. False

9. **You need to measure Mrs. Walden's height, but she cannot stand and is confined to bed. What must you do to obtain an accurate measurement of her height?**

   a. Have her assume the fetal position.

   b. Take her measurements in three segments.

   c. Measure from her head to her shoulder and her shoulder to her heel, then add the two together.

   d. Mark the bedsheet at her head and heel and measure the distance between the two marks.

10. **Height and weight are recorded in the resident's medical chart.**

   a. True   b. False

MEASURING VITAL SIGNS

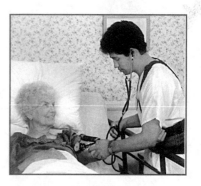

 Watch step-by-step demonstrations of the procedures discussed in this chapter in the Medcom videotape "The New Nursing Assistant 2000: Vital Signs: Temperature, Pulse, Respiration and Blood Pressure" (CNA502).

In this chapter... you will learn about:

▶ The importance of taking vital signs.

▶ How to take a temperature.

▶ How to take a pulse.

▶ How to count respirations.

▶ How to take blood pressure.

DEFINITIONS

Apical (Apical Pulse):	Heart rate measured with a stethoscope near the heart.
Axillary:	Relating to the armpit.
Baseline Measurements:	The first recording of vital signs taken when a resident comes into a healthcare facility.
Blood Pressure:	Force of blood against artery walls.
Brachial Pulse:	Pulse measured on the arm.
Bulb:	End of thermometer containing mercury.
Celsius:	The system of temperature measurement used in the metric system.
Centigrade:	A former name for Celsius.
Diastolic Pressure:	Blood pressure when the heart relaxes.
Expiration:	Breathing out.

Definitions Continued...

Fahrenheit:	A system of temperature measurement used mainly in North America.
Hypertension:	High blood pressure.
Hypotension:	Low blood pressure.
Inspiration:	Breathing in.
Prehypertension:	Blood pressure higher than normal, but below hypertension.
Pulse (Pulse Rate):	The rate the heart is beating.
Radial (Radial Pulse):	Heart rate measured at the inner wrist.
Respiration:	The act of breathing.
Sphygmomanometer:	The instrument for measuring blood pressure.
Stethoscope:	The instrument for listening to sounds in the resident's body such as heart beat.
Systolic Pressure:	Blood pressure when heart contracts.
Tympanic:	Measured in the ear (body temperature.)
Temperature:	Balance between the heat produced by the body and the heat lost by the body.
Vital Signs:	Temperature, pulse, blood pressure, respiration.

VITAL SIGNS

Blood pressure, temperature, pulse, and ***respiration*** are the ***vital signs***. They are called this because the information they produce is vital in judging the condition of a resident.

The charge nurse or physician will determine how often you will observe and record the vital signs for each resident. It is then your responsibility to correctly measure and record these signs.

When a resident is first admitted to a facility, the vital signs are recorded as ***baseline measurements***. The doctor can compare these to later readings to assess the resident's progress.

Chapter 26: Measuring Vital Signs

The following are situations in which you will take vital signs or assist the nurse in taking vital signs:

- Upon admission to the facility.

- During a physical examination of the resident.

- Before and after surgery.

- At specific times, as ordered by a doctor.

- When the resident complains of any event that could affect blood pressure, pulse, temperature or respirations.

TEMPERATURE

The body temperature is a measure of the amount of heat in the resident's body. It is a balance between the amount of heat generated by the body and the amount of heat lost to the environment. A number of things can affect the resident's body temperature:

- ▶ The time of day.

- ▶ The state of health or illness.

- ▶ Medicines being taken.

- ▶ The weather.

- ▶ Recent exercise.

- ▶ Age.

Body temperature can be measured in either **Fahrenheit (F)** or **Celsius (C)**, which was formerly called Centigrade. Normal body temperature in Fahrenheit is 98.6 degrees and in Celsius it is 37 degrees. Temperature is measured by a clinical thermometer. This can be a glass thermometer filled with mercury or an electronic or battery-operated digital thermometer. Temperature can be measured by four methods:

▶ *Oral* - in the mouth.

▶ *Axillary* - in the armpit.

▶ *Rectal* - in the rectum.

▶ *Tympanic* - in the ear.

All these areas have a rich blood supply near the surface and can produce an accurate measurement of body temperature if it is observed properly.

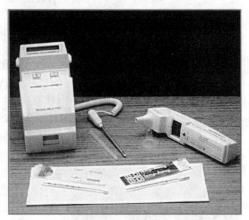

Thermometers and sleeves: *Clockwise from bottom right:* **oral, rectal, digital, tympanic.**

Thermometers

A. Glass Thermometers

You will most often be using a glass thermometer. Glass thermometers are marked with lines to indicate different degrees. On Fahrenheit thermometers, the scale runs from 94 degrees to 108 degrees F. The long lines indicate one (1) degree, and the short lines indicate two tenths (0.2) of a degree. *Normal oral body temperature of 98.6 degrees F. is indicated by an arrow.*

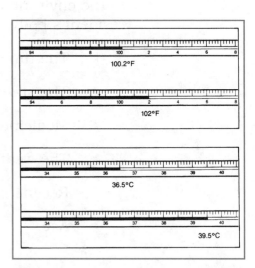

Thermometers with sample readings. Fahrenheit above, Celsius below.

The Celsius thermometer is scaled from 34 degrees to 43 degrees C. The long lines indicate one (1) degree, and the short lines indicate one-tenth (.1) of a degree. *Normal oral body temperature of 37 degrees C. is indicated by an arrow.*

The glass thermometer used for oral and axillary temperature readings has a long, narrow **bulb** filled with mercury at one end. It is always used with a disposable sleeve to prevent contamination or infection. The rectal thermometer has a short, round bulb.

B. Electronic Thermometers

The electronic digital thermometers are portable, hand held and battery operated. The temperature is displayed quickly in easy-to-read numbers on a small display screen. Electronic thermometers are usually very accurate and can be either oral or rectal.

The probe of an oral/rectal electronic thermometer is always covered by a disposable sleeve before it is used with a resident to prevent contamination or infection.

C. Tympanic Thermometers

A tympanic thermometer is a special kind of digital electronic thermometer that measures the temperature of the membrane in the ear. It is battery operated, quickly read and often used on children. The probe has a covering that is disposable after each use to prevent contamination or infection.

Normal Readings

What is considered a normal temperature reading depends on how the temperature is taken. Following are normal readings for all three sites:

	Oral	Rectal	Axillary
Fahrenheit	98.6°	99.6°	97.6°
Celsius	37.0°	37.5°	36.4°

Oral Temperature

Do not take an oral temperature within 10 minutes of the resident drinking hot or cold liquids or smoking. This would result in an inaccurate reading. The proper procedure for measuring an oral temperature with a glass thermometer is as follows:

1. Assemble the necessary equipment: an oral thermometer, paper towel, a disposable sleeve, pen and paper.

2. Wash your hands.

3. Explain to the resident what your are going to do and put on disposable gloves. Provide privacy for the resident.

4. If the thermometer has been soaking in disinfectant, rinse it with cool water and dry it with a paper towel.

5. Inspect your thermometer. NEVER use a chipped or cracked thermometer.

6. Shake the mercury down by holding the thermometer between your thumb and forefinger and shaking it with a snapping motion of the wrist, away from furniture or equipment.

7. Holding the end of the thermometer that is away from the bulb, insert the bulb end into a disposable sleeve. Remove any pull-off covering from the sleeve. Do not touch the end of the thermometer that goes into the resident's mouth.

8. Place the bulb end of thermometer under the resident's tongue and ask the resident to keep his or her mouth closed. Leave it in place for at least three minutes. The temperature is more accurate if left in place for five minutes. NEVER leave the resident with a thermometer in place.

9. Remove the thermometer from the resident's mouth and observe the tip of the column of mercury. It will be easier to read if you hold it at eye level and stand with your back to a light source.

10. Remove and discard your gloves. Discard the sleeve.

11. Immediately write down the temperature readings. Then transfer this information to the resident's medical chart and wash your hands.

12. Report to the charge nurse any abnormal temperature readings.

Using a Digital Thermometer

Using a digital thermometer is the same except for the following differences:

- Cover the probe with a disposable sleeve.

- Leave it in place until it beeps or buzzes.

- Simply read the digital display and make a note of it.

- Discard the disposable sleeve.

Rectal Temperature

The proper procedure for measuring a rectal temperature is as follows:

1. Assemble the necessary equipment: rectal thermometer, paper towel, gloves, lubricating jelly, pen and paper.

2. Wash your hands.

3. Explain to the resident what you are going to do and provide for privacy.

4. Inspect the thermometer. NEVER use a chipped or cracked thermometer.

5. If necessary, shake the thermometer down.

6. Put a sleeve over the thermometer.

7. Place a small amount of lubricating jelly on the paper towel and use it to lubricate the bulb end of the rectal thermometer. This will make insertion easier and more comfortable. (There may be lubrication inside the sleeve also.)

8. Turn the resident to the side. Put on protective gloves, and lift the upper buttock until the anus is exposed. Gently insert the bulb end of the thermometer about one inch into the rectum.

9. Hold it in place three minutes. NEVER leave the resident with a thermometer in place.

10. Remove the thermometer and discard the sleeve. Read the temperature.

11. Remove and discard your gloves.

12. Write the temperature down on paper immediately, using the letter "R" after the temperature to indicate it was taken rectally.

13. Record it in the resident's medical chart and wash your hands.

14. Any abnormal reading must be reported to the charge nurse immediately.

Axillary Temperature

You will only measure an axillary temperature when the charge nurse or physician has decided it is necessary and ordered it. The following is the proper procedure for measuring an axillary temperature:

1. Assemble the necessary equipment: an oral thermometer, paper towel, pen and paper.

2. Wash your hands.

3. Explain to the resident what you are going to do and provide privacy.

4. If the thermometer has been soaking in disinfectant, rinse it with cool water and dry it with a paper towel.

5. Inspect the thermometer. NEVER use a chipped or cracked thermometer.

6. Shake the mercury down and put on a disposable sleeve.

7. Remove the resident's garment from one arm. Dry the underarm with a towel, if necessary.

8. Place the thermometer bulb in the center of the axilla and place the resident's arm across the chest to hold the thermometer in place.

9. Leave the thermometer in place for 10 minutes. NEVER leave the resident with a thermometer in place.

10. Remove the thermometer, and dispose of the sleeve. Observe the mercury, and make a written note of the temperature reading. Write an "A" after the reading to indicate it is an axillary temperature.

11. Record the reading in the resident's medical chart and wash your hands.

12. Notify the charge nurse immediately of any abnormal temperature reading.

Tympanic Temperature

You will use a tympanic thermometer if the charge nurse decides it is necessary. This temperature is measured in the resident's ear. Use the following procedures:

1. Assemble the necessary equipment: a tympanic thermometer, disposable cover, pen and paper.

2. Wash your hands.

3. Explain to the resident what you are going to do and provide privacy.

4. Put a disposable sleeve on the probe of the thermometer.

5. Have the resident turn his or her head so an ear is facing you.

6. Insert the probe gently. Pull down and back on the earlobe so the probe can enter the ear more easily.

7. When the instrument buzzes or flashes a light to indicate the reading is complete, remove the probe.

8. Observe the display screen, and make a written note of the temperature reading. Write a "T" after the reading to indicate it is an tympanic temperature.

9. Record the reading in the resident's medical chart.

10. Discard the cover and return the tympanic thermometer to its charging unit.

11. Wash your hands.

12. Notify the charge nurse immediately of any abnormal temperature reading.

PULSE

One measure of how the circulatory system is functioning is the pulse. As the heart beats, it pumps blood through the arteries, causing them to expand. Between heartbeats, the arteries contract. This expansion and contraction rhythm is the pulse. The pulse tells us how fast or slow the resident's heart is beating.

There are certain points on the body where arteries are close to the skin. These points are where the pulse can be felt most easily.

Taking a Radial Pulse

The wrist is the easiest point to use to measure a pulse. This is called the **radial pulse** because you are using the radial artery beneath the wrist. Following is the procedure for measuring a radial pulse:

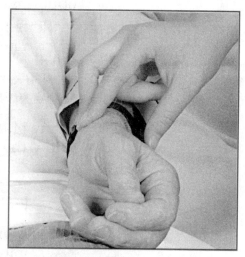

Taking a radial pulse.

1. Assemble the necessary equipment: a watch with a second hand, pen and paper.

2. Wash your hands.

3. Explain to the resident what you are going to do.

4. Position the resident's arm so that it is supported and comfortable.

5. Place your middle the fingers on the palm side of the resident's wrist in line with the thumb. Press gently to feel the pulse. If you press too hard, you may stop the flow of blood. Do not use your thumb to check a pulse as your thumb has its own pulse and will confuse your measurement.

6. When you have located the pulse, note the rhythm of the beats. Is it steady or irregular? Is the force of the beat strong or weak?

7. If the pulse is steady, you can take a 30-second reading. Noting the position of the second hand on your watch, count the pulse beats for 30 seconds. Then multiply this number by two. This will give you the measurement of the pulse for one minute. If required by your facility or if there are any abnormalities noted, count the beats for a full 60 seconds.

8. Make a written note of the pulse rate. Transfer this information to the resident's medical record and wash your hands.

9. If any of the following conditions are observed, notify the charge nurse immediately:

   • A change in rate, force, or rhythm from previous measurement.

   • A pulse rate of over 90 or under 60 beats per minute.

   • An irregular rhythm.

   • A weak or racing pulse.

Taking an Apical Pulse

The charge nurse may ask you take an **apical pulse** instead of a radial pulse. The apical pulse is measured with a **stethoscope** on the chest directly over the heart. Use the following procedures.

1. Assemble the necessary equipment: a stethoscope, alcohol wipes, a watch with a second hand, pen and paper.

2. Wash your hands.

3. Explain to the resident what you are going to do and provide privacy.

4. Clean the earpieces and diaphragm of the stethoscope with alcohol wipes. Put the earpieces into your ears.

5. Uncover the left side of the resident's chest. Place the bell or diaphragm of the stethoscope on the left side of the chest, below the nipple.

6. When you have located the loudest sounds of the heart beat, count the beats for a full minute.

7. Make a written note of the apical pulse rate. Also make a note of any irregular heart sounds you notice.

8. Transfer this information to the resident's medical record and wash your hands.

9. If any of the following conditions are observed, notify the charge nurse immediately:

   • A change in rate, force, or rhythm from previous measurement.

   • A pulse rate of over 90 or under 60 beats per minute.

   • An irregular rhythm.

   • A weak or racing pulse.

BLOOD PRESSURE

The blood being pumped through the circulatory system causes pressure against the walls of the arteries. This **blood pressure** is influenced by the rate of the heartbeat and the condition of the arteries. When the heart contracts, blood is forced through the arteries. The high pressure this creates is called **systolic pressure**. The normal range of systolic pressure for a healthy adult is below 120 millimeters (mm) of mercury.

When the heart relaxes between contractions, the pressure of the blood in the arteries is lower. This is called **diastolic pressure**. For a normal, healthy adult, the diastolic pressure should be below 80 millimeters (mm) of mercury.

When a blood pressure reading is taken, the systolic pressure is always written or given first, and then the diastolic; for example, 119/78.

Factors Affecting Blood Pressure

The following factors can affect a resident's blood pressure:

- Age.
- Sex.
- Body build.
- Pain or disease.
- Heredity.
- Exercise and diet.
- Medications.
- Emotions or stress.

Blood pressure in the range of 120/80 to 139/89 is classified as **prehypertension**, and indicates the need for steps to be taken to lower the blood pressure. Blood pressure of 140/90 or higher is a condition called **hypertension**. Readings far below the normal range are referred to as **hypotension**.

Physical exercise, illness, stress, emotional turmoil, and certain medications can raise the blood pressure. The process of aging causes the arteries to lose some of their elasticity, and this results in higher blood pressure for many older adults. Blood pressure is lowered with rest and certain medications. Very low blood pressure can also be the result of shock.

Things to Consider when Taking Blood Pressure

A resident's blood pressure should always be taken with the resident in the same position. Lying down raises the pressure, while sitting or standing lowers it. For comparison purposes, always use the same position. The charge nurse may ask you to take a blood pressure reading with the resident in a sitting, standing or lying position. You may also be asked to use a particular arm or both arms.

Always take the reading in a quiet area away from distractions or activity. On a very thin resident, you may use a smaller child's cuff. For an obese resident, you may need to use a thigh cuff.

Never take blood pressure on an arm with an IV, cast, injury or paralysis. Also, never take a blood pressure reading immediately after exercise. Allow the resident to rest for 10 to 20 minutes first. Do not apply the cuff over clothing. This could cause an inaccurate reading. Don't overinflate the cuff, as this can be painful.

If you are unsure of a reading, always repeat the procedure. If you are still unsure, ask for help from the charge nurse.

Taking a Blood Pressure Reading

The procedure for taking a resident's blood pressure is as follows:

1. Assemble the necessary equipment: a blood pressure cuff *(sphygmomanometer)*, a stethoscope, alcohol wipes, pen and paper.

2. Wash your hands.

3. Explain to the resident what you are going to do and provide privacy.

4. The resident may be either lying down or sitting up.

5. Remove or roll up the resident's sleeve and rest the forearm on the bed or chair arm.

6. Unroll the blood pressure cuff, loosen the valve on the bulb, and then squeeze the cuff to release any air. Clean the earpieces and diaphragm of the stethoscope with alcohol wipes.

7. Place the cuff snugly around the resident's arm one inch above the elbow, with the arrows on the cuff pointing toward the elbow.

8. Locate the **brachial pulse** (inside the elbow) with your three middle fingertips. Place the diaphragm of the stethoscope on the brachial pulse, but not touching the cuff.

9. Put the earpieces of the stethoscope in your ears.

10. Turn the thumbscrew of the valve clockwise to tighten it. Be careful not to turn it too tightly.

11. Holding the stethoscope diaphragm in place over the brachial artery, repeatedly squeeze the bulb to inflate the cuff until you no longer hear a pulse. This should be when the mercury reaches 30 mm beyond the point where you last heard a pulse.

12. Slowly turn the thumbscrew on the valve counterclockwise, allowing air to escape. After a few seconds, you should hear a pulse.

13. As you hear the first sound, note the point on the scale. This is the systolic reading.

14. Allow air to continue to escape. When the sounds change or disappear, note the point on the scale. This is the diastolic reading.

15. Deflate the cuff completely and remove it from the resident's arm. Remove the stethoscope from your ears.

16. Record the person's name and the blood pressure on your notes.

17. Return the equipment to its proper place and wash your hands.

18. Report the blood pressure and any abnormalities observed to the charge nurse.

Respiration is both breathing in, referred to as **inspiration**, and breathing out, or **expiration**. The following are some things that can affect the respiration rate.

- ▶ Age and sex.

- ▶ Emotions and stress.

- ▶ Medications.

- ▶ Exercise.

- ▶ Respiratory illness.

- ▶ Heat and cold.

- ▶ Disease, especially cardiac illness.

Observing a resident's respiration can alert the nursing assistant to possible respiratory problems. To count respiration, you can either watch the resident's chest rise and fall or you can place your hand on the resident's chest and feel this movement. One rise and fall of the chest is counted as one respiration.

Usually, adults have a respiration rate of 16 to 20 per minute. Children breathe faster, and the elderly slower. Respiration can also be affected by temperature change, exertion, illness, stress, and medications. To get an accurate, normal measurement, it is best to count the respirations without telling the resident this is what you are doing.

While counting the respirations, you should listen to and observe the breathing. If you notice that the breathing is shallow, irregular, noisy, or difficult, notify the charge nurse immediately.

When charting respiration, note and record the following things:

- **Rate.** How many respirations per minute?

- **Rhythm.** Is the rhythm regular or irregular?

- **Character.** Is the respiration slow, fast, noisy, or irregular.

- **Color of skin.** Does the skin appear unusually pink or blue?

Vital signs are very important for determining a resident's medical condition and general health. You should always be careful to measure the vital signs as accurately as possible.

*Circle the correct answer. There is only **one** correct answer.*

1. **Which of the following signs is considered a vital sign?**

    a. Skin temperature.

    b. Blood count.

    c. Blood pressure.

    d. Urine test.

    e. None of the above.

2. **Body temperature is always measured in the mouth.**

    a. True   b. False

3. **On a Fahrenheit thermometer, what does a short line indicate?**

    a. 1 degree.

    b. 2 degrees.

    c. 0.1 degree.

    d. 0.2 degree.

4. **When measuring an oral temperature, how long should a glass thermometer remain in a resident's mouth?**

    a. 20 seconds.

    b. 2 minutes.

    c. 5 minutes.

    d. 60 seconds.

5. **When measuring a rectal temperature, how long should a glass thermometer remain in the rectum?**

    a. 15 minutes.

    b. 10 minutes.

    c. 3 minutes.

    d. As long as needed.

6. **Where is an axillary temperature measured?**

    a. Groin.

    b. Anus.

    c. Armpit.

    d. Mouth.

7. **In accurately measuring a radial pulse, you should**

    a. Press firmly on the wrist.

    b. Use your thumb on the wrist.

    c. Count the beats until they become irregular.

    d. Count the beats for 30 seconds, then multiply by two.

8. **Blood pressure should always be taken with the resident in the same position.**

    a. True   b. False

9. **In taking Mrs. White's blood pressure, you obtain a reading of 130/85. Which of the following is an accurate interpretation of this reading?**

    a. Mrs. White has hypertension.

    b. Mrs. White has hypotension.

    c. Mrs. White has prehypertension.

    d. Mrs. White's blood is normal.

10. **You can measure respiration accurately by**

    a. Counting each rise and fall of the chest separately.

    b. Counting each rise and fall of the chest as one respiration.

    c. Counting the number of breaths for 60 seconds and multiplying by two

    d. Telling the resident what you are doing.

Chapter 27

THE "FIFTH VITAL SIGN" — PAIN

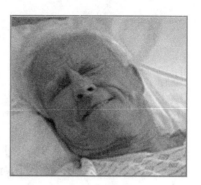

 Additional examples, descriptions and demonstrations of the concepts discussed in this chapter, are shown in the Medcom videotape, "Measuring Vital Signs Part II: Blood Pressure and Pain"(M220).

In this chapter... you will learn about:

▶ The importance of pain in a person's recovery and quality of life.

▶ How to recognize and report pain.

DEFINITIONS

Acute Pain:	Sudden onset not long lasting.
Chronic Pain:	Constant, long lasting and on-going, lasts over six months.
Intensity:	The strength or power of a feeling, such as pain.
Radiate:	To spread outward from a source.

INTRODUCTION

Pain has been called "the fifth vital sign" because it is so important to knowing about someone's health status and healing. An initial assessment of pain will be made and recorded with the initial physical assessment and history when a resident enters the facility. After that, you may be asked to recognize and report pain regularly to your supervisor. In this way the medical team can track any changes in the resident's pain that might indicate serious problems.

RECOGNIZING PAIN

Signs of pain can sometimes be observed in a resident, such as cries or moans or a facial expression that indicates pain. However, asking a resident to give a self-report is the best and most reliable way to recognize the existence and intensity of pain.

The goal, especially with a continuing or chronic pain, is to recognize and communicate three main things about the pain:

- ▶ Its intensity

- ▶ Its location

- ▶ Its nature

RECOGNIZING THE INTENSITY OF PAIN

The best way of recognizing the intensity of pain is to use a pain scale. A variety of pain scales are available. Some scales simply list numbers from zero to 10, with zero indicating no pain, 5 indicating moderate pain, and a 10 indicating the worst pain possible.

Some scales use words, such as "no pain," "mild pain," etc. For those who may be mentally confused, you may need to use a visual scale made up of faces that show different degrees of pain. Most facilities should have a variety of pain scales available for use with various resident populations.

Explain the scale carefully to the resident the first time you use it. Then have the resident indicate the intensity of the pain by pointing to the number, or the word, or the face that best represents the intensity of what they feel.

RECOGNIZING THE LOCATION OF PAIN

Have the resident indicate the location of pain by pointing to the site on their body. If the resident is shy about the body or for some other reason cannot point to her own body, use a diagram of a body and have her point to the place of the pain on the diagram or mark it.

RECOGNIZING THE NATURE OF PAIN

Finally, ask questions about the nature of the pain. Ask the resident what the pain feels like. You may need to use some sample questions, such as:

- ▶ Did the pain start suddenly?

- ▶ Does it feel like a burning pain?

- ▶ Does it feel like a pinching pain?

- ▶ Does it feel like a stabbing pain?

RECOGNIZING NEW PAINS

There are some other things you may need to ask the resident, especially if the resident is complaining of a new pain or a pain that has changed.

- When did it start?
- Have you felt it before?
- How long does it usually last?
- Does it seem to radiate, such as, pain moving through a shoulder and down an arm?
- Does change of position help or hinder it?
- Does anything make it worse?
- Does anything you do make it better?
- Does it interfere with your sleep or any other activities (appetite, emotions, concentration)?

When you have completed discussing the pain with the resident, be sure to communicate or note what you have found out, following the charge nurse's instructions.

AFTER PAIN INTERVENTION

Usually pain interventions will be decided by the physician or charge nurse. These can include medications, hot or cold pads, change of position, and various activities. After a pain intervention is made, allow sufficient time for the treatment to work and then return to check on the degree of pain intensity. Follow the recommendations of the charge nurse on timing.

By recognizing and reporting pain you will help you and other members of the healthcare team provide the highest quality of care to your residents.

Safety measures are equally as important when a patient has received pain medication:

1. Put the bed in its lowest position.
2. Put the side rails up.
3. Check often on the patient.
4. Assist the patient out of bed, etc. when sedated.
5. Put the call light at the patient's fingertips.
6. Provide a quiet, restful environment.

*Circle the correct answer. There is only **one** correct answer.*

1. **Pain has been called the _____ vital sign.**

    a. Most important.

    b. Least important.

    c. Fifth.

    d. First.

2. **Who will determine how often you need to recognize and report on a resident's pain?**

    a. The patient.

    b. The charge nurse or physician.

    c. Another CNA.

    d. The resident's family.

3. **The best way of recognizing the intensity of pain is to _____.**

    a. Listen for moans.

    b. Watch a resident's face.

    c. Ask the family.

    d. Ask the patient to use a pain intensity scale.

4. **In recognizing chronic or continuing pain, one of these three things is less important than the others:**

    a. How intense is it?

    b. Where is it?

    c. What is it like?

    d. Have you felt it before?

5. **If the resident cannot point to herself or her body, you may use _____.**

    a. A pointer stick.

    b. A diagram of the body.

    c. different words for the body parts.

    d. a crayon to draw on the body.

6. With a new pain it is NOT important to know if it interferes with sleeping or eating.

      a. True   b. False

7. When you have recognized a new pain or a change in pain, the last step is usually _____.

      a. Washing your hands.

      b. Documenting what you found out.

      c. Asking about pain again immediately.

      d. Calling the physician.

8. Who will select the pain intervention?

      a. The patient.

      b. The charge nurse or physician.

      c. The CNA.

      d. The resident's family.

9. One common pain intervention is _____.

      a. Surgery.

      b. Ignoring it.

      c. Medications.

      d. As an extra meal.

10. Pain intensity scales usually run from _____.

      a. 0 to 5.

      b. 0 to 10.

      c. 0 to 25.

      d. 0 to 100.

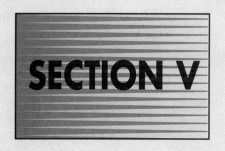

SECTION V

CARING FOR DAILY ACTIVITIES

Chapter 28

ACTIVITIES OF DAILY LIVING

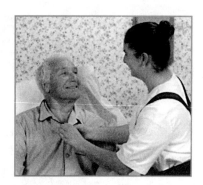

 Watch step-by-step demonstrations of the procedures discussed in this chapter in the Medcom videotape "The New Nursing Assistant 2000: Personal Care" (CNA505).

In this chapter... you will learn about:

▶ Activities of daily living.

▶ How you can assist a resident with the activities of daily living.

▶ How to assist an uncooperative resident.

DEFINITIONS

Activities of Daily Living (ADL):	Ordinary activities of daily living, including bathing, dressing, eating and toileting.
Alzheimer's Disease:	Chronic degenerative brain disease resulting in loss of memory, personality, and judgment.
Arthritis:	Chronic disease of the joints resulting in stiffness and pain.
Cerebral Palsy:	Chronic disease of the nervous system resulting in uncontrolled movement.
Chronic:	Ongoing.
Confrontation:	Argument.
Cutlery:	Knives, forks and spoons used for eating.
Learned Helplessness:	Belief that you have no effect on what happens to yourself.
Multiple Sclerosis:	Chronic degenerative disease of the nervous system resulting in decreased ability to move.
Parkinson's Disease:	Disorder of the nervous system resulting in body stiffness and uncontrolled shaking.

The **activities of daily living (ADL)** are all those chores we do routinely each day to care for ourselves. Chores like bathing, dressing, eating, shopping, and paying bills are all examples of activities of daily living. Some are common to most people, like brushing the teeth and bathing, while others apply only to some people. Shaving may be an ADL for most adult men, but for those who wear full beards it is not. If you live alone, cooking may be an ADL. If you live with someone who cooks for you, it is not an ADL for you.

Being Independent

Being independent means being able to take care of all of your ADLs without assistance. In our culture, independence is very much prized, and the loss of it is keenly felt. As we grow to maturity, all of us strive to be independent, to be able to take care of ourselves. Accidents and illness can limit a person's independence at any age. Automobile accidents, falls, and diseases such as **multiple sclerosis** and **cerebral palsy** limit many younger adults' ability to be independent. Many **chronic** conditions which are associated with aging also result in a loss of some independence. The crippling of **arthritis** or stroke may impair a person's ability to dress or shave unassisted. The tremors of **Parkinson's Disease** may prevent cooking safely. Residents who have always done these activities for themselves must now accept help to accomplish them.

Loss of independence can also be the result of depression or confusion. Depression robs the resident of the desire to do the ADLs, and confusion robs the resident of the ability to accomplish them. Inactivity for long periods of time can also result in increased dependence. Muscles become weak without activity, and tasks become more difficult. Residents who have been dependent may believe that they can no longer do anything for themselves. This is called **learned helplessness.** In this case, the residents must be remotivated to accept more responsibility for their own daily activities.

Since independence is valued in our culture, it greatly influences our feelings of self-esteem. Therefore, helping residents become more independent in their ADLs will also help them feel better about themselves. The nursing assistant is responsible for the ADLs of the residents, and has the opportunity to assist residents in regaining at least some of their independence. There are four main ways in which you will help residents become more independent in ADLs: physical strength and ability, special training, assistive devices, and adaptive equipment.

Physical Strength and Ability

Many residents have special programs of physical therapy to regain strength and ability. The nursing assistant can encourage the residents in these programs. Praise residents for their efforts and progress. For residents who are able, walking is an important way a nursing assistant can help residents increase their strength and endurance. Walking also gives the resident a sense of independence.

The nursing assistant should encourage residents to do as much for themselves as possible. It is often faster for you to do the task for the resident yourself, but if you have the patience to let residents do what they can, you will be helping the resident gain independence and self-esteem.

A single task can often be broken down into numerous smaller tasks, some of which the resident may be able to do. For instance, the resident may not be able to dress without assistance, but may be able to choose which clothes to wear. The resident may be able to pull up a pair of pants, but be unable to fasten them. Some residents may be able to put their arms into a shirt, but unable to manage the buttons. It is important to encourage the residents to do those tasks they are able to do and to reinforce this effort with recognition and praise. The residents may become frustrated and discouraged. The nursing assistant can help them by handling these situations matter-of-factly, providing temporary assistance, and reinforcing the belief that soon they will be able to do the task without assistance.

Special Training

Some residents may have disabilities that prevent them from performing some tasks in the usual way. There are usually a number of different ways to do something. The nursing assistant can be creative in figuring out another possible way of accomplishing a task, a way which will allow the resident to do the task independently. For example, a resident may not be able to hook her bra in the back, but she may be able to hook it before putting it on, then step into it, and pull it up. Don't assume there is only one way to do something. Be creative.

Adaptive Equipment

Adaptive equipment enables residents to perform bodily functions they would otherwise be unable to do. The resident who is unable to walk may be able to ambulate with a leg brace, walker, or cane. Mobility can also be attained with the use of a wheelchair. A hearing aid may increase the independence of the resident who is hard of hearing; eyeglasses may increase the function of those with loss of vision.

ASSISTIVE DEVICES

There are many devices available to assist the physically impaired with otherwise impossible or difficult tasks. These are used to assist in eating, dressing, or grooming and bathing. Be sensitive about suggesting their use because some people may be embarrassed about losing some of the hand control they used to have.

Eating

There are many devices available to help those who cannot easily grasp cutlery, cannot rotate their wrists easily, or who lack the steadiness with their hands to scoop food off a plate.

- ▶ *Cutlery with big rubber handles or ridged handles.* This cutlery is easier to hold onto.

- ▶ *Cutlery with handles that clip onto the person's hand.* This cutlery is for those who cannot grip at all.

- ▶ *Cutlery with angled or swivel ends.* This is for people who cannot rotate their wrists easily.

- ▶ *Gripping devices.* Regular cutlery can be inserted into these devices so a person can hold the cutlery.

- ▶ *Plates with high edges or lips, or snap-on food guards.* A person with limited hand control can push food against the raised edge to load it onto a fork or spoon.

- ▶ *Non-skid plates and dishes.* These help keep dishware from being pushed off the tray.

- ▶ *Spill-proof cups.* These have a cover and a built-in drinking spout.

- ▶ *Easy-grip cups with large handles.* These help prevent dropped cups and spills.

Dressing

Dressing, too, can be a problem. Think of the skill needed to push a button through a buttonhole, or to fasten a tiny hook. Many devices or special items of clothing can help.

- ▶ *Buttonhooks.* These devices are like a needle-threader. They have a large handle with a wire loop that can be used to reach through a button hole, grasp the button and pull it through.

▶ **Blouses, dresses and bras with front closures.** These make it easier to reach many fasteners to dress.

▶ **Velcro fasteners instead of zippers and hooks.** These are much easier to use.

▶ **Soft, roomy, pullover clothing.** This clothing makes dressing easier.

Grooming and Bathing

▶ **Brushes, razors, toothbrushes and denture brushes with big handles.** These allow the person with reduced gripping skill to continue ordinary grooming activities.

▶ **Long-handled bathing sponges.** These allow the person to wash areas that are hard to reach.

▶ **Long handled shoe-horn.** These make it easier to put on shoes without bending over.

There are many other devices that can assist physically impaired people with many tasks. There are lap desks that can prop up a book on a person's lap, page turners to help turn book pages, and grasping poles to help pick up items off the floor. You should become familiar with the devices available in your facility.

THE UNCOOPERATIVE RESIDENT

So far we have discussed residents who are incapable of performing some daily activities because of disability, weakness, illness or some other physical cause. You will also deal with cases in which the residents simply do not want to do things for themselves or are too confused to do their ADLs.

Residents who are depressed will have no motivation nor energy for doing ADLs. Some residents, like those with Alzheimer's Disease, may be too confused to cooperate, while others may decide that it is the nursing assistant's job to do everything for them. Since they are paying for care, they may assume this means they will not have to do anything.

These situations require patience and consistency on the part of all the nursing staff. The charge nurse should develop a plan for handling these residents and all nursing staff must follow the plan for it to work. It is important not to argue or get into a **confrontation** with the resident. This almost always leads to a situation where nothing is accomplished. Usually, being firm but pleasant is the best approach with uncooperative residents.

The charge nurse should be kept informed of the resident's level of independence in ADLs and any changes in the level should be noted in the resident's chart.

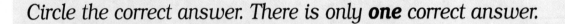
*Circle the correct answer. There is only **one** correct answer.*

1. **Bathing, dressing, and eating are all activities of daily living.**

    a. True   b. False

2. **Chronic conditions associated with aging rarely result in a loss of independence.**

    a. True   b. False

3. **Physical strength and agility and assistive devices are areas in which a nursing assistant can help a resident become more independent.**

    a. True   b. False

4. **Residents who no longer believe they can do anything for themselves have a condition known as**

    a. Arthritis.
    b. Confrontation.
    c. Cerebral palsy.
    d. Learned helplessness.

5. **When dealing with dependent residents, it is helpful if the nursing assistant**

    a. Does all tasks for the residents.
    b. Discourages the resident from doing anything.
    c. Encourages the residents to do tasks they are able to do.
    d. Doesn't do anything.

6. **Special training includes finding other creative ways to accomplish a task.**

    a. True   b. False

7. **Few assistive devices are available to help dependent residents accomplish otherwise impossible tasks.**

    a. True　(b.) False

8. **Adaptive equipment enables residents to perform bodily functions they**

    (a.) Would otherwise be unable to do.
    b. Have never done before.
    c. Can still do.
    d. Don't want to do.

9. **Mrs. Lowery is suffering from Alzheimer's disease. How should the nursing assistant care for her?**

    a. Argue with her whenever possible.
    (b.) Be patient and consistent.
    c. Be spontaneous; don't follow any set plan.
    d. Ignore her.

10. **When trying to help an uncooperative resident, it is best to be firm but pleasant.**

    (a.) True　b. False

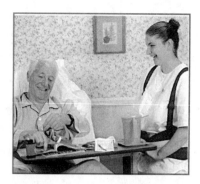

Chapter 29

RESIDENT ACTIVITY NEEDS

In this chapter... you will learn about:

▶ Recreational and social activity needs of resident.
▶ Your role in assisting with activities.

DEFINITIONS

Activity Coordinator: Staff member responsible for planning and carrying out social activities for the residents.

Interaction: Conversation, communication relating to others.

RESIDENT ACTIVITIES

We all have the need for interaction with other people. And we need hobbies or interests or recreations to keep our minds and bodies active. Most of us do this every day without planning or even thinking about it. But for a resident in a long-term care facility, the opportunities for **interaction** and activity may be very limited. This is particularly true if the resident is confused or confined to bed.

The Activity Coordinator

Every long-term care facility is required to have an **activity coordinator**. It is the coordinator's responsibility to plan and carry out activities to meet the social needs for every resident in the facility. This is a big job because every resident has different interests and capabilities. The activity coordinator tries to offer a wide range of activities to meet these needs. These activities could include arts and crafts, music, sports, games, parties, movies, cooking, outings, classes, discussion groups, and exercise.

YOUR ROLE IN RESIDENT ACTIVITIES

Even though you do not plan and carry out these recreational and social activities, you will probably have a role in assisting with resident activities. This will be true for both residents who can ambulate and for residents confined to bed.

You can facilitate resident attendance at activities in a number of ways:

▶ You can keep the residents informed of current activities along with the date, time, and place.

▶ You can encourage, but not force, the resident to try new things and attend appropriate activities.

▶ You can assist the resident in being groomed and dressed appropriately and on time for the activity.

▶ You can be interested in the resident's activities and provide reinforcement for participation.

▶ You can assist the resident in getting to and from the activity.

Residents Confined To Bed

Not all residents are able to attend activities. However, residents who are confined to their beds still have the same social and recreational needs as the more active residents. The activity coordinator also has a responsibility to provide appropriate activities and social stimulation for these residents.

The nursing assistant's role in this situation may include helping the resident to participate as well as encouraging and reinforcing participation. Special celebrations can be brought to a resident's room. Other activities could include reading, listening to music, visiting with others, arts and crafts, and adaptive exercise.

The confused resident is probably the one in most need of social stimulation. The confused person is often unable to concentrate on an activity for more than short periods of time. Also, many people are embarrassed by the confusion, do not know how to react, and avoid interacting with the confused person.

The nursing assistant is usually the most familiar staff member for the confused person. The nursing assistant can provide the one-to-one attention that the confused resident needs to stay with an activity and to enjoy it. Confused residents also need someone to listen to them, to be interested in them, and to help them feel worthwhile.

Activities which are suitable for confused residents may include simple games and puzzles, listening to music, singing, talking about familiar people and situations, sports and exercises.

Activities are not just a nice extra. They are an important part of a resident's care plan. Recreational and social activities are also an essential component in maintaining the resident's self-esteem and ability to interact with others.

*Circle the correct answer. There is only **one** correct answer.*

1. **Long-term care facilities do not need to hire an activity coordinator.**

    a. True   b. False

2. **The activity coordinator is responsible for the recreational and social program in a long-term care facility.**

    a. True   b. False

3. **Arts and crafts, movies, and exercise classes are some of the recreational and social activities offered by a long-term care facility.**

    a. True   b. False

4. **It may be the nursing assistant's responsibility to keep the resident informed of current activities and their dates, times, and locations.**

    a. True   b. False

5. **The nursing assistant should not do one of the following things. Which?**

    a. Assist the resident in grooming and dressing.

    b. Make sure the resident is on time for an activity.

    c. Force the resident to try a new activity.

    d. Provide reinforcement for resident participation in activities.

6. **Residents who are confined to their beds have the same social and recreational needs as more active residents.**

    a. True   b. False

7. **When residents are confined to bed, they are unable to take part in activities.**

   a. True   (b.) False

8. **Since confused residents are unable to concentrate for very long, they don't really need social activities.**

   a. True   (b.) False

9. **Who is the most familiar staff member for the confused resident?**

   a. Activity coordinator.

   b. Charge nurse.

   c. Therapist.

   (d.) Nursing assistant.

10. **Recreational and social activities in a long-term care facility are an important part of a resident's care plan.**

   (a.) True   b. False

Chapter 30

PHYSICAL NEEDS OF THE RESIDENT

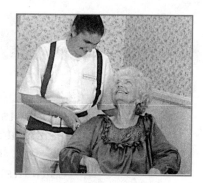

In this chapter... you will learn about:

▶ The resident's physical needs.

▶ The nursing assistant's responsibility in caring for the resident's physical needs.

DEFINITIONS

Elimination: Process of removal of waste products from the body.

Residents have many physical needs and it is the nursing assistant's responsibility to see that many of these needs are met. The basic physical needs of everyone, including residents, are:

▶   Sleep.

▶   Exercise.

▶   Food.

▶   Elimination.

▶   Cleanliness.

We all have these physical needs. Most adults fulfill these needs for themselves; however, illness, age, and handicaps can interfere with the person's ability to take care of these needs without assistance. This chapter will introduce you to these physical needs and later chapters will explain in more detail how to assist the residents with these needs.

Sleep

Sleep is necessary for our bodies and minds to rest and be able to continue with the demands of the next day. Rest is particularly important for people who are ill or weak. Much of their energy is directed toward healing and overcoming the weakness. Rest and sleep renew energy; therefore, the person who is weak and ill will need more rest.

The nursing assistant can help the residents by providing regular periods of quiet, uninterrupted time. Help make the resident comfortable. The bed should be neat and unwrinkled. If the resident is resting while dressed, the shoes should be removed and any belts loosened. A light cover should be provided to prevent chilling as the body temperature lowers slightly while the resident sleeps.

Exercise

Bodies were designed to move, and residents need regular exercise. They should be encouraged by the nursing assistant to move within their physical limits. Walking is one of the best forms of exercise. Residents who are able to do so should be encouraged and praised for walking. You will learn how to assist a resident with walking, or ambulation, in Chapter 44.

Assisting the resident daily with range-of-motion exercises helps the resident maintain the ability to move. You will learn how to assist with range of motion exercises in Chapter 36.

Food

Food provides the energy for our bodies. Eating is also enjoyable and often a time to be with other people. The nursing assistant can encourage residents to eat and can help make meal times relaxing and pleasurable.

Some residents need assistance in cutting their food or in eating. The nursing assistant can provide this help in a pleasant, cheerful manner. You will learn how to assist a resident at mealtimes in Chapter 44.

Elimination

All body processes produce waste materials. These must be eliminated from the body through urine and feces. Many residents need assistance with these **elimination** processes. Helping the resident remember to use the toilet, assisting when necessary, and cleaning up accidents in a matter-of-fact manner eases the resident's embarrassment. You will learn more about assisting residents with their elimination needs in Chapters 46 and 47.

Cleanliness

The nursing assistant is responsible for keeping residents clean. They may need assistance in bathing, teeth and nail care, and hair care. Keeping residents clean promotes physical health by killing bacteria and germs. It also helps residents feel good about their appearance. You will learn more about assisting residents in bathing and personal hygiene in Chapters 39 and 40.

The nursing assistant fills many roles and does many tasks for residents. One of the most important jobs is letting the residents do as much for themselves as possible. This provides residents with exercise and feelings of independence and self-esteem.

By cheerfully assisting residents with tasks they are unable to do, the nursing assistant helps fulfill residents' physical needs.

*Circle the correct answer. There is only **one** correct answer.*

1. **There are five basic physical needs for everyone, two of which are food and sleep. What is another basic physical need?**

    a. Laughter.

    b. Entertainment.

    c. Excitement.

    d. Exercise.

2. **A person who is weak and ill needs more rest than the average person.**

    a. True   b. False

3. **To help residents get their rest, the nursing assistant can.**

    a. Make them stay in bed even if they aren't tired.

    b. Make sure the bed is neat and unwrinkled, and provide a light cover to prevent chilling.

    c. Make them keep their shoes on and tighten belts.

    d. Remove any covers.

4. **Walking is one of the best forms of exercise.**

    a. True   b. False

5. **Only residents who can walk need regular exercise.**

    a. True   b. False

6. **Energy for the body is provided by:**

   a. Water.

   b. Fresh air.

   c. Food.

   d. Sunlight.

7. **Only one of the body processes produces waste materials.**

   a. True   b. False

8. **The nursing assistant can help ease embarrassment by:**

   a. Helping the resident remember to use the toilet.

   b. Refusing to clean up any toilet accidents.

   c. Scolding residents for toilet accidents.

   d. Completely ignoring the resident.

9. **Keeping a resident clean promotes physical health.**

   a. True   b. False

10. **Letting the residents do as much for themselves as possible** _____.

   a. Is the responsibility of the charge nurse.

   b. Should only be done on special occasions.

   c. Provides the resident with exercise and feelings of independence.

   d. Is not a good idea.

Chapter 31

RESIDENT BELONGINGS AND PROSTHESES

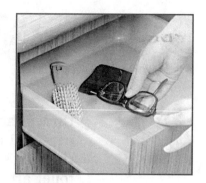

In this chapter... you will learn about:

▶ How to care for a resident's belongings.

▶ The different kinds of prostheses and their care.

DEFINITIONS

Ambulation Device: A device used to assist in walking; a cane, crutch, walker, physical therapy bars, or quad cane.

Prosthesis: Artificial body part.

PERSONAL BELONGINGS

Under the law, all residents' belongings are protected. All personal belongings should be clearly marked with the resident's name and room number. This includes clothing, toilet articles, **ambulation devices**, appliances, televisions, radios, and **prostheses**. Each resident must have a specific place in which to keep clothing and personal items.

VALUABLE BELONGINGS

Expensive items, such as jewelry, should be kept by the resident's family or in the facility safe. If kept in the safe, the item should be placed in an envelope clearly marked with the resident's name, room number, item in envelope, and sealed. Items taken home by the family or locked in the safe should be carefully recorded in the resident's chart. You should become familiar with your facility's policy regarding valuable property and where it is stored.

PROSTHESES

A prosthesis is an artificial replacement for a body part which no longer functions properly. The prostheses can be an artificial limb, an artificial eye, eyeglasses, contact lenses, or a hearing aid. The nursing assistant is responsible for the care and cleaning of the residents' prostheses.

Artificial Limb

A resident may have an artificial arm or leg due to a birth defect or amputation. The prosthesis is attached to the limb stump with straps and/or laces.

To prevent swelling, the stump should always be protected with a stump sock when the resident is wearing the prosthesis. It is the nursing assistant's responsibility to handle the prosthesis carefully and to check it for loose, bent, or broken parts. These should be reported immediately to the charge nurse and noted in the resident's chart. The nursing assistant is also responsible for checking the stump for signs of swelling, bruising, or redness. This must also be reported and charted.

Artificial Eye

In rare cases, a resident may have had an eye removed and replaced with an artificial eye.

The artificial eye should be removed at bedtime and placed in a container filled with contact lens solution. Before reinserting the artificial eye, it must be rinsed with warm running water. It is the nursing assistant's responsibility to handle the artificial eye carefully to prevent scratching or breaking it.

Eyeglasses

Most older residents will wear glasses to improve their vision.

It is important to keep eyeglasses clean. The nursing assistant should wash the resident's eyeglasses under running water after placing a washcloth in the bottom of the sink to prevent breakage if glasses fall. Glasses should be stored in their case when they are not being used.

The glasses should be dried with a soft towel. While cleaning them, the nursing assistant should inspect the glasses for loose or broken parts, or bad scratches on the lenses. These should be reported to the charge nurse and entered in the resident's chart.

Contact Lenses

Some residents may wear contact lenses in place of glasses or after cataract surgery.

Contact lenses should always be removed before sleeping, even before a nap. The lenses should be stored in a container filled with lens solution. Before reinserting lenses, they must be rinsed off.

Hearing Aid

Many older residents wear a hearing aid to compensate for impaired hearing. A hearing aid makes the sound louder.

The nursing assistant is responsible for helping the resident care for the hearing aid. When the aid is not in use, it should be turned off and kept in a safe place. The aid must be removed before the resident showers or bathes. Getting the wires wet could create a hazard for the resident or damage the hearing aid. Always keep the hearing aid away from moisture or heat. Store a hearing aid properly in a marked container when it is not in use.

Chapter 31: Resident Belongings and Prostheses

The need for repairs or new batteries should be reported to the charge nurse. The nursing assistant should keep the hearing aid clean and check the resident's ear for wax build-up or soreness. These conditions must be reported to the charge nurse.

All belongings of residents, including prostheses, must be treated with care and concern.

*Circle the correct answer. There is only **one** correct answer.*

1. **Mrs. Daniels, a resident, is forgetful and sometimes leaves her gold wedding band on the nightstand in her room. What is appropriate for the nursing assistant to do?**

    a. Don't allow her to take her ring off.

    b. Tell her not to wear her ring.

    c. Put it in the safe in a marked envelope.

    d. Don't worry about it; no one will take it from her room.

2. **Personal belongings should be clearly marked with the resident's name and room number.**

    a. True   b. False

3. **Who is responsible for cleaning and caring for a resident's prosthesis?**

    a. Resident.

    b. Charge nurse.

    c. Resident's family.

    d. Nursing assistant.

4. **When a resident has an artificial limb, why should a stump sock be worn?**

    a. To keep it clean.

    b. For privacy.

    c. To prevent swelling.

    d. To keep it warm.

5. **Artificial eyes should be removed at bedtime and placed in a container of contact lens solution.**

    a. True   b. False

6. **Before reinserting Mrs. Donley's contact lenses, what action should the nursing assistant take?**

     a. Dry them.

     b. Clean and rinse them.

     c. Wait two hours.

     d. Nothing.

7. **While cleaning eyeglasses, the nurse assistant should inspect them for loose or broken parts:**

     a. True   b. False

8. **Mrs. Murphy has trouble hearing and wears a hearing aid. What are the nursing assistant's responsibilities toward care of the hearing aid?**

     a. Reporting the need for repairs or batteries.

     b. Soaking it regularly in soapy water.

     c. Making sure the resident wears it during bathing..

     d. Replacing the batteries.

9. **When not in use, a hearing aid should be stored.**

     a. In the resident's ear.

     b. In the facilities safe.

     c. In a marked container.

     d. At the nursing station.

10. **Ambulation devices refers to artificial limbs.**

     a. True   b. False

Chapter 32

THE ENVIRONMENT OF CARE: RESIDENT SAFETY

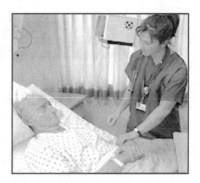

In this chapter... you will learn about:

▶ The importance of maintaining a safe environment for residents.
▶ Hazards to look for and eliminate

DEFINITIONS

Hazard: A danger that may cause an injury.

Oxygen: The gas in the air we breathe that supports
                                    fire.

Type A fire extinguisher: A fire extinguisher used for paper, wood or
                                    cloth.

Type B fire extinguisher: A fire extinguisher used for liquids

Type C fire extinguisher: A fire extinguisher used for electrical fires

GENERAL SAFETY

People in a long-term care institution often have special risks for their personal safety. Some of these residents have disabilities, vision or hearing problems, or general weakness. Some are taking medications that cause drowsiness or unsteadiness. Others have mental problems, confusion or dementia. These problems can help contribute to accidents and injuries. It is the responsibility of all healthcare providers to remain safety conscious at all times, and to actively search out and remove hazards in the environment.

Slips and falls alone, among people over 65, kill about 8,500 Americans every year. In institutions, more than half of those with high risk factors fall every year. And one out of ten of these falls results in a serious injury.

Other risks involve electrical safety, oxygen safety and fire safety. This chapter will identify some of these hazards and suggest practical steps you can take to protect resident safety.

SAFETY INSPECTION

If your institution has a safety inspector or safety committee, you should work with them to identify and report any hazards you see. Look around you as you visit residents and do your daily job. Many simple hazards, such as spills, can be corrected right on the spot. Others, such as broken equipment, may need to be reported to your supervisor so repairs can be made.

The safety team may make regular studies of incident reports to try to identify any areas of special danger in the facility, or any types of patients who may have an increased risk for falls. If you are asked, make suggestions to the committee on hazards you have noticed.

The next sections will suggest some of the hazards to look for, in halls, rooms and other areas.

Corridors

In a safe environment, every area should have enough light, including night lights so the patients will be able to see where they are going. If you notice any lights that are out, report them immediately.

The corridors should not have any objects standing around that could trip a patient. Floors should not be so brightly polished that they are slippery or cause a blinding glare. If you see something that doesn't belong on the floor, pick it up. Housekeepers may only clean an area once a day.

When traveling through corridors or moving patients through corridors, you should keep to the right and take special care at intersections or turns. Also take special care when opening doors so that you do not hit someone.

Resident Rooms

The rooms should be well lit. The patient needs a secure bedside light, and visible wall switches. Report any bulbs that are out.

The patient's belongings should be in easy reach so she does not have to stretch far out of bed to get them. The same is true for any call switches and controls for televisions. Make sure items are not lying on the floor that may cause a resident to trip. There should be no throw rugs that can move as they may cause a fall.

Most rooms and bathroom have sturdy grab bars. The patients should be shown where they are and how to use them. Raised toilet seats fixed in place can also help when appropriate.

Another help can be non-skid shoes and slippers, which should fit well on a patient's feet. Floppy shoes and slippery soles can contribute to falls even for the most agile patients. Make sure that shoes and slippers, when not worn, are kept in a regular place where the resident can get them easily and won't trip over them.

In storage rooms, you should be sure all equipment is in working order without obvious hazards such as broken parts or sharp edges. Report any hazards immediately to your supervisor and do not use this equipment.

Never use the contents of an unlabeled container, whether you think it is a medication or a cleaning solution. Keep all cleaning items and medications in their separate assigned areas, and make sure that these items are properly labeled.

Safety in the use of restraints and bed rails will be discussed in later chapters.

IF A FALL HAPPENS

You should also know what to do if you witness a fall in your facility or you come upon a person who has fallen.

If you are caring for a resident who is starting to fall, you shouldn't try to stop the fall by yourself. You might hurt yourself and both of you might go down and make the situation worse. Ease the person to the floor as gently as you can, and then call for help. Always stay with a fallen patient until assistance arrives.

Do not try to lift a resident who has fallen until someone has assessed whether there are any injuries. Be sure to notify your supervisor of the incident immediately. You might make an injury worse by trying to pick her up.

Once the resident is safely cared for your supervisor will probably ask you to assist her in writing out an incident report. Be as accurate as you can. This may help prevent falls in the future.

ELECTRICAL HAZARDS

To maintain the safety of the environment, there are several other special areas you should be aware of. Faulty electrical equipment can cause electrical shock or fire to a resident, to yourself or to other healthcare workers. This can include items as complex as portable respirators or as simple as a resident's own table radio.

Always check electrical equipment to see if there are any obvious problems, such as broken plugs or worn wires. Do not use equipment in this condition. Report it immediately to your supervisor.

Also, you should never unplug equipment by pulling on the cord. Always grasp the plug and pull firmly. Make sure electrical wiring is not lying where someone could trip over it. Except in emergencies, you should not use extension cords. They increase the danger of tripping and of overloading the wires with too much electrical current.

OXYGEN HAZARDS

When oxygen is in use for a resident, there is a special danger of fire. Ordinary room air contains about 20% oxygen. Pure oxygen can cause a fire to ignite much more easily and burn much faster than room air.

An "OXYGEN IN USE" sign must be posted on the door of the room. Be especially alert for any electrical equipment near the oxygen, even something as simple as a radio. The tiniest electrical spark can start a fire in the presence of pure oxygen. Most facilities now ban smoking completely, but be watchful for any matches or cigarettes that visitors or residents may try to bring into the facility. Report this to your supervisor immediately.

FIRE SAFETY

Your residents rely on you especially to prevent fires and to take quick action if fire should happen. Imagine how terrifying fire can be for someone who is bedridden.

First, you should stay alert for any hazards that might cause a fire. Look for:

- Oily rags
- Paper products left lying around
- Faulty electrical equipment
- Overheated equipment
- Oxygen near anything that could cause a spark

Report any fire hazards immediately to your supervisor.

You should also learn the location of all fire alarms and fire extinguishers. Learn the three types of fire extinguishers and what sorts of fire they are good for:

▶ **TYPE A:** for paper, wood or cloth

▶ **TYPE B:** for liquids such as grease or oil

▶ **TYPE C:** for electrical fires

▶ **TYPE ABC:** for all fires

If a Fire Happens

There is a simple reminder-word that you should remember in case of a fire: RACE.

R — Rescue residents near the fire. Move anyone who is in immediate danger

A — Activate the alarm

C — Contain the fire by closing doors and windows

E — Extinguish the fire if it is small. Use the appropriate fire extinguisher.

Remember that many residents are vulnerable to hazards, especially slips and falls. Keeping the environment as safe as possible should be your concern at all times.

Procedures for Using a Fire Extinguisher

1. Pull the fire alarm.

2. Set the fire extinguisher and upright.

3. Remove the latch safety.

4. Point the nozzle low at the base of the fire.

5. Push down on the handle and water or foam will come out.

*Circle the correct answer. There is only **one** correct answer.*

1. **You should be safety conscious mainly _____.**

    a. When you are with residents
    b. In resident rooms
    c. At all times
    d. On regular safety inspections

2. **The most common hazards facing residents are _____.**

    a. Terrorism
    b. Slips and falls
    c. Electrical shock
    d. Fire

3. **If you see something that doesn't belong on a corridor floor _____.**

    a. Report it to housekeeping.
    b. Report it to your supervisor.
    c. Ignore it
    d. Pick it up immediately

4. **If you find someone who has fallen, you should _____.**

    a. Pick the person up immediately
    b. Find someone to help you pick her up
    c. Walk away and ignore it
    d. Do NOT move her before she is checked for injuries

5. **To pull out an electrical plug you should pull by _____.**

    a. The cord
    b. The plug only
    c. The apparatus itself
    d. The cord and the plug both

6. **Pure oxygen causes a fire to burn faster than room air.**

    a. True   b. False

7. **A TYPE A fire extinguisher is used for _____.**

    a. Electrical fires
    b. Paper, wood and cloth
    c. Oil and grease
    d. Any fire

8. **A resident's belongings should be stored _____.**

    a. In a locked area
    b. Within easy reach
    c. In the office
    d. With the resident's family

9. **If you find an unlabeled container of liquid, you should _____.**

    a. Smell it to find out what it is
    b. Taste it to find out what it is
    c. Properly dispose of it immediately
    d. Light with a match

10. **The letter R in the memory aid for fire stands for _____.**

    a. Run
    b. Rescue
    c. Resident
    d. Report

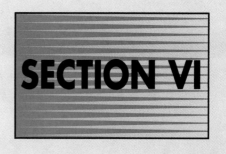

SECTION VI

SKILLS FOR ASSISTING
THE RESIDENT

Chapter 33

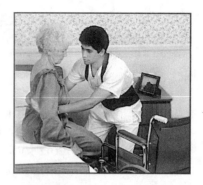

✳ MOVING A RESIDENT

 Watch step-by-step demonstrations of the procedures discussed in this chapter in the Medcom videotapes "The New Nursing Assistant 2000: Moving and Turning" (CNA503), and "The New Nursing Assistant 2000: Transfer and Ambulation" (CNA504).

In this chapter... you will learn about:

▶ How to lift a heavy object safely.

▶ How to move a resident safely.

DEFINITIONS

Base of Support:	The area on which an object rests. Relating to your body, the base of support is your feet when standing and your hips when sitting.
Center of Gravity:	Place where the mass or weight of an object is centered (for example, your center of gravity is higher when you are standing up then when you are lying on the ground).
Gait Belt:	A belt placed around the resident's waist used to assist in transfer.
Posture:	Alignment of the skeletal body as a whole.

BODY MECHANICS

How you use your body affects how you feel, how much strength you have, and how you look. Good **posture** helps you look better and, together with proper lifting and moving techniques, will result in fewer back pains and injuries and increased strength.

Posture

The rules of good posture are to stand with your feet facing forward, your knees slightly flexed, your chest up, shoulders back, and chin parallel to the floor. Good sitting posture includes keeping your feet flat on the floor with your knees, ankles, and hips at right angles, and your chin parallel to the floor. These rules of posture apply to both you and your resident.

The foundation of an object is its **base of support**. For people, this base is the feet when standing and the hips when sitting. Standing with your feet spread apart will give you a wider base, and the wider the base, the more stable you are. Your **center of gravity** is in your hip area. You are usually more stable when your center of gravity is low, for example, when you are sitting or lying down.

General Rules for Lifting and Moving

* ▶ Always wear a support belt to help protect you from injury when lifting.

  ▶ Use good posture, keeping your body properly aligned. Keep your back straight, knees bent, and your weight evenly balanced on both feet. When lifting, your feet should be about 12 inches apart.

  ▶ Get as close as possible to the object you are lifting.

Chapter 33: Moving A Resident

- ► Use your arms to support the object and your legs to lift.

- ► Bend your knees and keep your back straight as you lift smoothly to avoid strain. Pivot with your feet, taking short steps. Be careful not to twist or turn your back.

- ► If the object is too heavy for you to move, **GET HELP**. Then coordinate your efforts by counting out loud: "One, two, three . . . **lift**."

- ► When moving a heavy object, if you have a choice, push, pull, or roll rather than lift.

- ► Use a *gait belt* for lifting and transfer of a resident.

Understanding and practicing these rules for lifting and moving will help you make the best use of your strength and avoid fatigue.

RESIDENT ALIGNMENT AND TRANSFER

Many of the nursing assistant's duties involve lifting and moving residents who cannot do this by themselves. It is important to remember and use the rules of body mechanics for lifting and moving so that this can be done without injury. If you cannot move the resident by yourself, ask for help. But, before you ask for help, be sure you and the resident are ready. Then decide whether you or your partner will count "1, 2, 3" to coordinate your efforts. Be sure to tell the resident what you are going to do. Use a gait belt on the resident for lifting, transfer, and support.

Alignment

Residents who cannot reposition themselves need to have their position changed often. Proper alignment of the resident's body is important. The body should be straight and properly supported.

Moving a Resident in Bed

If the resident is able to assist with the move, encourage him or her to do so. The procedure for assisting a resident to move up in bed is as follows:

   * 1.   Explain to the resident what you are going to do and wash your hands.

     2.   Place the resident's pillow upright on the headboard to protect the resident's head from injury.

     3.   Stand next to the bed with your feet about 12 inches apart. The foot that is closer to the head of the bed should be pointed in that direction.

     4.   Place a hand under the resident's shoulders and one under the buttocks.

     5.   Ask the resident to bend the knees and brace his or her feet firmly against the mattress.

     6.   On a count of "three" have the resident push toward the head of the bed with the feet as you support and move the resident. Remember to keep your back straight and knees bent.

     7.   Wash your hands.

Moving a Resident with a Lift Sheet

It is easier to move some residents with a "lift" or "turn" sheet. This is a folded sheet placed under the resident from shoulders to knees. The procedure is as follows:

   Chapter 33: Moving A Resident

1. Ask for help from another healthcare worker.

2. Explain to the resident what you are going to do and wash your hands.

3. Place the resident's pillow upright on the headboard to protect the resident's head from injury.

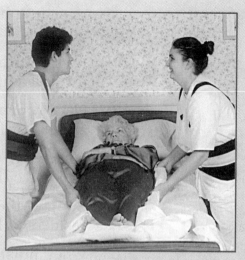

Using a lift sheet.

4. With one person on each side of the bed, roll both sides of the lift sheet as close as possible to the resident's body.

5. Stand straight, with your feet 12 inches apart and pointed in the direction of the move. Keep your body turned slightly toward the head of the bed.

6. Grasp rolled sheet at resident's shoulders and hip. Ask the resident to raise his or her head on count of "three."

7. Count "One, two, three . . . **lift**," and then lift.

8. When lifting, keep your back straight and your knees bent and support the resident as you shift your weight from one foot to the other.

9. When finished, wash your hands.

Moving a Resident Without a Lift Sheet

The procedure for moving a resident to one side without a lift sheet is as follows:

1. Explain to the resident what you are going to do and wash your hands.

2. With your hands under the knees and ankles, move the resident's feet and legs toward you.

3. Place your forearms under the small of the back and buttocks and move the resident toward you.

4. Place your hands under the resident's shoulders and move the resident toward you.

5. Support the resident's back with a pillow when the resident is lying on his or her side.

6. When finished, wash your hands.

Turning a Resident Away from You

The procedure for turning a resident away from you is divided into two parts, beginning with moving the resident toward you:

1. Explain to the resident what you are going to do and wash your hands.

2. With your hand under the knees and ankles, move the resident's feet and legs toward you.

3. Place your forearms under the small of the back and buttocks and move the resident toward you.

4. Place your hands under the resident's shoulders and move the resident toward you.

5. If possible, bend the resident's knee nearest you. If the knee cannot be bent, cross the near leg over the far leg.

6. Place one hand on the knee and one on the hip. Roll the resident over.

7. Move your hand from the knee to the hip and from the hip to the shoulder to complete the turn.

8. Support the resident's back with a pillow.

9. When finished, wash your hands.

Chapter 33: Moving A Resident

Turning a Resident Toward You

The procedure for turning the resident toward you is as follows:

1. Explain to the resident what you are going to do and wash your hands.

2. Cross the leg farthest from you over the leg closest to you.

3. Cross the resident's arms over the chest.

4. Reach across the resident and put one hand behind the shoulder. Place your other hand behind the hip and gently roll the resident toward you.

5. Support the resident's back with a pillow.

6. When finished, wash your hands

Turning a Resident Using The Log-Rolling Technique

Some residents must be moved without disturbing the alignment of the body. They must be moved as one unit rather than in sections. This technique is called log-rolling.

1. Ask another health care worker to help you.

2. Explain to the resident what you are going to do and wash your hands.

3. Use a lift sheet rolled up as close as possible to both sides of the resident's body.

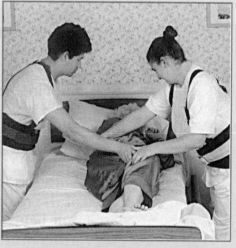

Turning a resident using log-rolling.

4. Coordinate your movements by counting. Keeping your knees bent and your back straight, lift and move the resident to one side of the bed.

5. Using the lift sheet, roll the resident onto his or her side, turning the body as one unit without bending the joints. Your helper can support the resident's legs during the roll

6. Make sure the resident is in correct body alignment. Properly position pillows for support and wash your hands before leaving the resident.

Pivot Transfer from Bed to Wheelchair

This technique is used for a resident with a paralyzed or severely weakened extremity.

1. Explain to the resident what you are going to do and wash your hands.

2. The resident should be wearing shoes with nonskid soles.

3. Position the wheelchair on the resident's nonparalyzed side. Place the chair at a 45 degree angle to the bed with the brakes locked and the pedals up.

4. Help the resident sit on the edge of the bed with legs and feet hanging over the edge. Put a gait belt on the resident.

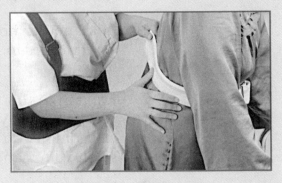

Using a gait belt.

5. Stand in front of the resident. With your hands, firmly grasp the gait belt. The resident should not put his or her arms around your neck. Have the resident put his or her arms at your waist.

6. Stand so your feet are about 18 inches apart and so the resident's paralyzed or weakened leg is between your knees.

7. Help the resident stand, supporting the paralyzed leg with your knees.

8. Have the resident use the nonparalyzed hand to grasp the armrest of the wheelchair.

*9. Pivot your body, helping the resident to pivot toward the nonparalyzed leg.

10. Bend your knees, keep your back straight, and help the resident sit in the chair.

11. When finished, wash your hands.

Transferring the Dependent Resident

You will need help to transfer residents who cannot help themselves. There should be at least two persons to perform the transfer. When you have the resident ready to move, ask for help.

1. Explain to the resident what you are going to do and wash your hands.

2. Place the wheelchair at a 45 degree angle to the bed and facing the foot of the bed. Lock the brakes.

3. The taller person should be at the head of the bed and the shorter at the resident's knees.

4. Help the resident to sit up in bed, keeping legs and feet on the bed. The nursing assistant at the head will reach around resident, cross resident's arms, and grasp the wrists. The other person reaches under resident's knees and thighs.

5. On a count of "three," lift and move the resident to the edge of the bed.

6. Adjust your base of support. On a count of "three," lift the resident into the wheelchair, keeping your back straight and your knees bent.

7. When finished, wash your hands.

Using a Mechanical Lift

If a resident is too heavy for the nursing assistants to lift and move, a mechanical lift may be used. The procedure for using this lift is as follows:

1. Ask another healthcare worker to help you.

2. Explain to the resident what you are going to do and wash your hands.

3. Place the wheelchair next to the bed with the back of the chair in line with the headboard.

4. Turn the resident from side to side on the bed while sliding the sling under the resident.

5. Attach the sling to the mechanical lift with the hooks in place through the metal frame.

6. Have the resident fold both arms across the chest, if possible.

7. Lift the resident out of bed by turning the crank.

8. Have the other person guide the resident's legs.

9. Lower the resident into the wheelchair.

10. Remove the hooks from the frame and leave the sling under the resident for use when lifting him or her back into bed.

11. When finished, wash your hands.

After any transfer or repositioning, you should perform the following steps before leaving the resident.

1. Make sure the call bell is within the resident's reach.

2. Make sure the side rails of the bed are up.

3. Make sure the bed is lowered to its lowest position.

4. Thank the resident for cooperating and wash your hands.

All of these techniques for lifting, moving, and transferring residents will need to be practiced many times in order for you to do them properly and easily. This practice will result in safety for both you and your residents.

Circle the correct answer. There is only **one** *correct answer.*

1. **Where is your center of gravity?**

    a. Hip
    b. Ankle
    c. Shoulders
    d. Knees

2. **When lifting heavy objects, carry them as far away from the body as possible.**

    a. True   b. False

3. **The rules of good sitting posture state that you should keep your feet flat on the floor, and your knees, ankles, and hips at right angles.**

    a. True   b. False

4. **When moving a heavy object by yourself, what should you do?**

    a. Pull it or roll it.
    b. Bend from the waist.
    c. Lift rather than push the object.
    d. Straighten your knees.

5. **Your resident, Mrs. Stone, must be turned in bed without bending her ankles, knees, or hips. The technique you should use is called**

    a. Using a mechanical lift.
    b. Pivot transfer.
    c. Log-rolling.
    d. Sliding.

6. **When moving a resident in bed, you should not encourage him or her to assist with the move.**

    a. True   **b.** False

7. **When lifting and moving residents, always explain to them what you are going to do.**

    a. True   b. False

8. **When moving a resident with a lift sheet,**

    a. You do not need help from another nursing assistant.

    b. Put the resident's arms around your neck.

    c. Roll the lift sheet as close as possible to the resident's body.

    d. Have the resident sit on the edge of the bed first.

9. **In a pivot transfer of a partially paralyzed resident from bed to wheelchair,**

    a. Put the resident's arms around your neck.

    b. Make sure the resident is barefoot.

    c. Position the wheelchair on the resident's nonparalyzed side.

    d. Do not tell the resident what you are going to do.

10. **The techniques for lifting, moving, and transferring residents require a lot of practice by the nursing assistant in order to be done properly and easily.**

    a. True   b. False

Chapter 34

AMBULATION

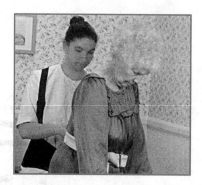

 Watch step-by-step demonstrations of the procedures discussed in this chapter in the Medcom videotape "The New Nursing Assistant 2000: Transfer and Ambulation" (CNA504).

In this chapter... you will learn about:

▶ Why ambulation is important to a resident.

▶ How to assist a resident with ambulation.

DEFINITIONS

Ambulation:	To walk in upright position, to assist someone to walk.
Ambulation Device:	A device used to assist in walking; including braces, cane, walker or crutches.
Incapacitate:	Disable.
Walker:	A portable frame that a person can move along as he or she walks to provide support.

Ambulation means walking, moving about in an upright position. It can also refer to helping a person walk. Ambulation is beneficial to a resident because it:

▶ Strengthens muscles.

▶ Improves circulation.

▶ Moves joints.

▶ Relieves pressure on other body parts.

▶ Bears weight on the leg bones.

▶ Helps urinary and bowel systems to function better.

▶ Provides independence.

▶ Improves self-esteem.

If there is any question about a resident's ability to ambulate, the resident's physician will make the decision, with input from the physical therapist and the nurse. If you are not certain about helping a resident ambulate, check with your supervisor. Never assume a resident cannot walk. In order to ambulate safely, a resident must be able to:

▶ Maintain sitting balance unassisted.

▶ Stand up.

▶ Maintain standing balance.

There are several **ambulation devices** that are useful to assist ambulation for patients with impaired strength or balance.

Gait Belt

A device called a gait belt, or a transfer belt, is used to assist a resident in ambulation. The belt is placed around the resident's waist. The nursing assistant stands behind or beside the resident and holds onto the belt with one or two hands. This allows the nursing assistant to help the resident remain steady, to prevent a resident from falling, and allows the resident better control over his or her own balance.

Braces

A resident may wear a leg or back brace to limit movement or to assist in movement. The nursing assistant is responsible for routinely checking the resident's skin under the brace for redness, irritation, sores, or blisters.

Cane

A cane can be a straight, single point cane or a quad cane which provides greater support. Both provide balance and confidence for the resident. The cane should be used on the strong side of the body. Canes must be inspected routinely to see if the rubber tips need to be replaced.

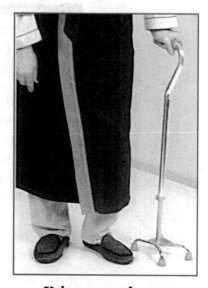

Using a quad cane.

Walkers are portable frames that provide stability and support to residents while ambulating. There are three types of walkers:

▶ Pick-up walker

▶ Rolling walker

▶ Wheeled walker

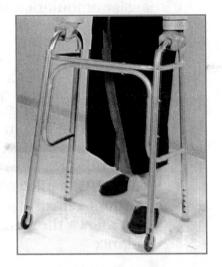

Using a walker.

Pick-up walkers have no wheels. They must be lifted and moved forward at each step. They provide the most stability, and are used for residents with weakness and balance problems.

Rolling walkers are used for residents with arthritis, Parkinson's Disease, and poor backward and forward balance. They have wheels on two or more of the legs.

Wheeled Walkers are similar to rolling walkers except they have a seat. This makes them appropriate for residents who are weak because they provide an immediate place on which to sit and rest.

Most residents want to ambulate and welcome the nursing assistant's help. Positive reinforcement is important to encourage the resident to continue ambulating. The nursing assistant can congratulate the resident on his or her progress and encourage the resident to set new goals and work toward them.

If a resident has not walked for a period of time or has some paralysis, he or she may be afraid when trying to walk again. You should reassure the resident that you will be there to help and prevent any injury. It is more reassuring to have two assistants when ambulating for the first time. The procedure for assisting a resident to ambulate is as follows:

1. Explain to the resident what you are going to do, what you expect the resident to do, and wash your hands.

2. Help the resident to sit up. Allow time for the resident to gain his or her balance.

3. Fasten a gait belt around the resident's waist.

4. Help the resident put on firm shoes.

5. Firmly grasp both sides of the gait belt to help the resident stand up and maintain his balance.

6. Stand on the unaffected (strong) side, and help the resident stand up. Remember to keep your own back straight.

7. Allow time for the resident to gain balance, but do not let go of the gait belt.

8. Remind the resident to stand as straight as possible with the chin parallel to the floor.

9. Walk along with the resident, providing support with the gait belt.

10. Be alert to signs of fatigue, such as rapid breathing, rapid heartbeat, sweating, or dizziness. If these are observed, stop and help the resident sit or lie down.

11. Be alert to hazards, such as spills, items on the floor, or untied shoelaces.

12. Return the resident to the chair or bed, remove the gait belt, and wash your hands.

13. In the resident's medical chart, note distance, time ambulated, and resident's response.

While ambulating, residents may lose their balance or their legs may become weak. When this happens, a fall can occur. Falls can further *incapacitate* a resident. This is why residents have a fear of falling and need a great deal of reassurance and assistance.

If a resident starts to fall while being ambulated, the nursing assistant should slowly ease the resident to the floor. Never try to stop the fall as this may result in personal injury or injury to the resident. Use good body mechanics to prevent injury to yourself. The nursing assistant should stay with the resident and call for help. Before moving or being moved, the resident must be checked for injury by a licensed nurse. Never try to lift a resident from the floor by yourself. Always ask for help.

*Circle the correct answer. There is only **one** correct answer.*

1. **Leg and back braces are worn to limit or assist in movement.**

    a. True   b. False

2. **When a resident wears a leg or back brace, what should the nursing assistant routinely do?**

    a. Check if rubber tips need to be replaced.

    b. Make sure the resident stays in bed.

    c. Nothing.

    d. Check the skin under the brace for signs of irritation.

3. **Mr. Wilson is very weak and has trouble supporting himself for long. Which type of walker is he most likely to use?**

    a. Cane.

    b. Pick-up walker.

    c. Rolling walker.

    d. Wheeled walker.

4. **Mrs. Mills is anxious about ambulating. How can the nursing assistant aid her?**

    a. Allow Mrs. Mills to ambulate unassisted.

    b. Discourage her from ambulating.

    c. Encourage her to set goals and move toward them.

    d. Confine her to a wheelchair.

5. **Ambulation is beneficial to a resident because it strengthens muscles and improves circulation, as well as improving self-esteem.**

    a. True   b. False

6. **Where is a gait belt worn?**

    a. Around the nursing assistant's waist.

    b. Around the resident's waist.

    c. Around the resident's stronger leg.

    d. Only on a resident confined to a wheelchair.

7. **When assisting a resident with some paralysis to stand, you should stand either in front of the resident or on the unaffected (strong) side.**

    a. True   b. False

8. **The resident should wear light slippers when walking.**

    a. True   b. False

9. **If a resident starts to fall, what should you do?**

    a. Try to stop the fall.

    b. Quickly grab the resident.

    c. Slowly ease the resident to the floor.

    d. Shout to warn the resident.

10. **It's okay to lift a resident from the floor by yourself.**

    a. True   b. False

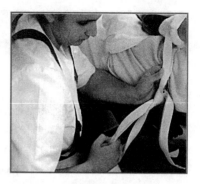

Chapter 35

SAFETY IN AMBULATION AND RESTRAINT

 Watch step-by-step demonstrations of the procedures discussed in this chapter in the Medcom videotape "The New Nursing Assistant 2000: Transfer and Ambulation" (CNA504).

In this chapter... you will learn about:

▶ How to help residents stay safe using ambulation devices.

▶ How to use protective devices and restraints.

DEFINITIONS

Limbs:	Arms and legs.
Mobility:	The ability to move about.
Postural Support:	Soft protective device used to protect a resident from injury.
Restraint:	Device that holds back or limits movements, which the resident cannot remove.

RESIDENT SAFETY

Every employee in a long-term care facility is responsible for the safety of every resident. The nursing assistant must know how to use equipment safely and must be alert to, and report, any hazardous situations.

All care facilities have special equipment and devices. As a nursing assistant, you are expected to use this equipment properly in order to prevent resident and staff injuries.

Identification

One primary safety responsibility is to know exactly who you are giving care to. Even simple nursing care given to the wrong resident can be extremely dangerous. Use the following rules for identification every time you are about to provide care:

1. Call the patient by name, but do not rely on this alone for identification.

2. Compare the name on the identification bracelet to any order for treatment. Every resident should have an ID bracelet that lists:

    - Name.

    - Room number and bed.

    - Age.

    - Sex.

    - Doctor's name.

    - Any allergies.

3. If there is any doubt at all, double check with the charge nurse before providing care.

Beds in care facilities are equipped with side rails. When these rails are up, the resident is protected from falling out of the bed. In most cases, the side rails will always be up at night. Residents who are at risk for falling out of bed or trying to walk unassisted may have their side rails up during the day. Individual instructions for when side rails are to be used should be in each resident's chart. It is the nursing assistant's responsibility to follow these instructions.

Safety precautions to remember when using side rails are:

1. Before raising or lowering side rails, check to be sure the resident's arms and legs are out of the way.

2. Side rails are to be securely locked into position, whether up or down.

3. **Restraints** are never to be tied to side rails.

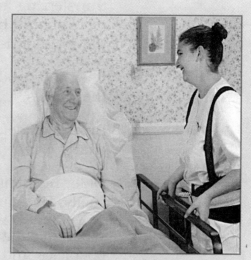

Raising the side rails.

4. Broken side rails are to be reported immediately to the charge nurse.

5. Side rail padding should be used to prevent injury to residents who thrash about in bed.

Wheelchair

Many residents in long-term care facilities depend on wheelchairs for **mobility**. Even residents who can walk may use a wheelchair because they may lack the strength or balance to ambulate safely.

Safety precautions to remember when using a wheelchair are:

1. Always lock the brakes before attempting to transfer a resident into or out of a wheelchair.

2. The foot rests should be up when a resident is transferring into or out of a wheelchair. The foot rests should be down for support for the feet when the resident is sitting in the wheelchair.

3. Keep the resident's **limbs** and clothing away from the wheels.

4. Broken or defective parts are to be reported to the charge nurse immediately.

5. Older residents have fragile skin which injures easily. Use care during wheelchair transfers.

6. When moving a resident in a wheelchair, be alert to obstacles and hazards.

Walker

Residents who have poor balance or general weakness often use a walker for safe ambulation. It takes some of the weight off the resident's legs and puts more on the arms. There are three types of walkers:

- Pick-up walker. This has no wheels and is picked up and moved forward at each step. It provides very firm support.

- Rolling walker. This has wheels on two legs. The other legs must be lifted at each step.

- Wheeled walker. This has wheels on the legs and usually a seat.

Safety precautions to remember when a resident uses a walker are:

1. Check the walker regularly and report immediately any broken or defective parts.

2. Keep the resident's path free of obstacles and hazards.

3. If the resident appears to be using the walker improperly, report this to the charge nurse immediately.

4. If the walker appears to be the wrong size for the resident, check with the physical therapist or charge nurse immediately.

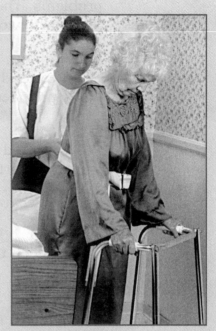

Using a walker.

Crutches

Crutches are used by residents to decrease the weight borne by one or both legs.

Safety precautions to observe when residents use crutches are:

1. Check the underarm padding to be sure it is adequate and in good repair.

2. Be sure there are no loose screws and the tips are in good repair.

3. Check the resident's underarm area for signs of pressure. If found, notify the charge nurse immediately.

4. If the resident appears to be having difficulty or uses the crutches improperly, notify the charge nurse immediately.

Canes offer some support for residents who have balance problems. The cane is used on the strong side of the body. There are two types of canes:

▶ *Straight single point.* This is the ordinary walking cane. It touches the ground at one point and provides little side-to side support.

▶ *Quad.* This type has four small feet and touches the ground at four points. It provides more side-to-side support.

Safety precautions for residents who use canes are:

1. Check the cane regularly for loose screws or cracks.

2. Rubber tips should be clean and in good repair.

3. Report to the charge nurse any difficulty the resident has using the cane.

SOFT PROTECTIVE DEVICES

Soft protective devices or **restraints** infringe on a resident's right to freedom of movement. Restraints can only be used if they are ordered by the resident's physician and only under certain conditions. These conditions are:

▶ To help the resident sit upright and prevent falls from a bed or wheelchair.

▶ To protect the resident while administering treatment (IV, feeding tube, or catheter).

▶ To protect the resident from injuring himself or herself or others.

There are several types of protective devices:

Vest Support

This is worn like a vest to provide **postural support.**

Pelvic Support

This is worn between the thighs to prevent the hips from slipping forward.

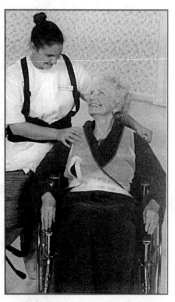

Mittens

These are worn on the hands to prevent scratching or removing dressings.

Resident wearing a vest support.

Limb Ties

These are used to immobilize a limb during treatment or to protect the resident from causing injury to himself, herself or others.

The Use Of Restraints

The use of restraints can cause the resident to be anxious and frustrated. The following guidelines should be followed when using restraints:

1. Approach the resident in a calm, unhurried manner. Make sure you have a physician's orders and you are approaching the correct resident.

2. Wash your hands and explain to the resident and his or her family what you are going to do in a simple, non-threatening way. Stress the protective purpose of the supports, using non-threatening terms such as "safety belt" and "postural support."

3. Restraints are to be used ONLY when the resident is in a bed or chair which has wheels. If there is an emergency, the resident will have to be moved quickly.

4. Restraints are NOT to be tied to side rails or parts of the bed that are raised or lowered. If the rails or parts of the bed were raised or lowered with the limb attached, the restraint might injure the resident.

5. Restraints are to be tied in simple, easy-to-release knots placed out of the resident's reach. NEVER use a slip knot as it can tighten when a resident moves.

6. The resident must be checked for proper positioning before a restraint is applied.

7. Restraints, when in place, should fit snugly, without binding. Check to see if you can slip two fingers under the edge of the restraint after it has been tied.

8. Restraints must never restrict the resident's circulation. Check the resident for the following signs of restricted circulation:

   a. Change in skin color.

   b. Change in skin temperature.

   c. Complaints of tingling, numbness, or pain.

   d. Swelling.

9. Protect the resident's skin from wrinkles, knots, and buckles. Use padded restraints or pad bony places to prevent pressure sores.

10. A resident in supportive restraints must be observed every hour, and the resident in treatment restraints must be observed every 15 minutes or as required by the Policies and Procedures of your facility. These observations must be entered in the Nurse's Notes at the end of each shift.

11. Restraints must be released every one to two hours for short periods, to allow for massage, exercise and movement. This also provides time for a position change.

12. The resident must always be able to reach and use the call button.

13. Restraints are NEVER used as punishment or for the convenience of the staff.

Restraints are considered the last resort. They are to be used to protect the resident, or to prevent him or her from harming others. When restraints are ordered by the physician and used by the staff, the resident's medical chart must contain the following information:

- Type of restraint used.

- Reason for restraint.

- Time restraint was applied and released.

- Effectiveness of restraint.

- Nursing care provided (massage, exercise, repositioning). Soft protective devices should not be used as a matter of routine. Alternative methods of protection should be tried first.

Some alternatives to restraints are:

▶ Placing the resident where he or she can be constantly observed.

▶ Keeping the resident dry, clean, and comfortable to reduce agitation.

▶ Responding promptly to the resident's needs.

▶ Diverting the resident's attention to safer, more meaningful activities.

▶ Taking time to provide special attention to the resident.

Ambulation and protective devices are very important to a resident's mobility and safety. It is the responsibility of the nursing staff to ensure their safe and proper use.

*Circle the correct answer. There is only **one** correct answer.*

1. **Every employee in a long-term care facility is responsible for the safety of every resident.**

    (a.) True   b. False

2. **Which of the following is true about side rails?**

    a. In general, side rails are up day and night for ambulatory residents.

    b. Side rails should not be locked into position.

    (c.) Instructions on when to use side rails should be in each resident's chart.

    d. Restraints can be tied to side rails.

3. **Few residents in long-term care facilities use wheelchairs.**

    a. True   (b.) False

4. **The cane is used on which side of the resident's body?**

    (a.) Strong   b. Weak

5. **If a resident needs to decrease the weight supported by one or both legs, what should he or she use?**

    a. Mittens.

    (b.) Walker.

    c. Limb ties.

    d. Crutches.

6. **Restraints can be used**

    a. To punish the resident.

    b. To immobilize a wanderer.

    c. To protect the resident, under physician orders.

    d. Whenever it is convenient to staff.

7. **A vest support**

    a. Prevents hips from slipping forward.

    b. Prevents the resident from scratching.

    c. Provides postural support.

    d. Immobilizes a limb during treatment.

8. **Application of restraints is considered the last resort - used to protect the resident, or to prevent him or her from harming others.**

    a. True   b. False

9. **An alternative to restraints is:**

    a. Punishment.

    b. Constantly observing the resident.

    c. Limb ties using slip knots.

    d. Ignoring the resident.

10. **Under which of these conditions should the nursing assistant report to the charge nurse the possible need for a postural support?**

    a. When a resident cannot sit upright and keeps falling out of the wheelchair.

    b. When a resident keeps walking in and out of a room.

    c. When a resident is wearing damp, soiled clothing.

    d. When a resident is very irritable and makes a lot of demands.

Chapter 36

INACTIVITY AND RANGE OF MOTION EXERCISES

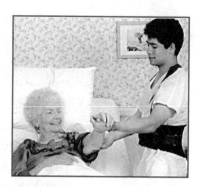

 Watch step-by-step demonstrations of the procedures discussed in this chapter in the Medcom videotape "Exercise Techniques" (CNA208).

In this chapter... you will learn about:

▶ The effects of inactivity on a resident.

▶ Assisting a resident with range of motion exercises.

DEFINITIONS

Active Range of Motion:	Range of motion exercises performed by the person himself or herself.
Abduction:	Moving arm or leg away from center of body.
Adduction:	Moving arm or leg toward center of body.
Atrophy:	Wasting away of muscle, with muscle becoming smaller and weaker.
Contracture:	An abnormal shortening of a muscle.
Degenerate:	To become worse.
Extension:	Straightening of an arm or leg.
Flexion:	Bending a joint.
Passive Range of Motion:	Range of motion exercises, as performed with the assistance of someone else.
Pronation:	Turning palms down.
Range of Motion:	Moving a joint through its normal range of activity.
Rotation:	Moving a joint in a circle.
Stasis:	Stoppage of the flow of body fluids.
Supination:	Turning palms up.

THE EFFECTS OF INACTIVITY

Our bodies are designed for movement. Long periods of inactivity can cause changes which harm tissues and may prevent future movement. Inactivity may be due to weakness, pain or paralysis.

Whatever the reason, the inactivity can lead to more problems. Since you will have the most contact with many residents, you may be able to observe and report early signs of problems with inactive residents.

Degeneration

When a resident is inactive, the body begins to **degenerate** and functions less efficiently. Muscles **atrophy** and become weak if they are not used, and muscle strength is lost. The muscles, tendons, and ligaments also begin to shorten, and **contractures** are the result. Contractures limit function and can be extremely painful. The nursing assistant should report to the charge nurse any changes observed in a resident, such as swollen or painful joints, increased weakness, decreased strength, and contractures.

RANGE OF MOTION EXERCISES

Many of these changes can be prevented with an increase in activity and movement. Residents must be repositioned often and assisted or encouraged to exercise. Residents who are able should be shown how to do **range of motion** exercises and should be encouraged to do them on their own. This is referred to as **active range of motion**.

Residents who are unable to do range of motion exercises on their own must be assisted by the nursing assistant. This is referred to as **passive range of motion**.

As you learn to perform range of motion exercises, there are a number of terms you should be familiar with. You may see these on doctor's orders or you may have to use some of them yourself in charting a resident's progress.

▶ **Abduction.** This is moving an arm or leg away from the center of the body. You are abducting your own arm when you reach out to pick up an object.

▶ **Adduction.** This is moving an arm or leg toward the center of the body. You are adducting your arm as you bring an object toward you.

▶ **Extension.** This the straightening of an arm or leg.

▶ **Flexion.** This is making any bend in a joint.

▶ **Pronation.** This is turning the palm down.

▶ **Rotation.** This is moving a joint in a circle. As you turn a doorknob, you are rotating your wrist.

▶ **Supination.** This is turning the palm up.

Passive Range of Motion Exercises

Range of motion exercises should start with the head and neck and work down the body to the feet. If you exercise in a set order, you won't forget any joints. Support the joint and gently move it through its normal range three times. The proper procedure for range of motion exercises is as follows:

1. Wash your hands and explain to the resident what you are going to do.

2. Provide privacy for the resident.

3. Place the resident in supine position with knees extended and arms at the side.

4. Raise the side rail on the far side of the bed.

5. Exercise the neck. Remember, throughout all these exercises, NEVER move a joint past the point of pain.

6. Exercise each shoulder.

7. Exercise each elbow.

8. Exercise each wrist.

9. Exercise each finger.

10. Exercise each hip.

11. Exercise each knee.

12. Exercise each ankle.

13. Exercise each toe.

14. Wash your hands.

15. Chart the time, what exercises were performed, whether active or passive, and any abnormalities or complaints. Report any abnormalities or complaints to the charge nurse.

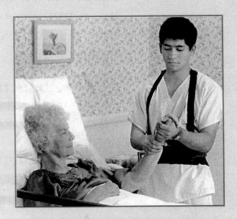

Exercising a resident's wrist.

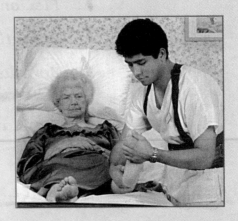

Exercising a resident's ankle

The purpose of these exercises is to increase the function of each joint and not to cause pain. If any joint is red and swollen, don't exercise it until it gets better.

Active Range of Motion Exercises

Residents who do their own range of motion exercises still need to be checked to see if they are doing them properly. Have them follow the same pattern as above. Watch them to see they learn the appropriate motion for each joint and complete the full range of motion series. Continued reinforcement and encouragement is also important.

OTHER PROBLEMS OF INACTIVITY

Stasis

When a resident is confined to bed, this can cause **stasis** or a fluid build-up in the body tissues. This can lead to swelling, edema, or pneumonia. When the resident does sit up, the body's blood pressure may drop. This can cause dizziness and the resident may feel cold and clammy. The inactive resident may easily develop a cough or have difficulty breathing. These observations should be reported to the charge nurse.

Preventing Problems of Stasis

Stasis can be minimized by frequently repositioning the residents and assisting them into sitting and standing positions. The nursing assistant can encourage residents' deep breathing and coughing to help clear fluids from the lungs and help prevent pneumonia.

Urinary Problems and Constipation

Inactivity can also cause urinary problems. The resident may have difficulty urinating and may develop infections of the urinary tract.

Constipation can be another problem of inactivity. Any problems a resident has with urination or elimination should be reported to the charge nurse.

Preventing Urinary Problems and Constipation

Increasing fluid intake and frequently changing position can help prevent urinary problems. Constipation can be reduced by encouraging the resident to eat more cereals, fruits, and vegetables, to drink more fluids, and to increase exercise.

Pressure

Lying in one position for long periods of time increases the pressure on bony areas of the body. The pressure cuts off the flow of blood to the area, the body tissue dies, and pressure sores (decubitus ulcers) develop.

Preventing Pressure Sores

Pressure sores are prevented by relieving pressure on the bony areas of the body. This is done mainly by frequent changes of position. Keeping the skin clean and dry also helps. In the next chapter you will learn about these sores and about repositioning bed-ridden residents every two hours to help prevent them.

Continued activity is important for everybody. It is particularly important for the resident who is confined to bed or has limited mobility. Your role as a nursing assistant is to know what problems to look for and report, and to assist the resident in preventing tissue damage or a decrease in muscle and joint function.

*Circle the correct answer. There is only **one** correct answer.*

1. **Long periods of inactivity can cause bodily changes which may prevent future movement.**

    (a) True   b. False

2. **What are contractures?**

    a. Sores that develop where tissue has died.

    b. Joints that won't bend.

    c. Swollen joints.

    (d) Abnormally shortened muscles.

3. **What is the name of the procedure in which a nursing assistant helps a resident perform exercises at many body joints?**

    a. Degeneration.

    b. Rotation.

    (c) Passive range of motion.

    d. Active range of motion.

4. **In doing range of motion exercises, you should start with the feet and work your way up the body to the head.**

    a. True   (b) False

5. **To prevent pneumonia, the nursing assistant can encourage the resident to**

    a. Lie down.

    (b) Do deep breathing and coughing.

    c. Stop drinking so many fluids.

    d. Lie in one position for long periods of time.

6. **Which of the following reduces constipation?**

    a. Decreasing exercise.

    b. Drinking less fluids.

    c. Staying in the same position for long periods of time.

    d. Eating more cereals, fruits, and vegetables.

7. **The purpose of range of motion exercises is to decrease activity and movement.**

    a. True   b. False

8. **When a resident is in bed for long periods, urinary infections may result.**

    a. True   b. False

9. **What can the nursing assistant do to help a resident prevent urinary problems?**

    a. Increase the resident's fluid intake.

    b. Keep the resident in one position.

    c. Keep the resident's skin clean and dry.

    d. Decrease the resident's fluid intake.

10. **Lying in one position for long periods of time increases pressure on bony areas of the body, sometimes resulting in pressure sores.**

    a. True   b. False

Chapter 37

PRESSURE ULCERS AND POSITIONING

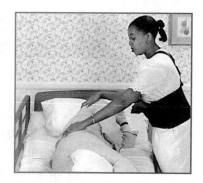

 Watch step-by-step demonstrations of the procedures discussed in this chapter in the Medcom videotapes "Positioning Techniques" (CNA209), and "Prevention, Assessment and Treatment of Pressure Ulcers in Long Term Care". (M176)

In this chapter... you will learn about:

▶ Pressure ulcers (decubitus ulcers).

▶ Positioning a resident to prevent pressure ulcers.

DEFINITIONS

Coccyx:	The tailbone.
Decubitus Ulcer (Pressure Sore):	An open sore on the skin caused by tissue breakdown due to pressure and reduced blood flow.
Edema:	Swelling due to increased fluid in the tissues.
Prone:	Face down.
Sacrum:	The rear pelvic bone.
Supine:	Face up.

One of the serious effects of immobility is the risk of developing **decubitus ulcers**, which are also called pressure ulcers, pressure sores, or bedsores. When a resident sits or lies in one position for several hours, the pressure against certain areas of the body can disrupt the flow of blood. The tissue dies from lack of oxygen, falls off, and leaves an open sore. This open sore provides a way for microorganisms to enter the body and cause infection. Once a sore has developed, it is very painful and often difficult to heal.

The body areas most likely to develop pressure sores are those which have little fat between the skin and bone, such as the toes, heels, ankles, knees, hips, elbows, shoulders, **coccyx**, spine, shoulder blades, ears, and the back of the head.

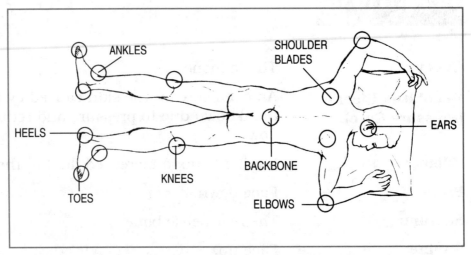

Pressure points susceptible to pressure ulcers.

Residents who are most likely to develop decubitus ulcers are those who have difficulty moving or cannot move. This could be due to paralysis, extreme weakness, coma, pain, or depression. Residents at particularly high risk are those with poor circulation, diabetes, anemia; those who are underweight or overweight; and those who are in casts, braces, or splints.

Residents who are at risk should be examined several times in every 24-hour period for signs of the beginning of pressure sores. If unnoticed and untreated, pressure sores normally go through the following four stages of development:

▶ ***Stage 1 — Reddened skin.*** The first sign is a redness which does NOT disappear with gentle massage. In a dark-skinned person, the area becomes darker than the surrounding skin. The reddened or darker area is warm and tender when touched.

▶ ***Stage 2 — Blistering or breakdown of top layer of the skin.*** If the pressure is not removed after the first stage, a white blister will form. The blister will break and leave an opening that may grow larger.

▶ ***Stage 3 — Breakdown of the lower tissue.*** The tissue under the top layers of the skin may begin to break down. If the sore becomes infected, a foul smelling drainage will be evident.

▶ ***Stage 4 — Involvement of muscle, bone, nerves and blood vessels.*** Sores that reach this stage are extremely painful and difficult to heal. Prevention is much easier.

The certified nursing assistant, who is the person responsible for giving a lot of hands-on care to residents, must recognize the importance of his or her role in the recognition, reporting, and prevention of pressure ulcers. Almost all pressure ulcers can be prevented by responsible nursing care!

Be alert, observe early signs of skin breakdown and report them to the charge nurse. Carefully observe the resident's skin for changes in color, any torn skin, places where skin is worn away, redness or blueness, drainage, odors, and swelling.

It is important to protect the resident's skin in order to prevent skin breakdown. Following are things that the nursing assistant can do to help prevent pressure sores:

> ▶ Keep the resident's skin clean and dry.
>
> ▶ Protect the skin from scratching and rubbing.
>
> ▶ Give gentle massages.
>
> ▶ Apply lotion to the skin to prevent dryness.
>
> ▶ Keep the bedding wrinkle free.
>
> ▶ Check the clothing, shoes, and any braces for signs of rubbing or pressure.

There are a number of devices which can be used to relieve pressure:

▶ Eggcrate cushions and mattresses provide cushioning, air and light pressure relief.

▶ Water mattresses and chair pads redistribute pressure.

▶ Air mattresses provide timed, automatic pressure redistribution.

▶ Sheepskin pads reduce friction, but not pressure.

▶ A foam ring reduces pressure in the center of the ring only. It raises pressure around the edges. Do NOT use inflatable rubber or plastic rings. These increase pressure.

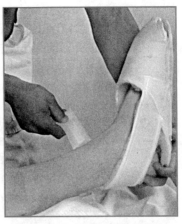

Sheepskin foot protection.

▶ Heel or elbow pads are used to decrease friction.

▶ A foot elevator is a foam casing for the foot to reduce heel pressure.

▶ A foot cradle is a tent-like frame at the foot of the bed to keep covers off the legs and feet to reduce friction and pressure.

POSITIONING

All of these treatments and devices help prevent decubitus ulcers, but by far the most important treatment is changing the immobile resident's position AT LEAST once every two hours. Residents who are seriously ill or extremely frail may need to have their position changed more often. If this is not done, the following complications could occur:

▶ Decubitus ulcers.

▶ Contractures.

▶ *Edema*.

▶ Pneumonia.

▶ Pain.

There are four basic positions for bedridden residents: *supine*, *prone*, semi-supine, and side-lying. Bedridden resident's position should be turned every 2 to 3 hours.

This is the position in which most bed-ridden residents spend the most time. The following guidelines should be followed when positioning a resident in the supine position:

1. Explain to the resident what you are going to do and wash your hands.

2. Place the pillow so that it is under the head, and slightly under the shoulders. Using two pillows should be avoided as it can lead to neck contractures and pain.

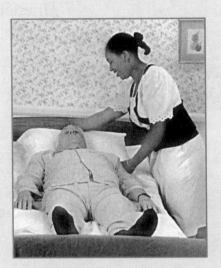

The supine position.

3. Place the resident's arms away from the body to allow air circulation in the axilla (armpit). Alternate palms up and then palms down.

4. To prevent or lessen hand contractures, place a small towel or piece of foam rubber in the resident's hand to prevent fist closure.

5. Place the resident's legs slightly apart to allow air circulation in the perineal area.

6 To prevent the legs from rotating outward, place a rolled towel or blanket at the hip joint.

7. Place the feet flat against a padded foot board to prevent foot drop, a contracture that occurs in residents who are bed-ridden. Place a small rolled towel or small piece of foam rubber under the resident's heels to elevate and prevent pressure on the heels. Use of a foot cradle can prevent additional pressure from bedding.

8. Change to another position every TWO hours.

9. When finished, wash your hands.

Semi-supine Position

This is a "tilt" position and not a true side-lying position. It can be used on both the right and left sides. It reduces direct pressure on the **sacrum** and coccyx without creating direct pressure on the hip. The correct procedure for positioning a resident in the semi-supine position is as follows:

1. Explain to the resident what you are going to do and wash your hands.

2. Roll the resident toward you.

3. Place one pillow behind the resident's back for support.

4. Take another pillow and place it under the resident's top leg, level with the hip joint.

5. Both legs should be straight with the top leg a little behind the bottom leg and supported by the pillow.

6. Check the lower shoulder placement. It should be forward so that pressure is distributed over the back of the shoulder rather than on one shoulder.

7. When finished, wash your hands.

8. Change to another position every *two* hours.

Prone Position - Lying on the Stomach

The prone position can offer relief to bedridden residents who have been in the supine position for two hours. It can also be a comfortable position for lower extremity amputees. However, some residents are never comfortable in this position, and the resident's preferences should be respected. The correct procedure to position a resident in a prone position is as follows:

1. Explain to the resident what you are going to do and wash your hands.

2. Roll the resident over onto the stomach.

3. Turn the head to one side without a pillow.

4. Align the body with the spine straight. The resident may be more comfortable with a flat pillow under the abdomen.

5. If the shoulders tend to roll forward, place shoulder rolls lengthwise under each shoulder.

6. Both the arms may be positioned down at the side, or one down and one flexed up, whichever is more comfortable. Both arms should not be flexed up as this puts strain on the shoulders.

7. It is best to position the feet so that the toes fall between the mattress and the footboard of the bed. Also, a rolled towel can be placed under the ankles to relieve pressure on the toes or the top of the foot.

8. When finished, wash your hands.

9. Change to another position every TWO hours.

Side-lying Position

This is a reversal of the semi-supine position. It is a comfortable position and reduces pressure and contractures. The proper procedure for positioning a resident in the side-lying position is as follows:

1. Explain to the resident what you are going to do and wash your hands.

2. From the prone position, lift the resident's shoulder closest to you and place a pillow under the chest and shoulder with the arm over the pillow. Position the other arm behind the resident.

3. Place a second pillow lengthwise under the top leg, making certain that the knees are slightly flexed, and that one leg is positioned in front of the other.

4. When finished, wash your hands.

5. Change to another position every TWO hours.

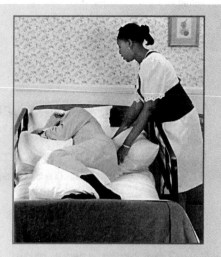

The side-lying position.

Completing a Transfer or Positioning

After any transfer or repositioning, you should perform the following steps before leaving the resident:

1. Make sure the call bell is within the resident's reach.

2. Make sure the side rails of the bed are up.

3. Make sure the bed is lowered to its lowest position.

4. Thank the resident for cooperating and wash your hands.

Proper positioning is the best prevention for decubitus ulcers. It is essential that immobile residents be repositioned at least every TWO hours.

Preventing skin breakdown and promoting healing are important responsibilities of the nursing assistant.

*Circle the correct answer. There is only **one** correct answer.*

1. **Decubitus ulcers, or pressure sores, develop when a resident sits or lies in one position for too long.**

    a. True   b. False

2. **The body areas most likely to develop pressure sores are**

    a. Where bones are near the skin.

    b. Areas of fatty tissue such as the buttocks.

    c. Hairy areas.

    d. Any area.

3. **Residents at particularly high risk for developing pressure ulcers are those who are immobile.**

    a. True   b. False

4. **What do air, water or gel mattresses and cushions do?**

    a. Reduce friction.

    b. Provide cushioning, air and light pressure relief.

    c. Encourage growth.

    d. Nothing.

5. **In what position do immobile, bed-restricted residents spend most of their time?**

    a. Supine.

    b. Prone.

    c. Semi-supine.

    d. Side-lying.

6. What is the first sign of a beginning bedsore?

    a. White blister.

    b. Contracture.

    c. Foul-smelling drainage.

    d. Redness or darkened area.

7. What can a nursing assistant do to prevent the resident from getting pressure ulcers?

    a. Remove the top sheet.

    b. Use an inflatable ring.

    c. Keep bedding wrinkle free.

    d. Keep the resident's skin moist.

8. Lying on either side is recommended for bedridden residents.

    a. True   b. False

9. It is easier to prevent pressure ulcers than it is to heal them.

    a. True   b. False

10. Immobile residents should be repositioned at least every two hours.

    a. True   b. False

BED MAKING AND COMFORT MEASURES

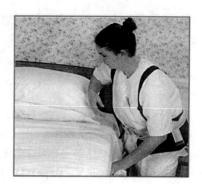

 Watch step-by-step demonstrations of the procedures discussed in this chapter in the Medcom videotape "Techniques in Bedmaking" (CNA212).

In this chapter... you will learn about:

▶ How to make an unoccupied bed.

▶ How to make an occupied bed.

▶ How to give a back rub.

▶ How to provide perineal care.

DEFINITIONS

Immobile:	Unable to move.
Miter:	A triangular fold at the foot or head of a bedsheet that produces a flat square corner.
Perineal Area:	In a female, the area between the vagina and anus. In a male, the area between the scrotum and anus.

The time and effort the nursing assistant spends making the residents comfortable will be rewarded by having healthier, happier residents. Making a bed properly is important to the comfort and well-being of the resident. Remember that the resident may be spending much or all of the day in the bed. Wrinkles in the sheets are very uncomfortable and can cause pressure sores and impaired circulation.

The proper technique for making an unoccupied bed is as follows:

1. Remove the soiled linens and place them in a dirty linen container.

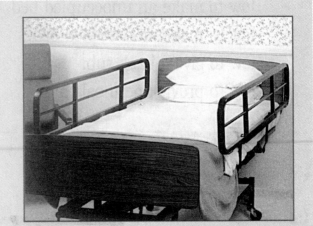

2. Wash your hands.

3. Obtain the clean linens.

4. Adjust the bed to a comfortable working height to protect your back and then unfold a bottom sheet lengthwise on the bed.

5. Starting at the foot of the bed, open the sheet. Make sure the sheet hangs evenly on each side of the bed. The hem at the foot of the bed should be even with the end of the mattress.

6. Raise the mattress and tuck in the sheet at the head.

7. Miter the corner. Pick up the edge of the sheet to make a triangle.

8. Lay the triangle on top of the bed and tuck the hanging portion under the mattress.

9. Holding the fold at the edge of the mattress, miter the corner by bringing the triangle down and tucking it under the mattress.

10. Tuck the hanging portion of the sheet all the way to the foot of the bed.

11. Place the draw sheet across the bottom sheet and tuck it under the mattress.

12. Lay the top sheet lengthwise on the bed. Leave enough sheet at the head of the bed to fold over the top of the bedspread later. Spread the sheet so it hangs evenly on each side of the bed.

13. Lay the bedspread and/or blanket over the top sheet. Open it so that it hangs evenly on each side of the bed.

14. Fold the hem of the top sheet over the top covers.

15. Tuck the top covers together at the foot of the bed and miter the corners but don't tuck them under the mattress.

16. Move to the other side of the bed.

17. Make a triangle tuck in the bottom sheet at the head. Then miter the corners of the sheet.

18. Tuck in the hanging portion of the bottom sheet and the drawsheet.

19. Miter the top covers at the foot of the bed.

20. Form a toe pleat at the foot of the bed. Grasp both sides of the top covers at the mitered corners and gently pull enough of the covers toward the foot to make a three- or four-inch fold at the foot of the bed. This is to prevent pressure on the resident's toes.

21. Hold the pillowcase at the center of the end seam and turn the case back over your hand.

22. Grasp the end of the pillow right through the pillowcase.

23. Bring the pillowcase down over the pillow and fit the corners of the pillow into the seamless corners of the pillowcase.

24. Fold the extra material from the side seam under the pillow.

25. Place the pillow on the bed with the open end away from the door. Place the call signal in position and return the bed to its lowest position.

26. When finished, wash your hands.

MAKING AN OCCUPIED BED

Some residents must remain in bed. It will then be necessary for you to change the linen with the resident in the bed. It is important to keep the resident comfortable and safe while this is done.

Following is the proper procedure for making an occupied bed:

1. Assemble the clean linens on a bedside chair.

2. Explain to the resident what you are going to do and wash your hands.

3. Provide privacy for the resident.

4. Raise the bed to a comfortable working height and bring the backrest and knee rest to a flat position.

5. Loosen the bed covers all around the bed, but leave the top covers over the resident for warmth and privacy. Raise the side rail for protection of the resident before going to the opposite side.

6. Turn the resident on his or her side. Make sure the pillow supports the resident's head.

7. Roll the used draw sheet and the full width of the bottom sheet against the resident's back and legs and tuck it there.

8. Unfold the fresh bottom sheet with its lengthwise center fold along the center of the bed. The bottom hem should be even with the mattress.

9. Place the draw sheet over the bottom sheet and tuck it against the resident's back.

10. Tuck the bottom sheet at the head of the mattress; miter the top corner, and then drop the side and tuck in the bottom sheet and the draw sheet all along the side of the bed.

11. Raise the side rail where you have been working and go around to the other side of the bed.

12. Lower the side rail and roll the resident onto the fresh linens.

13. Remove the soiled bottom sheet and soiled draw sheet, maintaining the resident's privacy, and put them into the soiled linen hamper.

14. Pull the clean bottom sheet and draw sheet toward you. Tighten the sheets, making them as wrinkle-free as possible.

15. Use a mitered corner at the top as you did on the other side. Then tuck in the bottom sheet and the draw sheet all along the side.

16. Roll the resident onto his or her back. Spread a clean top sheet over the resident and remove the blanket or bedspread.

17. Ask the resident to hold onto the fresh top sheet, if possible, and then pull the soiled top sheet out from under it.

18. Then place the blanket or bedspread over the resident; tuck in the top covers, mitering the corners at the foot of the bed.

19. Make a toe pleat (See Step 20 for Making an Unoccupied Bed).

20. Change pillowcase (See Steps 21-25 for Making an Unoccupied Bed).

21. Make sure the side rails are up before moving away from the resident.

22. Lower the bed and raise the head of the bed. Place the call signal within reach and make sure the resident is comfortable.

23. When finished, wash your hands.

BACK RUB

A back rub can be very beneficial to a resident. It helps the resident relax, releases the tension in the back and neck muscles, and increases circulation. If the resident is bedridden, these benefits are even more important.

A back rub is usually given right after the resident's bath; however, a back rub in the evening can help a resident relax and fall asleep. Sometimes the doctor will order back rubs when you are changing the position of *immobile* residents to increase circulation and comfort.

When giving a back rub, use the following procedures:

1. Assemble the necessary equipment: lotion, a basin of warm water (105 degrees F.), a towel

2. Explain to the resident what you are going to do and wash your hands.

3. Provide privacy for the resident.

4. Place the bottle of lotion in a pan of warm water.

5. Position the resident so that his or her back is toward you, or the resident is lying face down.

6. Place the towel lengthwise on the bed next to the resident's back.

7. Pour a small amount of lotion into the palm of your hand. Rub your hands together to warm the hands and lotion.

Chapter 38: Bed Making and Comfort Measures

8. Apply the lotion with long, firm strokes upward from the buttocks to the back of the neck and shoulders.

9. Use firm pressure as you stroke upward and gentle pressure as you stroke downward. Use a circular motion over the bony areas. As you go through the process, your hands should never leave the back as this can create a shock to the resident. It should be one continuous, flowing motion.

10. Continue for three minutes.

11. Pat the resident's back with the towel.

12. Assist the resident with dressing and position the resident comfortably.

13. When finished, wash your hands.

PERINEAL CARE

Cleansing the *perineal area* between showers or baths helps prevent irritation, infection, and skin breakdown as well as keeping the resident comfortable. Perineal care is especially important for residents who are *incontinent*. Urine and feces will cause skin breakdown. Bacteria in feces can cause urinary tract infections. The procedure for giving perineal care is as follows:

1. Assemble the necessary equipment: disposable bed protector, bedpan, basin, peri-wash solution if this is used by your facility, soap, two washcloths and towels.

2. Explain to the resident what you are going to do and wash your hands.

3. Provide privacy for the resident.

4. Offer the resident a bedpan or urinal.

5. Place the disposable bed protector under the resident's buttocks.

6. Assist the resident onto the bedpan.

7. Before continuing, put on protective gloves.

8. Position the resident's legs apart. Spray the peri-wash solution over the resident's perineal area.

9. Use a wet washcloth to clean the area. Rinse the washcloth and wipe the solution from the perineal area. Observe the resident's skin for any rashes or sores.

    •   For the female resident, spread the labia and be sure to wash from front to back.

    •   For uncircumcised males, retract the foreskin and wash the head of the penis thoroughly.

    •   If the resident is soiled with urine or feces, use soap and water before using peri-wash solution.

10. Dry the area with a soft towel.

11. Remove the bedpan and disposable bed protector.

12. Discard the bed protector and gloves according to the policies of your facility.

13. Empty, rinse and clean the equipment used. Deposit soiled linen in a soiled linen container.

14. When finished, wash your hands.

Your efforts in keeping your residents comfortable with neatly made beds, back rubs, and perineal care will be greatly appreciated.

*Circle the correct answer. There is only **one** correct answer.*

1. **Why aren't wrinkles acceptable in bedding?**

   a. They can cause pressure sores and they make the resident uncomfortable.

   b. They are unsightly

   c. They have to be ironed out.

   d. None of the above applies.

2. **How can the nursing assistant prevent pressure on the resident's toes from the bed covers?**

   a. Miter the corners.

   b. Tuck the bottom sheet under the mattress.

   c. Form a toe pleat across the foot of the bed.

   d. Use a draw sheet.

3. **The proper step to begin making an unoccupied bed is:**

   a. Obtain clean linen.

   b. Remove soiled linen.

   c. Wash your hands.

4. **When making an occupied bed, always put the side rail up on the side opposite you.**

   a. True   b. False

5. **The pillow should be removed from under the resident's head when making an occupied bed.**

   a. True   b. False

6. **A back rub may be ordered when changing the position of immobilized residents to increase circulation and comfort.**

    (a.) True   b. False

7. **One advantage of a back rub is**

    a. It increases circulation.

    b. It prevents infectious disease.

    c. It covers sores.

    d. None of the above.

8. **When giving the resident a back rub, in what order should the procedure be done?**

    a. Apply lotion, wash your hands, pat resident's back with towel.

    b. Pat resident's back with towel, wash your hands, apply lotion.

    c. Wash your hands, apply lotion, pat resident's back with towel.

    d. Pat resident's back with towel, apply lotion, wash hands.

9. **Cleansing the perineal area between showers or baths.**

    a. Is not a good idea.

    b. Helps prevent irritation and infection.

    c. Should not be done with immobile residents.

    d. Should not be done by the nursing assistants.

10. **Perineal care is especially important for incontinent residents.**

    a. True   b. False

Chapter 39

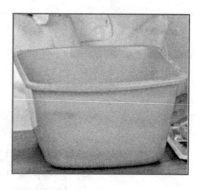

BATHING THE RESIDENT

 Watch step-by-step demonstrations of the procedures discussed in this chapter in the Medcom videotape "Techniques in Bathing" (CNA211).

In this chapter... you will learn about:

▶ How to assist a resident take a tub or shower bath.

▶ How to bathe residents who are confined to bed.

DEFINITIONS

Axilla:	Armpit.
Skin Integrity:	Good skin condition.
Umbilicus:	Navel.

The nursing assistant is responsible for bathing the residents or assisting them to bathe. Personal hygiene is necessary to stay clean and comfortable and for many people it is necessary to preserve a sense of dignity. The frequency of bathing varies widely from culture to culture and individual to individual. As a person ages, his or her skin often becomes thinner and dryer and the need for bathing may change. The charge nurse in consultation with the physician will decide how often to bathe each resident.

There are many health reasons why bathing is important:

> It restores cleanliness by removing dirt and body odors.

> It removes bacteria and germs from the skin.

> It cools and refreshes the skin.

> It promotes good *skin integrity*.

> It stimulates circulation.

> It provides movement and exercise.

> It provides the nursing assistant an opportunity to check the resident's body for changes, abnormalities, and skin integrity.

> It feels good and helps the resident relax.

Some areas of the body require frequent cleaning. These include the hands, face, underarms, perineal area, and any area where the body folds and creases. These areas should be washed, rinsed, and dried often.

SAFETY IN BATHING

The resident's safety while bathing is an important concern. Since older people are more sensitive to heat and cold, the water temperature must be carefully checked and monitored. Usually, the most comfortable temperature for bathing is between 105 and 110 degrees F. checked with a thermometer. However, you should not rely upon the thermometer alone. You should always personally test the water temperature using the inside of the wrist. After you test and judge the water temperature safe, ask the resident to test it for comfort.

Since slipping and falling are particular risks for the older resident, all showers and tubs should be equipped with grab bars, non-skid surfaces, and emergency call buttons. The resident must be instructed in how to use the grab bars and the emergency call button to summon help.

Unless a resident has demonstrated that he or she is totally independent in bathing, the resident should never be left unattended while bathing.

To protect the resident's skin from irritation, all soap should be rinsed off completely and the skin dried thoroughly. Lotion may be used on rough areas that have been cleansed and dried. toes and finger

PRIVACY

Bathing is a very personal activity which most people do in private. It is important to remember this when assisting with bathing. Calmly explain what you are going to do. Close the door or pull the curtains around the area to provide privacy. In a bed bath, uncover only the area being washed. As you move to another area, cover the area you have already washed.

There are four different ways for a resident to bathe:

- ▶ Shower.

- ▶ Tub.

- ▶ Complete bed bath.

- ▶ Partial bed bath.

Shower

If the resident is able to transfer and sit on a chair, the shower is the preferred method of bathing. A shower chair should be used for the resident to sit on. This eliminates the need for prolonged standing and reduces the risk of falls. Following is the procedure for assisting a resident to shower:

1. Assemble the bathing equipment on a shelf or regular chair near the shower: towel, soap, wash cloth, shower cap, and clean clothing.

2. Take the shower chair and a large sheet to the resident's bedside.

3. Explain to the resident what you will be doing, wash your hands and provide privacy.

4. Remove the resident's clothes and transfer the resident to the shower chair, making sure the wheels are locked.

5. Cover the resident, making sure that the entire body including the buttock area and limbs are covered.

6. Unlock the wheels and quickly transport the resident to the shower area.

7. Turn on and adjust the temperature of the water.

8. Give the resident soap and a wash cloth and encourage the resident to wash and rinse as much as possible. Assist when necessary. If you wash the perineal area or face, put on gloves first.

9. Turn off the water.

10. Assist the resident in drying thoroughly.

11. Assist the resident with dressing.

12. Return to the shower, clean it and remove any soiled linen.

13. Dispose of gloves, if you are wearing them, and wash your hands.

Tub Bath

Following is the procedure for assisting in a tub bath:

1. Assemble the bathing equipment on chair near the tub: towel, soap, wash cloth, and clean clothing.

2. Explain to the resident what you will be doing, wash your hands and provide privacy.

3. Fill the tub half full with water at 105 degrees F. Test the water with a thermometer and the inside of your wrist. Have the resident test it for comfort.

4. Place a towel or bath mat on the floor beside the tub to prevent slipping when getting out.

5. Assist the resident in removing clothing and jewelry.

6. Assist the resident into the tub.

7. Give the resident soap and a wash cloth and encourage him or her to wash and rinse as much as possible. Assist when necessary. Never leave the resident alone in the tub. If you wash the perineal area or face, put on gloves first.

8. Assist the resident out of the tub, encouraging the use of grab bars.

9. Assist the resident in drying thoroughly.

10. Assist the resident with dressing.

11. Wash the tub with disinfectant.

12. Place soiled linen in a covered dirty linen container.

13. Dispose of gloves, if you are wearing them, and wash your hands.

Complete Bed Bath

The resident who is unable to transfer to a shower or tub and unable to wash himself or herself must be bathed in bed. Only one part of the body is washed, rinsed, and dried at a time. That area is then covered before moving to the next part. The water in the basin should be changed as it becomes soapy, dirty, or cold. When not using the soap, place it in the soap container rather than leaving it in the water. The procedure for giving a complete bed bath is as follows:

1. Assemble the necessary equipment on the bedside table: soap in container, wash cloth, wash basin, and bath blanket (if available).

2. Explain to the resident what you are going to do and provide privacy.

3. Wash your hands and put on gloves.

4. Offer the resident a bedpan or urinal.

5. Remove and fold the bedspread and blankets.

6. Cover the resident with a bath blanket or top sheet.

7. Lower the head and foot of the bed to a flat position and raise the entire bed to a comfortable working height. Be sure the side rail on the opposite side is up. Position the resident comfortably for a bath.

8. Assist the resident in moving closer to you.

9. Remove the resident's clothing and jewelry. Keep the resident covered to prevent chilling.

10. Fill the wash basin two-thirds full with water at 105 degrees F. Test it with a thermometer and the inside of wrist. Then have the resident test it for comfort.

11. Lay a towel across the resident's chest and make a mitt with the wash cloth.

12. Begin by washing the eyes from the nose to the outside of face, using only water unless otherwise requested. Rinse and dry the face by patting gently with a towel.

13. Place a towel lengthwise under the arm farthest from you. Support the arm with your hand under the resident's elbow. Wash the shoulder, **axilla**, and arm with mild soap or special bathing preparation. Rinse and dry well.

14. Place a basin of water on the towel and place the resident's hand into the water. Wash, rinse, and dry the hand.

15. Repeat steps 12 and 13 with the arm nearest to you.

16. Fold the sheet down to the resident's abdomen. Wash, rinse, and dry the resident's ears, neck, and chest. For female residents, lift the breasts to wash, rinse, and dry thoroughly.

17. Cover the chest with a towel and fold the sheet down to the pubic area.

18. Wash, rinse, and dry the resident's abdomen being careful to include the **umbilicus** and skin creases.

19. Pull the sheet up over the abdomen and chest and remove the towel.

20. Empty the wash basin, rinse and refill it with clean water if it becomes soapy or cool. Be sure to raise the side rail if you leave the bedside. Test the water for proper temperature.

21. Fold the sheet back from the resident's leg farthest from you and place a towel lengthwise under the leg.

22. Bend the knee and wash, rinse, and dry the leg and foot. If the resident can bend the knee easily, place the basin on a towel and place the resident's foot in the water and wash it.

23. Cover the resident's leg and foot with a sheet and remove the towel.

24. Repeat steps 21 and 22 with the leg nearest you.

25. Empty the basin, rinse and refill it with clean water and test for proper temperature.

26. Assist the resident to turn on his or her side so the back is toward you.

27. Place the towel lengthwise on the bed near the resident's back. Wash, rinse, and dry the resident's back of neck, behind the ears, back, and buttocks.

28. Remove the towel and assist the resident in turning onto his or her back.

29. Empty the basin, rinse and refill it with clear water and test it for proper temperature. If the resident is able to wash his or her own perineal area, provide a soapy washcloth, then a clean, wet cloth for the rinse, and a towel to dry. If the resident is unable to do this, assist by washing the perineal area front to back to avoid infection. For female residents, spread labia and wash front to back. For uncircumcised males, retract the foreskin and wash the tip of the penis.

30. Assist the resident into clean clothing.

31. Remove the sheets and remake the bed with clean linen.

32. Dispose of your gloves and wash your hands.

The resident who is confined to bed but able to wash himself or herself must be partially assisted to bathe while in bed. The resident should be encouraged and allowed to do as much as possible for himself or herself. The following procedure is to be followed:

1.   Assemble the necessary equipment on the bedside table: soap in container, wash cloth, wash basin, towel, and bath blanket (if available).

2.   Explain to the resident what you are going to do and provide privacy.

3.   Wash your hands and put on gloves.

4.   Offer a bedpan or urinal.

5.   Remove and fold the bedspread and blankets. Cover the resident with a top sheet or bath blanket if available.

6.   Assist the resident in removing clothing and jewelry.

7.   Fill the basin two-thirds full with water at 105 degrees F. Test the water with a thermometer and the inside of your own wrist. Ask the resident to test the temperature for comfort.

8.   Ask the resident to wash areas of the body which he or she can easily reach.

9.   Ask the resident to signal with the call light when finished. Dispose of your gloves and wash your hands. Leave the resident to continue bathing.

10. When the resident signals, return to the room and wash your hands and put on gloves. Empty the basin, rinse, and refill it with clean water. Test it for proper temperature.

11. Wash, rinse, and dry the areas of the body the resident was unable to reach, following procedures outlined in Complete Bed Bath above.

12. Assist the resident in putting on clean clothing.

13. Remove the sheets and remake the bed with clean linen.

14. Dispose of your gloves and wash your hands.

OBSERVATION

Bathing or assisting in bathing provides an opportunity for the nursing assistant to check the resident's body for changes or problems. Observe for swelling, broken skin, redness, rashes, bruises, bleeding, or unusual odors. The nursing assistant should also check the resident's fingernails, toenails, and hair during bathing. Any changes or observations are to be entered on the resident's chart and brought to the attention of the charge nurse.

Bathing the resident is an important responsibility of the nursing assistant. Cleanliness is important for the resident's health, comfort, and sense of well being.

*Circle the correct answer. There is only **one** correct answer.*

1. **Bathing is important because it restores cleanliness, stimulates circulation, and provides movement and exercise.**

   (a.) True   b. False

2. **The nursing assistant is responsible for bathing the resident who is confined to bed.**

   (a.) True   b. False

3. **Older residents are usually given a complete bath no more than once a week.**

   a. True   (b.) False

4. **The temperature of the bath water should be about:**

   a. 98.6 degrees F.

   b. 100 degrees F.

   (c.) 105 degrees F.

   d. 110 degrees F.

5. **A resident should never be asked to check the temperature of the bath water.**

   (a.) True   b. False

6. **It is important to protect the resident's privacy when bathing by pulling the curtains or closing the door.**

   (a.) True   b. False

7. **Mrs. Olsen needs a bath but cannot leave the bed. The nursing assistant should**

   a. Take her to the tub anyway.

   b. Provide a full bed bath.

   c. Provide a shower.

   d. Not give Mrs. Olsen a bath.

8. **Genital areas should be washed from side to side to avoid infection.**

   a. True   b. False

9. **The different ways to bathe a resident are the complete bed bath, partial bed bath, tub, and shower.**

   a. True   b. False

10. **When bathing a resident, the nursing assistant should**

    a. Look for rashes, bruises, and broken skin.

    b. Never put fresh water in the basin.

    c. Not be concerned with the resident's body.

    d. Make sure to wash the face with soap.

Chapter 40

PERSONAL HYGIENE

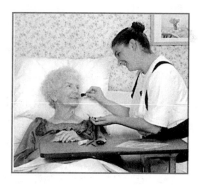

Watch step-by-step demonstrations of the procedures discussed in this chapter in the Medcom videotapes "The New Nursing Assistant 2000: Personal Care" (CNA505), and "The New Nursing Assistant 2000: Oral Care" (CNA506).

In this chapter... you will learn about:

▶ How to assist residents with dental, hair and nail care.

▶ How to assist residents with dressing and undressing.

DEFINITIONS

Emesis Basin:	Small, curved basin placed under resident's chin and used for resident to expectorate into.
Expectorate:	To spit.
Nasogastric Tube:	Tube inserted through the nose and into the stomach.
Oral Hygiene:	Care of mouth, teeth, gums, and tongue.
Personal Hygiene:	Grooming which includes oral hygiene, nail care, care of the hair, shaving, make-up, and dressing.
Plaque:	A film made up of saliva and microorganisms that sticks to the teeth.
Taut:	Tight.

Personal hygiene refers to keeping the residents' bodies clean and sanitary with regular care and cleansing. It includes the following areas:

- ▶ Oral and dental hygiene.

- ▶ Hair care.

- ▶ Shaving.

- ▶ Nail care.

- ▶ Dressing and undressing.

ORAL HYGIENE

It is important for residents to take good care of their teeth and gums. If teeth and gums are neglected, the results can include:

- ▶ Bad breath.

- ▶ Cavities.

- ▶ Gum disease.

- ▶ Lost teeth.

- ▶ Build-up of *plaque*, which can lead to gum disease and cavities.

It is equally important for residents with dentures to take good care of their mouth and gums as well as their dentures.

The purpose of *oral hygiene* is to keep the mouth, teeth, gums and tongue healthy. All residents should receive oral hygiene twice a day, in the morning and in the evening. In order to maintain moisture in the mouth, the following residents should receive oral hygiene every two hours:

- ▶ Those who are unconscious.

- ▶ Those unable to take fluids by mouth.

- ▶ Those who breath through the mouth.

- ▶ Those who receive oxygen.

- ▶ Those who are feverish.

- ▶ Those who are vomiting.

- ▶ Those who have a **nasogastric** or gastrostomy tube.

The nursing assistant is responsible for the oral hygiene of the residents. Residents who are able should be encouraged to brush their own teeth. Those who are unable to do this for themselves must be assisted by the nursing assistant using the following procedure:

Residents Who Still Have Their Teeth

1. Explain to the resident what you are going to do.

2. Wash your hands and put on gloves.

3. If the resident is in bed, place a towel on the resident's chest and an **emesis basin** under the resident's chin. Assist the resident in using the bathroom sink if possible.

4. Use a dry, soft bristle, junior size toothbrush held at a 45 degree angle to the teeth. Stimulate the gums by brushing in a circular motion where the teeth and gums meet.

5. Begin with the upper teeth and gums and then do the lower.

6. Place toothpaste on the toothbrush and repeat steps four and five, brushing first the outer surfaces, then the inner and chewing surfaces.

7. Have the resident rinse his or her mouth with warm water, and then **expectorate**, or spit the water out into the emesis basin if in bed.

8. If mouthwash is used, dilute with four parts of water to one part mouthwash.

9. Put all personal items away in the resident's drawer.

10. Dispose of the gloves and wash your hands.

Residents With Dentures

For residents with dentures, use the following procedures:

1. Explain to the resident what you are going to do.

2. Wash your hands and put on gloves.

3. If the resident is in bed, place a towel on the resident's chest and an emesis basin under the chin.

4. Place paper towels in the bottom of the sink to protect dentures from accidental breakage if dropped.

5. If the resident is able, ask him or her to remove the dentures. If the resident requires assistance, remove the dentures gently. To remove the upper plate, push down gently to break the suction.

6. Put the dentures in the basin and take it to the sink.

7. Brush the dentures with toothpaste and rinse them under running water.

8. Place the dentures in a clean, rinsed denture cup.

9. Encourage the resident to rinse his or her mouth with diluted mouthwash (one part mouthwash to four parts water).

10. Replace the dentures in the resident's mouth or store them in cold water in a denture cup.

11. Dispose of the gloves, and wash your hands.

Observation

While providing oral care, the nursing assistant should inspect the resident's mouth, teeth, gums, and tongue for any changes or signs of injury, such as:

▶ Bleeding.

▶ Sores.

▶ Loose or broken teeth.

▶ Dry, coated tongue.

▶ Mouth odor.

All changes or signs of injury must be reported to the charge nurse and noted in the resident's chart.

HAIR CARE

All of us like to look our best. Residents in long-term care are no exception; however, they often feel there is no point in making the effort or they may be unable to take care of their own personal grooming.

Residents who are physically able to do their own grooming should be encouraged to do so and then complimented on their appearance. For residents who are unable to care for themselves, the nursing assistant is responsible for providing their care.

Shampooing

Hair must be clean to be healthy and look its best. Residents should have their hair shampooed once or twice a week depending on the facility's policy. This is usually done while showering the resident. Some residents may have their hair shampooed weekly by a beautician or barber.

Following is the procedure for shampooing a resident's hair:

1. Assemble the necessary equipment: brush, comb, shampoo, creme rinse, and a towel.

2. Explain what you are going to do, and wash your hands.

3. Gently brush the hair to loosen dirt and tangles. Ask the resident to do this if he or she is able.

4. Wet the hair, apply shampoo, and wash thoroughly, being careful to keep shampoo out of the resident's eyes.

5. Rinse thoroughly, while protecting the resident's eyes.

6. Apply creme rinse to prevent tangles, then rinse thoroughly.

7. Dry the hair with a towel. Have the resident assist if possible.

8. Wash the resident's comb and brush and store them appropriately.

9. When finished, wash your hands.

Daily hair care is needed to keep a neat appearance. It is the responsibility of the nursing assistant to see that the residents' hair is brushed and combed daily. Residents who are able should be encouraged to do this for themselves and complimented on their appearance. The nursing assistant must do this daily hair care for those residents who are unable to do it for themselves. A simple, attractive hair style should be encouraged so that more residents will be able to care for their own hair.

While shampooing and performing daily hair care for residents, the nursing assistant should be alert to any changes in the scalp and hair or any signs of injury, such as:

- ▶ Sores.

- ▶ Crust.

- ▶ Dandruff.

- ▶ Excessive hair loss.

These changes should be reported to the charge nurse and entered in the resident's chart.

Shaving

Shaving must be done according to your facility's policy. Some facilities do not allow the use of safety razors.

For male residents, daily shaving is a part of their personal hygiene. Residents who are able to shave themselves should be encouraged to do so. If the resident cannot shave himself, the nursing assistant must provide assistance.

If the resident has his own electric razor, it may be used. However, an electric razor must never be used if the resident or a roommate is using oxygen, as this would present a fire hazard.

The procedure for shaving a resident with a safety razor is as follows:

1. Assemble the necessary equipment: a basin of warm water (105 degrees F.), shaving cream, the safety razor, a towel, washcloth, and aftershave.

2. Wash your hands and put on gloves.

3. Explain what you are going to do.

4. Place a towel under the resident's chin.

5. If the resident wears dentures, be sure they are in his mouth.

6. Put the washcloth in warm water, wring it out, and place it on the face to soften the beard.

7. Apply shaving cream to the face.

8. With the fingers of one hand, hold his skin **taut.** With the other hand shave in the direction the hair grows. Using short, firm strokes, shave under the sideburns, downward over the cheeks, over the chin, and upward on the neck.

9. Rinse the razor often.

10. Wash the remaining shaving cream off his face.

11. Apply aftershave, if the resident desires it.

12. Store all articles in the appropriate place.

13. When finished, dispose of the gloves and wash your hands.

If you nick the resident accidentally while shaving him, report it to the charge nurse immediately. If you contacted the resident's blood, follow your facility's procedure for exposure to blood.

Care and inspection of the resident's fingernails and toenails is also the responsibility of the nursing assistant. Residents who are able to take care of their own nails should be encouraged to do so. Many residents, however, are not able to do this, and their nail care will be provided by the nursing assistant.

Nails should be kept short, smooth, and clean. Daily nail care consists of keeping the nails clean and checking for torn nails, rough edges, and hang nails. Torn and rough nails should be trimmed and smoothed with an emery board. Hangnails should be carefully clipped to prevent further tearing.

Fingernails should be manicured regularly. You will not trim the resident's toenails. Small nicks or cuts around the toenails could be very dangerous to many older residents, and nail care will probably be done during regular visits by a podiatrist.

Older people often have thickened nails which are easier to cut after soaking in warm water. For this reason, nails are the easiest to trim immediately following a shower or bath.

Following is the procedure for cleaning and trimming nails:

1. Assemble the necessary equipment: nail clippers, an emery board, an orange stick, lotion, a basin of warm water, and a towel.

2. Wash your hands.

3. Explain what you are going to do.

4. Place the hands in a basin of warm water. If the resident has just had a shower or bath, this step may be omitted.

5. Clean the nails with an orange stick.

6. Push the cuticles gently back with the orange stick.

7. Dry the hands.

8. Trim the nails straight across with clippers. Scissors are NEVER used. Be very careful not to cause damage to surrounding tissue.

9. Smooth any rough or sharp edges with an emery board.

10. Apply lotion and massage the hands.

11. When finished, wash your hands.

While providing nail care, or when bathing, the nursing assistant should check the resident's hands and feet for any changes or signs of injury. Any changes or injuries should be reported to the charge nurse and noted in the resident's chart.

DRESSING AND UNDRESSING

Being appropriately and neatly dressed helps residents feel good about themselves. Some residents can dress and undress themselves, some need minimum assistance, while others are totally dependent. Residents who can partially or completely dress themselves should be encouraged to do so and be complimented on their appearance.

The nursing assistant is responsible for dressing the totally dependent resident. This is easier to do if the resident is lying on the bed. When dressing a resident who is paralyzed, injured, or wearing a cast, always dress the affected side first and undress it last.

Following is the procedure to follow to dress a resident who is lying on the bed:

1. Explain to the resident what you are going to do and wash your hands.

2. Provide privacy for the resident.

3. Help the resident select clothes for the day.

4. Be sure all buttons and hooks are undone and zippers are unzipped.

5. Remove the nightclothes and provide further privacy for the resident with a sheet, bath blanket, or spread.

6. Put on the underclothing.

7. To put on slacks or trousers, gather up the pant leg for the leg farthest from you.

8. Put your hand up through this pant leg and grasp the resident's ankle. Then pull the pant leg over your hand and the resident's leg. Repeat with the other leg.

9. Pull the pants up as far as possible. Have the resident raise his or her hips, if possible, so that you can pull the pants up and fasten them. If the resident is unable to do this, roll the resident to the side away from you, pull up the pants, and fasten them.

10. You can put on a shirt or dress in a similar way. Open the shirt or dress, put your hand backwards through the sleeve farthest from you and hold the resident's wrist. The pull the sleeve over your hand and the resident's arm.

11. Roll the resident toward you, smooth the garment across the resident's back, and then roll the resident back. Repeat step nine with the other sleeve and fasten it.

12. To put on a pullover garment, place both of the resident's arms in the sleeves. Pull the garment up on his or her arms, grasp the garment neck and slide it over the resident's head.

13. Have the resident sit up, if possible, and pull the garment down. If the resident is unable to do this, roll him or her from side to side while pulling the garment down.

14. Position the resident comfortably.

15. When finished, wash your hands.

Looking good helps a resident feel good. Careful attention and appropriate help can raise a resident's self-esteem. Since a nursing assistant is responsible for many tasks in the daily care of the residents, it is important to develop an individual routine to ensure that these important services are provided for all residents daily.

Circle the correct answer. There is only **one** *correct answer.*

1. **Mrs. Smith has a nasogastric tube. What is most important to remember in assisting her with oral hygiene?**

    a. It should be done twice daily.

    b. She should do it herself.

    c. It should be done only at night.

    (d.) It should be done every two hours.

2. **Residents who wear dentures should take good care of their mouth and gums as well as their dentures.**

    (a.) True   b. False

3. **What kind of toothbrush is recommended for residents?**

    a. A large, hard-bristled brush.

    (b.) A junior-size, soft-bristled brush.

    c. A junior size, hard-bristled brush.

    d. A large, soft-bristled brush.

4. **You should trim the toenails of residents regularly.**

    a. True   (b.) False

5. **Mr. Leslie has a cast on his left arm and is unable to dress or undress himself. In helping Mr. Leslie dress, what procedure should the nursing assistant follow?**

    a. Dress Mr. Leslie's left side last.

    b. Make him get out of bed before dressing him.

    (c.) Dress Mr. Leslie's left side first.

    d. Have him dress himself from the waist up.

6. **It is recommended that mouthwash be used full strength.**

   a. True   (b.) False

7. **The nursing assistant should inspect the resident's mouth, teeth, gums, and tongue for changes or signs of injury.**

   (a.) True   b. False

8. **Mr. Stanley owns an electric razor. Are there any restrictions regarding shaving with his electric razor?**

   a. No.   He can use it whenever he likes.

   b. Yes.   Only safety razors may be used.

   c. Yes.   It can only be used by the nursing assistant.

   (d.) Yes.   It may never be used if he or his roommate is using oxygen.

9. **For older residents hair care becomes unimportant and you can ignore it.**

   a. True   (b.) False

10. **If the nursing assistant nicks the resident while shaving, it should be reported.**

   (a.) True   b. False

Chapter 41

Dressings and Bandages

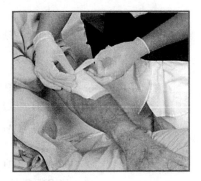

In this chapter... you will learn about:

▶ How to apply a clean, dry dressing.

▶ How to apply an elastic bandage.

▶ How to apply an elastic stocking.

DEFINITIONS

Dressing: Clean, cloth covering for a wound or sore.

Gauze: Thin, mesh-like cloth.

Applying both sterile and clean and dry **dressings** to open or closed wounds is the responsibility of the licensed nurse. However, nursing assistants may be allowed to place adhesive bandages over small closed wounds. The nursing assistant may be asked to apply an elastic bandage to a resident's limb or elastic stockings to a resident's legs.

Dressings are used to:

➤ Protect the wound area from germs and dirt.

➤ Protect the skin from pressure and rubbing.

Elastic bandages are used to:

➤ Support the muscle and tissue of the limb.

➤ Prevent swelling.

➤ Relieve pain.

➤ Hold a dressing in place.

Elastic stockings are used to:

➤ Support the veins of the leg.

➤ Reduce inflammation of the veins in the legs.

➤ Reduce the development of blood clots.

➤ Be sure you know and follow your facility's policies regarding the application of dressings and elastic bandages.

Applying a Dressing

Dressings come in several different sizes. The size used depends on the size of the area to be covered. **Gauze** is the most common type of dressing material. Rayon strips, absorbent cotton pads, and Telfa pads are also used.

Different types of tape are available to hold the dressing on the resident's skin. When applying a dressing to an older resident, choose the type of tape which is most easily removed to prevent damaging the fragile skin.

When applying a clean, dry dressing, the following procedure should be used:

1. Assemble the necessary equipment: a clean dressing, tape, scissors, and an infectious waste plastic bag.

2. Explain to the resident what you are going to do and provide privacy.

3. Wash your hands and put on disposable gloves.

4. Open the dressing package, being careful not to touch the dressing.

5. Cut strips of tape.

6. Remove the old dressing and dispose of it. NOTE: If it shows any signs of body fluids, place in an infectious waste bag for disposal.

7. Remove your gloves and dispose of them. Put on new gloves.

8. Thoroughly cleanse and dry the affected area.

9. Apply the new dressing, being careful not to touch the portion which will be in contact with the resident's sore skin.

10. Apply tape, covering the ends of the dressing. If the tape is applied over a joint, place it across the joint, not parallel to it.

11. Ask the nurse to dispose of the bag in the infectious waste container. Replace the equipment.

12. Remove and dispose of the gloves. Wash your hands.

13. Write on the chart that you changed the dressing. Also chart any skin abnormalities observed such as broken skin, redness, bruises, or sores.

14. Notify the charge nurse that you completed the procedure, and explain any abnormalities you observed.

Elastic bandages are applied only when ordered by the resident's doctor. These bandages come in different widths. The size chosen depends on the area to be bandaged.

Elastic bandages are to be applied according to the following procedure:

1. Select an appropriate size bandage.

2. Explain to the resident what you are going to do and wash your hands.

3. Provide privacy.

4. Elevate the limb to be wrapped.

5. Begin at the part of the limb which is farthest from the heart.

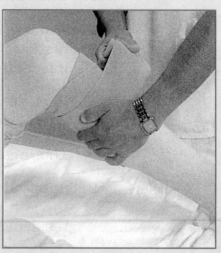

An elastic bandage.

6. Wrap the elastic bandage around the limb with firm, consistent pressure. Wrap from the area farthest from the heart and proceed toward the heart; for example, from the wrist toward the elbow.

7. Check with the resident to see if the bandage is comfortable. If the bandage is too tight, remove it and begin again.

8. When finished, wash your hands.

9. Chart the application of the bandage.

The wrapped limb must be observed frequently for signs of impaired circulation or swelling. If you observe signs of swelling, pain, or change in skin color or temperature, remove the bandage immediately and notify the charge nurse.

Elastic bandages must be removed at least every eight hours. When the bandage is removed, the affected area must be thoroughly cleansed and dried.

Elastic stockings are applied when ordered by the resident's doctor, often just before or just after an operation.

Apply elastic stockings according to the following procedure:

1. Select elastic stockings of the proper length and size.

2. Explain to the resident what you are about to do, and wash your hands.

3. Provide privacy.

4. The patient should be lying down. Expose one leg at a time.

5. Hold a stocking at the top with both hands and roll it down to the toe. Note that any raised seams should be on the outside.

6. Gently place the rolled stocking over the toes and begin to unroll. Position the toe opening at the base of the toes on top of the foot unless the toes are to remain covered.

7. Gently unroll the stocking up the leg. Be sure the stocking is smooth and free of wrinkles.

8. When the stocking is applied, cover the leg and repeat the procedure on the opposite leg.

9. When stockings have been applied to both legs, wash your hands and chart the procedure.

As with elastic bandages, elastic stockings should be removed at least every eight hours, or as ordered.

Be aware that in many cases where dressings, elastic bandages or elastic stockings are used, the resident's doctor will order the affected limb to be elevated to help prevent edema.

*Circle the correct answer. There is only **one** correct answer.*

1. **Signs of impaired circulation of a bandaged limb include swelling, pain and change in skin color.**

    a. True   b. False

2. **What is the most common type of dressing?**

    a Rayon strips.

    b. Elastic bandages.

    c. Telfa pads.

    d. Gauze.

3. **The nursing assistant is responsible for applying sterile dressings to open wounds.**

    a. True   b. False

4. **Tape should be applied parallel to a joint.**

    a. True   b. False

5. **How many pairs of gloves are necessary to change a dressing?**

    a. None.

    b. One.

    c. Two.

    d. Three.

6. **When applying a dressing,**

    a. Don't let the resident know what you're doing.

    b. Choose the tape which is not easily removable.

    c. It's okay to touch the dressing when you open the package.

    d. Place the used dressing in an infectious waste bag.

7. **When applying elastic bandages,**

    a. Lower the limb that is to be wrapped.

    b. Do not use any pressure.

    c. Begin wrapping the part of the limb farthest from the heart.

    d. There's no need to check with the resident to see if the bandages are comfortable.

8. **Elastic bandages must be removed at least every 8 hours.**

    a. True   b. False

9. **Dressings are used to protect the skin from drying out around a wound.**

    a. True   b. False

10. **A wrapped limb should be observed for signs of impaired circulation and swelling.**

    a. True   b. False

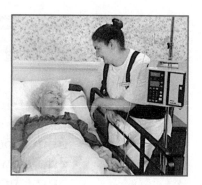

Chapter 42

IV CARE AND TUBE FEEDING

In this chapter... you will learn about:

▶ What an IV is.

▶ Assisting the nurse observing an IV.

▶ Changing the gown of a resident on an IV.

▶ Assisting the nurse observing tube feeding.

DEFINITIONS

Drip Chamber:
The small area under the IV bag or bottle that the fluid drips into. From the drip chamber the fluid goes down through a tube to the resident.

Feeding Pump:
A small machine used for tube feeding. It pumps liquid food slowly from a container to a resident.

Intravenous Infusion (IV):
Putting fluids directly into a resident's body through a vein.

Tube Feeding:
Putting liquid food directly into a resident's body through a tube inserted into the nose or a tube into a surgical incision into the stomach.

INTRAVENOUS INFUSION (IV)

An **intravenous infusion (IV)** is used to put fluid into a resident's body directly through a vein. The fluids come from a bottle or bag that is hanging from an IV pole. They drip slowly down a tube into a needle that the doctor or nurse has inserted into a vein, usually on the resident's arm. The fluid might be saline, blood, medication or liquid food.

The nurse is responsible for setting up the IV, but you may be asked to observe it and report anything wrong.

OBSERVING AN IV

▶ If the nurse asks you to do this, make sure the tube is not blocked or kinked or lying under the resident.

▶ Tell the nurse if the **drip chamber** is full or if the bag or bottle is nearly empty.

▶ Tell the nurse if the resident's skin near the IV needle is red or swollen.

CHANGING THE CLOTHING OF A RESIDENT ON AN IV

You will probably not be asked to perform any care on a person with an IV. This will normally be done by the nurse. However, if you are asked to assist the nurse, the following is the procedure for changing a gown or shirt for a resident on an IV. You have to take special care not to interfere with the IV tubing. Do NOT detach the tubing at any time.

1. Explain what you will be doing and wash your hands.

2. Provide privacy and lower the bed rail, just as you would normally for changing a resident's clothing.

3. Untie the gown or unbutton the shirt.

4. First remove the gown from the arm that does not have the IV needle.

5. Now carefully slide the gown down the arm that has the IV needle. Continue to slide the gown up the IV tubing to the IV bottle.

6. Temporarily lift the IV bottle off its hook and slide the gown over the bottle. Replace the bottle on its hook. Be sure to keep the IV bottle above the resident.

7. To put on the new gown, reverse this procedure: Temporarily lift the IV bottle off its hook, and slide the sleeve of the new gown down over the bottle. Continue to slide the sleeve down the tubing and then onto the resident's arm.

8. Put on the other sleeve and button or tie the clothing.

9. Make sure the IV tubing is not kinked or blocked.

10. Raise the bed rails again.

11. When finished, wash your hands.

TUBE FEEDING

Some residents who cannot take food by mouth are fed through a tube. The tube can be inserted through the resident's nose or through a small surgical incision directly into the stomach. The liquid food comes from a container like an IV container. It flows down a tube to a small machine called a **feeding pump**. The feeding pump puts the liquid food into the resident at a controlled rate.

The nurse will set up this equipment. You may be asked to observe a resident who is having **tube feeding**.

During tube feeding, a nursing assistant's duties may include:

1. Make sure the head of the bed is raised.

2. Make sure the pump is working properly and there is no alarm.

3. Make sure that the tubing is not kinked and hasn't come loose.

4. Report any problems immediately to the nurse.

Even though IVs and tube feeding are not part of the normal care you will be asked to provide, you should be aware of these procedures. And you should be aware of any problems that you might observe so you can report them immediately to the charge nurse.

*Circle the correct answer. There is only **one** correct answer.*

1. **An intravenous infusion (IV) is used to**

   a. Put food into a resident.

   b. Put fluid into a resident's vein.

   c. Make a surgical incision.

   d. Change a resident's gown.

2. **Setting up an intravenous infusion is the nursing assistant's responsibility.**

   a. True   b. False

3. **If a resident's skin near an IV needle is red or swollen, you should**

   a. Ignore it.

   b. Remove the needle.

   c. Tell the charge nurse.

   d. Change the drip rate.

4. **If you help change the clothing of a resident on an IV it is okay to detach the tubing briefly.**

   a. True   b. False

5. **If an IV bag or bottle is nearly empty, you should**

   a. Tell the charge nurse.

   b. Replace it.

   c. Refill it.

   d. Ignore it.

6. An IV bottle must always be

   (a) Above the resident.

   b. Below the resident.

   c. At the resident's chest level.

   d. At the resident's eye level.

7. If you are helping replace a gown on a person with an IV, which arm of the gown do you remove first?

   a. The arm with the IV.

   (b) The arm without the IV.

   c. Both arms together.

   d. It doesn't matter which arm is first.

8. Tube feeding is done through a tube inserted through the residents nose or

   a. Mouth.

   b. A vein.

   c. An artery.

   (d) A surgical incision into the stomach.

9. If a resident moves and causes a kink in an IV tube, you should immediately inform the charge nurse.

   (a) True   b. False

10. If a resident moves and causes a kink in a feeding tube, you should immediately inform the charge nurse.

   (a) True   b. False

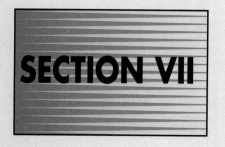

SECTION VII

FEEDING AND TOILETING

Chapter 43

BASIC FOODS AND FLUIDS

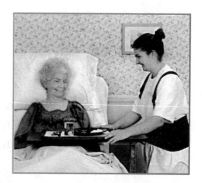

In this chapter... you will learn about:

▶ What are the basic substances in foods and fluids.

▶ Why the body needs these substances.

▶ Guidelines on diet for the older resident.

DEFINITIONS

Amino Acids:	Units of protein structure.
Carbohydrate:	Nutrient derived from plants sugars and starches.
Calorie:	Unit for measuring the amount of energy the body can get from a food.
Enriched:	Vitamins added to product.
Fat Soluble Vitamins:	Vitamins that dissolve in fat rather than water.
Fortified:	Vitamins and minerals added.
Genetic:	Inherited.
Hemoglobin:	Red substance in blood.
Macrominerals:	Nutritional minerals used by the body in relatively large quantities.
Nutrient:	Substance in food that supports life.
Nutrition:	Science of foods and how they affect health.
Pigment:	Substance that provides color.
Protein:	Nutrient derived from animals and some plants.
Trace Minerals:	Nutritional minerals used by the body in tiny quantities.
Water Soluble Vitamins:	Vitamins that dissolves in water instead of fat.

Proper **nutrition** is important for everyone. In order for our bodies to function properly, we must have certain basic foods and fluids. These foods and fluids:

- ▶ Provide energy for daily living and bodily functions.

- ▶ Promote growth and repair of tissue.

- ▶ Provide resistance to illness.

- ▶ Provide the necessary substances for bodily functions.

- ▶ Promote physical and mental health.

BASIC NUTRIENTS

Food provides the **nutrients** necessary for these functions. Nutrients are divided into different types:

- ▶ Carbohydrates.

- ▶ Proteins.

- ▶ Fats.

- ▶ Vitamins.

- ▶ Minerals.

- ▶ Fluids.

Carbohydrates

Carbohydrates provide the energy for the body to move, carry on the work of the cells, and maintain a steady body temperature. They are the fuel of the body.

Carbohydrates are found in cereals, breads, pasta, potatoes, vegetables, fruits, nuts, and sugars.

Proteins

Proteins are used to make body tissue, supply energy, and regulate bodily functions.

Proteins can be complete, partially complete, or incomplete.

Complete proteins contain all the nine **amino acids** necessary to maintain life and provide for growth. Complete proteins are found in foods from animals, such as meat, eggs, milk, poultry, fish, and cheese.

Partially complete proteins lack one or more of the amino acids and are able to support life, but unable to support growth. Partially complete proteins are found in some plant foods, such as dried beans and peas, whole grains, nuts, and soybeans.

Incomplete proteins are unable to support life or growth. Gelatin is an incomplete protein.

Fats

Fatty acids are necessary for the body to carry the fat-soluble vitamins, provide energy and heat, and arc necessary for growth and maintenance of tissue. Fats include vegetable oils, animal fat and butter, and foods such as meat, whole milk products, poultry, fish, and nuts.

Vitamins are substances found in small amounts in foods that are needed for specific actions in the body. Vitamins are divided into two main groups:

Fat-Soluble Vitamins

Fat-soluble vitamins are stored in body fat for later use, and since the body can store up a supply, they do not need to be consumed each day.

- Vitamin A is needed for healthy eyes, skin, hair, nails, gums, bones, and teeth. It also helps prevent infection. Vitamin A is found in dark green and deep yellow vegetables and fruits such as carrots, spinach, broccoli, and cantaloupe, plus liver, kidney, milk, eggs, *fortified* margarines, and fish liver oils.

- Vitamin D helps build and maintain teeth and bones. Foods rich in vitamin D are cod liver oil, sardines, salmon, egg yolks, and fortified milk. Exposure to sunlight enables the body to make its own vitamin D.

- Vitamin E helps form red blood cells, muscles, and other tissues. It is found in vegetable oils and whole wheat products.

- Vitamin K is needed for normal blood clotting and bone metabolism. Foods rich in vitamin K are leafy green vegetables, liver, egg yolks, oatmeal, and cauliflower.

Water-Soluble Vitamins

Water-soluble vitamins are not stored in the body and, therefore, must be consumed every day.

- B Vitamins (B1, B2, B3, B5, B6, and B12) are necessary for many body functions. They regulate appetite and digestion. They maintain a healthy nervous system. They also assist with food metabolism, the manufacture of hormones, the formation of red blood cells, brain function, and the building of *genetic* material. The B vitamins are found in many foods: whole grain and *enriched*

Chapter 43: Basic Foods and Fluids

grain products, red meat, fish, poultry, eggs, milk products, and dark green vegetables.

- Vitamin C helps bind cells together, strengthens the walls of blood vessels, promotes healing, helps to resist infection, and keeps gums healthy. Foods high in vitamin C are citrus fruit, cantaloupe, strawberries, dark green vegetables, tomatoes, and potatoes.

Minerals

In addition to vitamins, the body needs many different minerals to perform vital body functions. Some of these minerals are needed in relatively large quantities. These are called the **macrominerals**. Others are needed in very small amounts, and these are called the **trace minerals**. Following are some of the minerals needed for body functions:

Macrominerals

These are the major minerals that the body uses in the largest quantities.

- Calcium helps build strong bones and teeth. It also is involved in muscle and nerve functions, blood clotting, and in converting food to energy. Milk and milk products are our main sources of calcium. Canned sardines and dark green vegetables are other sources.

- Phosphorus works with calcium in building bones and teeth in nerve and muscle functions. Many foods contain phosphorus: meat, poultry, fish, eggs, whole grains, milk products, dried beans and peas, and nuts.

- Magnesium is involved in the release of energy and bone growth. Magnesium is found in whole grains, nuts, and dark green vegetables.

- Potassium helps regulate the body's fluid balance and is needed for nerve and muscle function. Potassium is found in fruits, nuts, potatoes, dried beans, and dark green vegetables.

Trace Minerals

These are minerals that the body uses in tiny quantities, but they are still important.

- Iron is essential to the production of **hemoglobin**, which carries oxygen to body cells. The food sources of iron are: meat, egg yolks, whole grains and enriched grain products, dried fruits, and dark green and yellow vegetables.

- Iodine is important to the function of the thyroid gland. Our main sources for iodine are fish and iodized salt.

- Zinc is involved in digestion and metabolism. It is found in red meat, fish, whole grains, and peanuts.

- Copper is needed to build red blood cells, tissue, nerve fibers, and **pigments** for hair and skin. Copper is found in seafood, raw mushrooms, dried beans and peas, nuts, and bananas.

Fluid

About seventy percent of our body weight is water. It makes up most of the volume of our blood. Water contains mineral elements, carries nutrients to the cells through the bloodstream, and carries waste materials away from the cells. It regulates temperature, lubricates joints, and aids in digestion.

You can survive several months without food, but only three days at most without water. For good health, the body requires about 8 glasses (2000 to 3000 cc or about 2 to 3 quarts) of fluids a day. At least 1000 cc of this fluid consumed should be water. Making certain your residents receive enough fluids daily is one of the most important caregiving functions. Fresh drinking water should always be available at every resident's bedside.

Dietary fiber, or roughage, is the indigestible portion of the food we eat. It is necessary for healthy, efficient elimination of waste products, and it helps prevent constipation. Fiber is found in all plant foods: fruits, vegetables, whole grains, and nuts. It is now thought that daily ingestion of fiber is absolutely essential for optimum health.

Nutrition scientists used to talk about "The Four Food Groups." These were dairy, vegetables and fruits, meat and fish, and breads and cereals. More recently, research has shown that this old-style grouping did not promote good nutrition. It tended to encourage people to eat equal amounts of each group, which meant they were consuming far too much fat and too little grains and vegetables.

To help people eat a balanced, nutritional diet, scientists have developed the Dietary Guidelines for Americans, and the Food Guidance System. The Food Guidance System has four overall recommendations for promoting healthy eating habits:

- Variety Eating foods from a variety of food groups.

- Proportionality Eating more of some foods, like fruits and vegetables, and less of others, like foods high in fats and added sugar.

- Moderation Choosing foods that limit saturated fats, added sugar, salt and alcohol.

- Activity Being physically active every day.

The Food Guidance System uses 12 daily calorie intake levels and seven food groups to create personalized diets to promote healthy eating. The seven food groups are:

- Fruits
- Vegetables
- Grains
- Meat and beans
- Milk
- Oils
- Discretionary calories

The 12 daily calorie intake levels start at 1,000 calories a day and progress to 3,200 calories a day, increasing in 200 calorie increments. Age, sex, and whether a person has an active or sedentary lifestyle determine the appropriate calorie level. For example, a sedentary 70-year-old woman would have a lower recommended calorie intake level than an active 18-year-old male. The Food Guidance System defines an active lifestyle as one that includes physical activity equivalent to walking more than 3 miles every day at 3 to 4 miles per hour, in addition to normal day-to-day activity.

Because the Food Guidance System is so personalized, the new food pyramid used to illustrate the principles of the Food Guidance System is now called MyPyramid. The federal government has created the website www.MyPyramid.gov to help people determine what suggested diet is right for them.

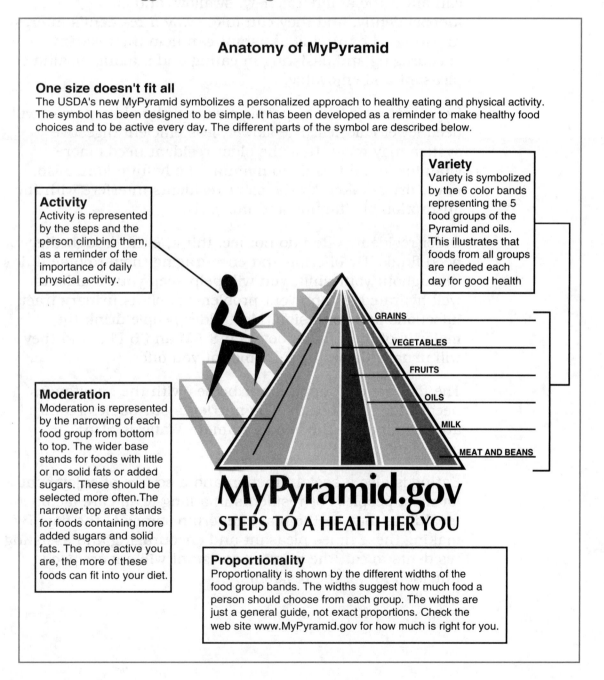

Anatomy of MyPyramid

One size doesn't fit all
The USDA's new MyPyramid symbolizes a personalized approach to healthy eating and physical activity. The symbol has been designed to be simple. It has been developed as a reminder to make healthy food choices and to be active every day. The different parts of the symbol are described below.

Variety
Variety is symbolized by the 6 color bands representing the 5 food groups of the Pyramid and oils. This illustrates that foods from all groups are needed each day for good health

Activity
Activity is represented by the steps and the person climbing them, as a reminder of the importance of daily physical activity.

GRAINS
VEGETABLES
FRUITS
OILS
MILK
MEAT AND BEANS

Moderation
Moderation is represented by the narrowing of each food group from bottom to top. The wider base stands for foods with little or no solid fats or added sugars. These should be selected more often. The narrower top area stands for foods containing more added sugars and solid fats. The more active you are, the more of these foods can fit into your diet.

MyPyramid.gov
STEPS TO A HEALTHIER YOU

Proportionality
Proportionality is shown by the different widths of the food group bands. The widths suggest how much food a person should choose from each group. The widths are just a general guide, not exact proportions. Check the web site www.MyPyramid.gov for how much is right for you.

AGE-RELATED CHANGES AFFECTING DIET

A well-balanced diet is just as important for an older person as it is for a younger person. There are some changes as a person ages which affect nutrition.

Many chronic diseases affect appetite. Chronic diseases can affect the ability to chew, swallow, and eat independently, and they can take away a resident's interest in eating. The nursing assistant can help the resident by encouraging and assisting in eating and making mealtimes pleasant and enjoyable.

Body systems slow as people age, and the older person will need fewer calories. The slower, less efficient digestive system may mean that the older resident needs more vitamins and minerals to maintain body functions. Also, many drugs taken by the older residents interfere with the absorption of vitamins and minerals.

Older residents often do not feel thirst, even though they need fluids. By offering and encouraging them to take fluids throughout your shift, you will help keep your residents well hydrated and prevent problems such as urinary tract infections and confusion. Most older people drink the majority of their fluids between 8 AM and 6 PM, and they will usually drink the full amount you offer.

The food we eat supplies our bodies with the substances needed for good health. The nutrients our bodies require are contained in the Food Pyramid. Water is also important.

Eating is also a social function and a source of enjoyment for most people. For residents in a long-term care facility, mealtimes may be the most important times of the day. By making these times pleasant and encouraging and assisting residents to eat, the nursing assistant will ensure good nutrition for all the residents.

Circle the correct answer. There is only **one** *correct answer.*

1. **Carbohydrates, fats, and proteins are nutrients.**

    a. True   b. False

2. **Partially complete proteins contain all nine amino acids necessary to maintain life and provide for growth.**

    a. True   b. False

3. **Gelatin is an example of**

    a. A complete protein.
    b. A partially complete protein.
    c. An incomplete protein.
    d. A vitamin.

4. **Fats are not necessary to the body and need to be eliminated.**

    a. True   b. False

5. **Water soluble vitamins, such as the B vitamins and vitamin C need to be consumed:**

    a. Daily.
    b. Hourly.
    c. Once a week.
    d. Once a month or so.

6. **You can survive three months without food, but only about how long without water?**

    a. Three minutes.

    b. Three hours.

    (c.) Three days.

    d. Three weeks.

7. **What is an advantage of fiber in the diet?**

    a. Helps build strong bones and teeth.

    b. Is used to make red blood cells.

    c. Helps regulate the body's fluid balance.

    (d.) Helps prevent constipation.

8. **What food group should we eat only sparingly?**

    (a.) Fats, oils and sweets.

    b. Dairy products.

    c. Meats and nuts.

    d. Vegetables.

    e. Fruits.

    f. Grains.

9. **What food group should we eat the most from?**

    a. Fats, oils and sweets.

    b. Dairy products.

    c. Meats and nuts.

    d. Vegetables.

    e. Fruits.

    (f.) Grains.

10. **The nursing assistant should discourage residents from taking too many fluids during the day.**

    a. True   (b.) False

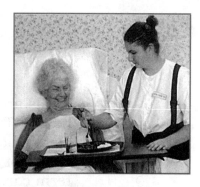

Chapter 44

FEEDING A RESIDENT

Watch step-by-step demonstrations of the procedures discussed in this chapter in the Medcom videotape "Feeding" (CNA216).

In this chapter... you will learn about:

▶ How to assist a resident at mealtimes.

▶ How to feed a resident who needs assistance eating.

▶ How to prevent choking.

DEFINITIONS

Heimlich Maneuver: Application of abdominal thrusts to clear an obstruction from the airway.

Interaction: Conversation, communication relating to others.

Socialization: Talking with and listening to others.

Unconscious: Unaware of surroundings or environment.

Meals are an essential part of maintaining and restoring health. They often mean pleasure, comfort, and companionship if shared with others. Mealtimes are often the most enjoyable part of the day for residents in long-term care facilities. In order to keep these times pleasant, the nursing assistant needs to provide a comfortable, enjoyable atmosphere by properly serving and assisting residents. Illness, disability, depression, and medications can all affect appetite. It is particularly important to maintain a positive attitude when residents have lost their interest in and appetite for food.

SERVING RESIDENTS IN THE DINING ROOM

Many residents in long-term care facilities eat together in a dining room. This provides a social atmosphere and the opportunity to be with and talk to other people. If it is possible for the residents to eat in the dining room, they should be encouraged to do so. Following are guidelines for serving residents in the dining room:

1. Wash your own hands. Assist the resident in washing and care for the face and mouth, if needed.

2. Assist the resident to the proper place in the dining room.

3. Protect the resident's clothing with a napkin or bib.

4. Remind the resident of the names of those sitting nearby. Encourage *interaction* among the residents at the table.

5. Check the tray to be sure it is the proper diet and meal intended for a particular resident.

6. Check to see that the resident has all the necessary silverware, food, and assistive eating devices if needed. Wash your hands.

7. Help the resident set up the tray, cut up the food and butter the bread. Identify the food for the resident, and assist only if necessary. It is important to encourage independence in eating.

8. If residents can feed themselves, observe to see if they are able to complete the meal, or provide assistance as needed.

9. It is important to prevent residents from taking food from each other's plate or tray. Certain food may not be on the resident's diet.

10. When feeding a dependent resident sit beside him or her so that you are at eye level. If you are at a feeding table, sit down facing the resident.

11. When the resident has finished eating, write down the percentages of food eaten and fluids drunk. Do not trust your memory; write it down immediately. Transfer this information to the resident's chart.

12. Assist the resident from the dining room.

13. Assist the resident in handwashing and caring for his or her face and mouth.

14. When finished, wash your hands.

SERVING RESIDENTS IN THEIR ROOMS

Some residents will not be able to come to the dining room to eat. They must eat in their rooms. The following guidelines should be used when feeding residents in their rooms:

1. Explain to the resident what you will be doing and wash your hands.

2. Assist the resident to an upright position in bed or in a chair.

3. Assist the resident in handwashing and caring for his or her face and mouth, if needed.

4. Wash your own hands.

5. Protect the resident's clothing or bed linen with a napkin or bib.

6. Place a tray on the bedside table, checking to see that all the necessary silverware and food are on the tray.

7. Verify that the resident is getting the proper tray and diet.

8. Place the table in front of the resident.

9. Remove the plate covers and arrange the dishes and silverware so they are convenient for the resident to use.

10. If necessary, identify the food for the resident, cut up the food, and butter the bread. Assist only as much as necessary. Encourage independent eating.

11. If the resident needs assistance in eating, sit at eye level next to the resident.

12. If the resident can feed himself or herself, make sure the resident has begun eating before leaving the room.

13. When the resident has finished eating, remove the tray and make a written note of the percentage of each food eaten and beverages drunk. Transfer this information to the resident's chart.

14. Assist the resident with handwashing and face and mouth care, then return the resident to a comfortable position.

15. When finished, wash your hands.

PROVIDING FEEDING ASSISTANCE

Some residents may need a great deal of assistance in eating. This requires patience and understanding on the part of the nursing assistant. When feeding dependent residents, remember they are adults, not children. Carry on a pleasant conversation as you feed them. This will provide the natural *socialization* that usually occurs during mealtimes. When feeding a resident, follow these guidelines:

1. Identify the foods on the plate or tray so the resident will know what he or she will be eating.

2. Ask the resident the desired order for eating the different foods and wash your hands.

3. Test the temperature of the food by feeling the container and testing a small amount against your inner wrist. Foods that are too hot may burn a resident's mouth. Foods which are too cold may startle the resident.

4. Use a spoon, filling it only half full and placing the food at the tip of the spoon.

5. Place the food on the center of the resident's tongue with a slight downward pressure. If the resident is paralyzed on one side, place the food on the unaffected side of the tongue.

6. Allow sufficient time for the resident to chew and swallow the food before putting more in the mouth.

7. Alternate solid food and fluids. If the resident has difficulty drinking from a cup, use a flexible straw. Place the straw between the resident's lips, not the teeth.

8. When finished, wash your hands.

The most frequent cause of airway obstruction is choking on large or poorly chewed portions of food. Some residents who have difficulty chewing and swallowing require close supervision while eating. Be certain the resident's individual feeding plan is followed.

The food should be cut in small pieces and offered in small amounts. Wait until each portion is chewed and swallowed before more is given. If choking does occur there may be partial or complete blocking of the airway.

Partial Obstruction

In partial obstruction, some air may be passing to the lungs. Signs of partial obstruction are:

▶ Wheezing or gurgling in the throat or airway.

▶ Unusual breathing, difficulty breathing.

▶ High pitched noise caused by a spasm in the larynx.

If the resident is conscious and can breathe, assist with coughing to force the obstruction from the airway.

Total Obstruction

In a total obstruction, the airway is completely blocked. The signs are:

▶ Clutching the throat.

▶ Sudden inability to speak or breathe or cough.

The resident may quickly become **unconscious**: IMMEDIATE ACTION IS NECESSARY! Shout for help and begin to assist in clearing the obstruction.

The **Heimlich Maneuver** is a method used to clear a blocked airway. The procedure is:

1. Stand behind a resident who is standing or sitting and place your arms around the resident's waist.

2. Make a fist with one hand and place the thumb side at a point in the middle of the abdomen half way between the resident's navel and the sternum.

3. Place the other hand over your fist.

4. Grasp your fist with the other hand and apply a hard upward thrust with both hands into the resident's abdomen.

The Heimlich Maneuver

5. Perform 6 to 10 rapid abdominal thrusts like this until the object is expelled.

6. When the object is partially or completely dislodged, use your fingers and sweep the resident's mouth to remove the food or other material causing the choking.

7. If the attempts to remove the object are unsuccessful, or the resident becomes unconscious, call for assistance and begin CPR.

Mealtimes are an important time of day for the residents and they should be assisted and encouraged to eat their appropriate diet.

*Circle the correct answer. There is only **one** correct answer.*

1. **Illness or disability, depression, and medication can all affect appetite.**

    (a.) True   b. False

2. **When possible, residents should eat in their own rooms, not the dining room.**

    a. True   (b.) False

3. **When residents eat in the dining room, you should be sure they do not**

    a. Speak to their neighbors.

    b. Eat with assistive devices.

    (c.) Eat off other residents' trays.

    d. Leave any food uneaten.

4. **When residents eat in the dining room, you should never help them by cutting up food.**

    a. True   (b.) False

5. **When feeding residents in their rooms, the nursing assistant should encourage independent eating.**

    (a.) True   b. False

6. **Mr. Wilson can feed himself in his own room. The nursing assistant should**

    (a.) Sit at eye level next to the resident.

    b. Bring the food and leave the room immediately.

    c. Watch the resident begin eating before leaving the room.

    d. Not do anything.

7. **When feeding a dependent resident, the nursing assistant should**

    a. Have the resident eat all the solid food first.

    b. Have the resident drink all the fluids first.

    c. Alternate solid food and fluids.

    d. Never offer fluids.

8. **When feeding a dependent resident, the nursing assistant should**

    a. Treat the resident like a child.

    b. Use only a fork.

    c. Carry on a pleasant conversation.

    d. Place the food on the back of the resident's tongue.

9. **Choking is commonly caused by**

    a. A portion of food caught in the airway.

    b. A cold or flu.

    c. Medications.

    d. Clothing that is too tight.

10. **In the Heimlich Maneuver, the nursing assistant should**

    a. Stand in front of the resident.

    b. Give a hard, upward thrust against the resident's abdomen.

    c. Have the resident lie down.

    d. Never repeat the maneuver.

Chapter 45

SPECIAL DIETS

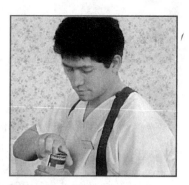

In this chapter... you will learn about:

▶ Special diets.

▶ Which residents get special diets.

▶ How to monitor food consumption.

DEFINITIONS

Allergy:	Hypersensitive reaction of the body to a specific food or substance.
Therapeutic:	Pertaining to or useful in treatment of a disease.

The law requires all long-term care facilities to have a registered dietitian to plan, review, and revise diet orders for residents. Regular diets are planned by the dietitian to provide the recommended daily amounts of basic foods as suggested by the Food Pyramid and nutritional science. In a regular diet, there are no restrictions on food choices.

Some residents will require special diets that eliminate some foods or are prepared in special ways. A part of each resident's care plan is a diet order. The physician will specify the type of diet for the resident. This special diet is called a ***therapeutic*** diet. It consists of special types and amounts of food that are specifically designed for that resident's physical condition. The following are several types of special therapeutic diets:

Low Sodium Diet

There are certain diagnoses, such as high blood pressure, for which a low sodium diet is usually ordered. Since the main source of sodium in our diets comes from salt, foods which contain large amounts of salt will be restricted. Residents on a low sodium diet will not be served ham, sausage, corned beef, bacon, lunch meats, frankfurters, pickles, potato chips, pretzels, or salted nuts. Also, there will be no salt packets with the resident's food tray.

Diabetic Diet

Residents with diabetes will be on a special diet. Sugar will be eliminated and an artificial sweetener or fruit juice will be substituted. Desserts and snacks will usually be fruit rather than cake, pie, cookies, candy, or pudding. Regular ice cream will be replaced with diabetic ice cream.

Low Calorie Diet

This may be ordered for residents who are overweight. The types of food remain in balance according to the Food Pyramid, but calories and amounts are controlled to help cut down the resident's weight.

High Calorie Diet

This may be ordered for residents who would benefit from weight gain. The amounts are increased to help raise the calorie count.

Low Fat Diet

A low fat diet, or low cholesterol diet, may be ordered for residents with high cholesterol levels, coronary artery disease, or who are overweight. A low fat diet eliminates fried foods, gravy, cream sauces, luncheon meats, and whole milk products. Low or nonfat milk and milk products will be substituted.

Bland Diet

Residents with digestive problems may be placed on a bland diet. This diet eliminates gas-producing foods, such as beans, cabbage, and onions. It also eliminates strong spices, pepper, coffee, and tea. Decaffeinated coffee, herb tea, and salt are not restricted.

Mechanical Soft Diet

The resident who has difficulty chewing because of poor or missing teeth may be placed on a mechanical soft diet. This means that the food is cut in very small pieces before it is served, making it easy to chew and digest.

Pureed Diet

The resident who cannot chew at all or who is at high risk for choking may be placed on a pureed diet. Food is placed in a blender and reduced almost to a liquid state so that it requires no chewing. Foods which are already soft and smooth, such as puddings, soups, and eggs are served in their normal form.

Clear Liquid

This may be ordered for a resident who has a digestive illness or following surgery. It does not provide adequate nutrition for a long period. This diet mainly consists of broth, tea, ginger ale or gelatin.

Full Liquid

This may be prescribed for a resident with a digestive illness. It does not provide adequate nutrition for a long period. It includes liquids such as broth and tea, plus custards, ice cream and soft cooked eggs.

Tube Feeding

A liquid diet containing all the necessary nutrients is given by tube through the nose (nasogastric tube) or through a surgical opening in the abdomen (gastrostomy tube). The nursing assistant will not administer a tube feeding. This will be done by a licensed nurse for those residents who cannot swallow food.

Food Allergies

Some residents are allergic to specific foods. This will be noted in the resident's chart and must be considered when planning a diet. Foods which cause an allergic reaction must be avoided. The nursing assistant should be aware of any food allergies residents may have.

In order to ensure adequate nutrition, the resident's doctor may order a nutritional supplement. This is usually in the form of a high protein drink. The doctor's order will be in the resident's chart and will contain the name of the supplement, how much, and when it should be given. The nursing assistant will be responsible for seeing that the resident receives and drinks the supplement. Nourishment refusals are to be reported to the charge nurse immediately.

The nursing assistant is responsible for seeing that residents receive the diet ordered. Most facilities have a system for identifying residents with special diets. This could be on a color-coded name tag or arm band. Be sure you understand the system used in your facility.

In addition to diet restrictions ordered by the physician, each resident will have a set of particular likes and dislikes. Eating patterns are established early in life, and people tend to eat the same types of food throughout their lives. There are also cultural differences, with people from different cultures liking different types of foods. It is very difficult to change the eating habits of residents. Therefore, the dietitian will take these likes and dislikes into consideration when planning individual menus. For example, liver is very nutritious, but many people do not like it. If it goes back to the kitchen untouched, all those nutrients go into the garbage rather than into the resident. Every effort should be made to provide foods which the residents will eat.

Some residents find it difficult to be on a special diet. They may take restricted foods from other residents, or family and friends may provide it. The nursing assistant should be alert to these incidences and report them to the charge nurse. The nursing assistant can also explain to the resident and the family the importance of staying on the prescribed diet even though it may be difficult.

The nursing assistant is responsible for charting the amount of food and fluid consumed by the resident. This is done by observing the resident's tray or plate after the meal and noting how much was eaten. The amount eaten is charted in terms of calories eaten. The charting guides of calories for sample meals will be posted at the nurse's station. It will probably be similar to the following guide.

Note that the percentage given is based on a total of 100% for the calories that one resident would get from all foods in one meal. The percentage listed for each food indicates the amount of that 100% that the resident gets from that type of food. For example, if the resident ate the full breakfast shown, 20% of the resident's calories at breakfast would come from cereal.

MEAL	FOOD	PERCENTAGE OF CALORIES
Breakfast	Cereal	20%
	Egg	20%
	Toast & Margarine	30%
	Milk	20%
	Juice	10%
	TOTAL:	100%
Lunch/Dinner	Meat, Fish, Fowl	40%
	Potato, Pasta	10%
	Vegetable	5%
	Bread & Margarine	20%
	Milk	15%
	Dessert	10%
	TOTAL:	100%

Coffee and tea (without sugar) have no calories; therefore, they are not counted.

If the main dish is a combination of foods, such as spaghetti, the percentages of each type of food are added together (meat 40% + starch 10% = 50%).

The total percentage of calories eaten is computed by using simple arithmetic. If Mr. Wilson, for example, ate half his meat at dinner, he ate half his meat calories, or 20% (half of 40%) of the allocated calories for meat. If all of the bread and margarine was eaten for lunch, he ate 20% of the calories allocated for bread. These percentages are added together to produce the totals consumed by the resident at each meal. It is important to remember that you are calculating the percentages of the allocated calories, not the actual amounts of food consumed. (You could, for example, eat everything but the meat and potato at dinner. It might seem like you ate most of the food, but in fact you consumed only 50% of the calories allocated.)

If a resident's intake suddenly changes or a resident is not eating well, the charge nurse must be notified.

The diet prescribed for the individual resident is as necessary for the resident's health and functioning as prescribed medications. The nursing assistant must be sure the resident is receiving the diet ordered, and encourage the resident to stay on the diet. Remain alert to any change in eating habits or reactions to foods.

*Circle the correct answer. There is only **one** correct answer.*

1. **The nursing assistant specifies the type of diet most therapeutic for the resident.**

   a. True   b. False

2. **In which type of diet is sugar eliminated?**

   a. Bland.

   b. Low sodium.

   c. Diabetic.

   d. Low fat.

3. **Which diet has no restrictions?**

   a. Bland.

   b. Pureed.

   c. Mechanical soft.

   d. Regular.

4. **Mrs. Johnson has coronary artery disease and is not allowed to eat fried foods, gravies, or foods using whole milk. What type of diet is she on?**

   a. Low fat.

   b. Low sodium.

   c. Diabetic.

   d. Pureed.

5. **The resident who is unable to chew at all may be placed on a pureed diet.**

   a. True   b. False

6. **When planning a resident's diet, the nutritionist does not take into account the residents likes and dislikes.**

    a. True   (b) False

7. **It is very difficult to change the eating habits of residents.**

    (a.) True   b. False

8. **How does the nursing assistant chart the amount of food and fluid consumed by the resident?**

    a. By asking the resident how much was eaten.

    (b.) By observing the resident's tray after the meal and noting how much was eaten.

    c. By asking one of the nurses on duty what the resident ate.

    d. By asking family or friends of the resident what the resident ate.

9. **For lunch, Mrs. Block ate half of her spaghetti and meatballs, none of the salad, and all of the bread and margarine, milk, and dessert. Using a guide in which meat = 40%, pasta = 10%, salad = 5%, bread and margarine = 20%, milk = 15%, and dessert = 10%, what is the total percentage of the allocated calories eaten by Mrs. Block?**

    a. 100%.

    b. 75%.

    (c.) 70%.

    d. 50%.

10. **Changes in a resident's eating habits must be reported by the nursing assistant to the charge nurse.**

    (a.) True   b. False

Chapter 46

ELIMINATION NEEDS

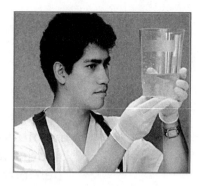

 Watch step-by-step demonstrations of the procedures discussed in this chapter in the Medcom videotape "Specimen Collection and Urinary Care" (CNA213).

In this chapter... you will learn about:

▶ How to care for an incontinent resident.

▶ How to measure fluid intake and output.

▶ How to care for a catheter.

DEFINITIONS

Abnormality:	The state of being unlike the usual or normal condition.
cc:	Cubic centimeter, a metric unit for measuring fluids; 1000 cc's = roughly 1 quart.
Closed Urinary Drainage System:	The complete catheter drainage unit which connects the catheter, drainage tube, and collection container.
Dehydration:	Condition in which fluid output is greater than fluid intake.
Edema:	Collection of excess fluid in tissue.
Labia:	Folds of skin surrounding the female genital area.
Leg Bag:	A urine collection bag attached to a catheter and worn on the leg.
Measuring Graduate:	Container with markings to measure fluids.
Mucus:	Secretion from the mucous membrane.
Mucous Membrane:	Moist tissue that lines the mouth, nose, eyes, rectum, urethra and vagina.
Sediment:	Material which settles to bottom of liquid.
Spasm:	Involuntary muscle contraction.
Urethral Meatus:	Opening at the end of the urethra to the body surface.

INCONTINENCE

Many of the elderly residents you will take care of will be incontinent. This means they are unable to control their bladder and or bowels. Some residents have control of their bowel and not their bladder, and some are just the opposite. Some will be incontinent all the time, and some will only be incontinent occasionally. Incontinence can have many different causes:

- ► Urinary tract infection (UTI).

- ► Stress, anxiety, frustration.

- ► Progressive chronic disease processes.

- ► Fear, worry.

- ► Central nervous system (CNS) injury.

- ► Tumors or **spasms** of the bladder.

- ► Confusion, memory loss.

- ► Loss of muscle control.

- ► Medications.

Whatever the cause, incontinence is embarrassing and frustrating to residents and their families. Since the nursing assistant is the one who provides the most direct care to residents, the way the nursing assistant reacts to incidents of incontinence is very important. The nursing assistant should:

1. Handle the incident in a calm, professional manner.

2. Never punish, shame, or scold the resident.

3. Provide privacy for the resident as care is being given.

4. Wear gloves whenever handling any body fluids.

The incontinent resident is at risk for skin breakdown. Urine and feces will destroy skin tissue if not promptly removed and the perineal area kept clean and dry. The nursing assistant must check incontinent residents frequently to ensure that they are not wet or soiled.

Every time the incontinent resident is changed, perineal care must be given. (See Chapter 38). Frequent clothing changes, turning, and perineal care will prevent skin breakdown and possible infection for the incontinent resident.

CATHETER CARE

Some residents who are having difficulty with urination have an indwelling catheter prescribed by their doctor. The catheter is a thin, sterile tube inserted through the resident's urethra into the bladder. The catheter remains in place and is connected to a drainage tube which drains the urine from the bladder into a bag or plastic container. This is called a ***closed urinary drainage system.***

Danger Points

Residents with catheters are very susceptible to infection. Germs and bacteria can enter the closed system at four points. They are:

- The ***urethral meatus***, the opening where urine leaves the body. In the male, this is at the tip of the penis. In the female, it is inside the folds of the ***labia***.

- The connection between the catheter and the drainage tube.

- The connection between the drainage tube and the collection bag or container.

- The drain spout of the collection bag or container.

Residents with a catheter in place must be given daily catheter care and special precautions must be taken to prevent germs and bacteria from entering the closed urinary drainage system.

Perineal Care

Good perineal care as a regular part of the morning and evening hygiene is essential for residents with indwelling catheters. Since feces always contain bacteria and germs, it is extremely important to prevent feces from coming in contact with the urethral meatus where infection is very likely to occur.

Always wear gloves when providing perineal care. For the female resident, spread the labia and be sure to wash from front to back, TOWARD the rectum. For uncircumcised males, retract the foreskin and wash the head of the penis thoroughly. For complete instructions on perineal care, refer to Chapter 38.

Always make sure the patient has privacy and time to ensure dignity and comfort.

Daily Catheter Care

An indwelling catheter is cleaned when a resident bathes. For residents unable to bathe themselves, the nursing assistant will provide routine catheter care when perineal care is given:

1. Assemble equipment as described below: disposable bed protector, bedpan, basin of warm water (about 105° F), peri-wash solution (if used by your facility), soap, at least four washcloths, towels, a bath blanket, and protective gloves.

2. Explain to the resident what you are going to do. Position the resident on his/her back.

3. Provide privacy for the resident

4. Perform hand hygiene and put on gloves.

5. Offer the resident a bedpan or urinal.

6. Place the disposable bed protector under the resident.

7. Drape the resident with the bath blanket and pull bed linens to the foot of the bed.

8. Flex the resident's legs and position them apart.

9. Wet the washcloths; wring out excess water.

10. Apply soap to a wet washcloth and clean the area thoroughly.

    - Men: wash the penis, scrotum and perineal area. With uncircumcised men, retract the foreskin and wash the head of the penis.

    - Women: spread the labia and wash from front to back.

11. Use a clean wet washcloth to rinse the area.

12. Dry the area by gently patting with a towel.

13. Observe the area around the catheter for sores, crusting, leakage or bleeding. Report any unusual observations to your supervisor immediately.

14. Apply soap to a new, clean, wet washcloth to clean the catheter. Starting from where the catheter leaves the body, clean four inches of the catheter tubing.

    - Retract the foreskin of uncircumsized men.

    - Females gently separate the labia with your thumb and forefinger, then clean the catheter moving away from the body.

15. Use a clean wet washcloth to rinse the catheter.

16. Remove the bed protector and discard it.

17. Make sure the catheter tubing isn't kinked or pulling. Check to ensure that the tubing is not left under any part of the body, to prevent skin breakdown due to pressure.

18. Discard the protective gloves.

19. Remove the bath blanket and replace bed linens over the resident. Make sure he/she is comfortable. Raise the side rail if ordered by the physician, and leave the call signal and any personal items requested within reach.

20. Empty, clean and store the wash basin. Gather the towels and washcloths and place them in a dirty linen container according to your facility's policy.

21. Perform hand hygiene.

When the urinary system is closed, there is less risk of infection; therefore, the system should be opened only when necessary. Each time the system is opened, the chance of infection increases. When it becomes necessary to open the system to replace the drainage tubing and collection container, the following procedure must be followed:

1. Assemble the necessary equipment: new sterile tubing and collection container, catheter clamp, antiseptic solution packet, sterile catheter plug, sterile drainage tubing cap, disposable bed protector, and disposable gloves.

2. Wash your hands.

3. Provide privacy for the resident.

4. Explain to the resident what you are going to do.

5. Place a disposable bed protector under resident.

6. Open the antiseptic packet.

7. Put on disposable gloves.

8. Be sure the new tubing and container are securely connected. Place them beside the old tubing and container.

9. Clamp the catheter shut with a catheter clamp.

10. With the applicator wipe the junction of the drainage tubing and the catheter with antiseptic solution.

11. Carefully disconnect the tubing. *Do not allow any object to touch either the catheter or the end of the drainage tubing.*

12. If the resident is going to be disconnected for a period of time, such as during bathing, insert a sterile catheter plug into the end of the catheter. Cover the end of the drainage tubing with a sterile drainage tube cap. *Do not allow the drainage tubing to touch the floor.*

13. Disconnect the clamp.

14. If the resident is to be connected to the new tubing and container immediately, eliminate steps 12 and 13 and attach the new tubing and container, being sure to maintain the sterile condition. Then disconnect the clamp.

15. Remove the disposable bed protector and your gloves and discard them.

16. Cover and position the resident for comfort.

17. Wash your hands.

Positioning A Closed Urinary Drainage System

To keep a free-flowing system going, the catheter drainage tubing and collection bag or container must be properly placed. The collection bag or container must always be below the level of the bladder to allow the urine to drain. If the drainage tubing is too long and allowed to hang down, urine will pool in the tubing, blocking drainage. Germs and bacteria grow very quickly in urine. If urine is allowed to pool or if the collection container is above the level of the bladder, these germs and bacteria can travel back into the body to cause illness.

Positioning A Closed Urinary Drainage System On A Bed

For a resident in bed, the drainage tubing should be long enough to reach the collection container and allow movement, but not so long as to allow the urine to pool. The drainage tubing should be taped to the inner side of the resident's thigh to prevent tension, then placed over the resident's leg. The drainage tubing should then be coiled on the bed and attached to the bed linen with the attachment device provided. The collection container should be attached to the bed frame, below the level of the resident.

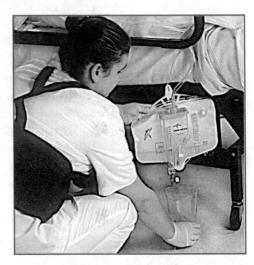

Emptying a drainage bag.

Positioning A Closed Urinary Drainage System On A Wheelchair

Before transferring a resident from the bed to the wheelchair, release the tubing from the bed linen and release the container from the bed. Transfer the resident, being careful NOT to pull on or increase the tension on the catheter and NOT to raise the collection container above the level of the bladder.

When the resident is in the wheelchair, pass the collection container under the wheelchair seat and fasten it behind the wheelchair below the level of the resident's bladder.

Positioning A Closed Urinary Drainage System for Walking

When walking, most residents prefer to use a urine collection bag called a **leg bag**, which is worn on the leg under the resident's clothes. The bag must be positioned so that the inlet of the bag is on top. Straps are always attached to the collection bag before putting it on the resident's leg. The straps should be next to the resident's leg and NOT over the bag. Putting a strap over the bag might compress the bag and prevent its filling. The collection bag should be emptied before the resident gets up to avoid pulling and tension on the catheter.

MEASURING INTAKE AND OUTPUT

Fluid is eliminated from the body through perspiration, breath, feces, and vomit, as well as through urine. Urine is the most easily measured and can be accurately measured if the resident is not incontinent. This is the most reliable measurement of fluid output.

The average resident in a long-term health care facility requires about two quarts (or about 2000 *cc's*) of fluid in a 24-hour period. If residents take in more fluid than they excrete, *edema* occurs. The signs of edema are:

- ▶ Weight gain.

- ▶ Swelling of feet, ankles, face, and fingers.

- ▶ Decreased urinary output.

- ▶ Fluid collection in abdomen.

If residents excrete more fluid than they take in, *dehydration* occurs. The signs of dehydration are:

- ▶ Thirst.

- ▶ Constipation.

- ▶ Decreased urinary output.

- ▶ Decreased blood pressure with weak, rapid pulse.

- ▶ Confusion or disorientation.

- ▶ Lethargy.

- ▶ Dry lips and mucous membranes.

- ▶ Rapid weight loss.

If the doctor suspects there is a fluid imbalance in a resident, an intake-output record will be requested.

All residents with catheters should have their intake and output of fluid monitored and recorded every 24 hours. Monitoring (observing and recording) this intake and output is the responsibility of the nursing assistant.

Measuring Intake

To measure fluid intake, it is necessary to accurately measure and record EVERY fluid a resident takes by mouth (water, tea, coffee, milk, juice, broth). Foods such as gelatin and ice cream which become fluid at room temperature must also be included. Fluids taken through tube feedings are also included in fluid intake measurements.

You must know how much fluid the containers used in your facility hold. After the resident has finished with the drink or meal, measure the fluid left in the container. It is important to measure what is left BEFORE the dishes are removed. (Some might be spilled or discarded before you can measure it.) Then subtract this amount from the amount offered and record the result as intake. These quantities should not be estimates, but actual measurements. It is your responsibility to record this figure immediately on the intake-output record used by your facility.

Measuring Output - A Resident Without A Catheter

If the resident uses a bedside commode or a bedpan, the urine can easily be collected and measured. The resident who uses the toilet must be given a special collection container which fits inside the toilet seat. The resident must be instructed not to empty the container, but to call the nursing assistant. The procedure for measuring fluid output is as follows:

1. Explain to the resident what you will be doing and provide privacy.

2. Wash your hands and put on disposable gloves.

3. Pour the urine into a **measuring graduate**.

4. Set the graduate on a flat surface at eye level and read and record the amount of urine.

5. Observe the urine for any signs of blood, dark color, mucus, **sediment**, or any change from its characteristic odor. Report any of these **abnormalities** to the charge nurse.

6. Empty the urine into the toilet and flush it.

7. Rinse the bedpan, urinal, commode pan, special container, and graduate, and store them in the appropriate area.

8. Remove and dispose of the gloves.

9. Wash your hands.

10. Record the amount and date and time the specimen was measured.

Measuring Output - A Resident with A Catheter

To measure fluid output for a resident with an indwelling catheter, follow the procedure below:

1. Explain to the resident what you will be doing and provide privacy.

2. Wash your hands and put on disposable gloves.

3. Place the graduate below the collection container.

4. Carefully open the drain outlet from the collection container. Be sure the drain outlet does not touch the container or the floor. Bacteria could be introduced into the container and passed to the resident, causing an infection.

5. Allow the container to drain completely.

6. Reattach the drainage outlet to the collection container.

7. Place the graduate on a level surface at eye level. Read and record the amount on the intake-output record.

8. Observe the urine for any abnormalities and report them to the charge nurse.

9. Discard the urine in a toilet and flush it.

10. Rinse out the graduate and store it properly.

11. Remove and dispose of the gloves.

12. Wash your hands.

Maintaining accurate intake and output records is an important function of the nursing assistant.

Circle the correct answer. There is only **one** *correct answer.*

1. **At dinner, Mrs. Flanagan eats soup, salad, chicken, jello, and ice cream. Which of these foods should be recorded as her fluid intake?**

    a. Only the soup.

    b. The soup and the jello.

    c. The soup, jello, and the ice cream.

    d. All of the above foods.

    e. None of the above foods.

2. **Mr. Jackson has a catheter. In monitoring intake and output of fluids, when is it best to record his fluid intake?**

    a. Three hours after drinking.

    b. At bedtime.

    c. When the liquids are brought to him.

    d. As soon as he drinks the liquids.

3. **Mrs. Johnson drinks an 8-oz. glass of milk, an 8-oz. cup of coffee, a 6-oz. glass of juice, and a 10-oz. bowl of soup. What is her total fluid intake measured in cc's? (Hint: 1000 cc's = 1 qt. = 32 oz.)**

    a. 600 cc.

    b. 750 cc.

    c. 1000 cc.

    d. 1200 cc.

4. **Perineal care is essential every time an incontinent resident is changed.**

    a. True   b. False

5. **Residents with catheters are usually not susceptible to infection.**

   a. True   (b.) False

6. **What must the nursing assistant do when caring for a female resident who has an indwelling urinary catheter?**

   (a.) Clean the area around the catheter.

   b. Apply lotion to the area where the catheter enters the urethra.

   c. Make sure the drainage tube touches the floor.

   d Retract the foreskin and apply solution.

7. **The collection bag or container should always be above the level of bladder.**

   a. True   (b.) False

8. **What is a result of decreased urinary output?**

   a. Dehydration.

   b. Infection.

   (c.) Edema.

   d. Bacteria.

9. **Abnormalities in urine are to be reported to the charge nurse.**

   (a.) True   b. False

10. **Dry lips and mucous membranes are signs of**

    a. Fluid retention.

    b. Edema.

    (c.) Dehydration.

    d. Decreased urinary output.

Chapter 47

BLADDER AND BOWEL CARE

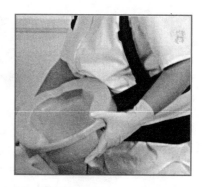

 Watch step-by-step demonstrations of the procedures discussed in this chapter in the Medcom videotape "Specimen Collection and Urinary Care" (CNA213) and "Techniques in Toileting and Incontinent Care" (CNA214).

In this chapter... you will learn about:

▶ How to assist a resident with a bedpan, urinal and commode.

▶ How to collect urine, stool, and mucus specimens.

▶ How to assist the resident with bowel and bladder training.

DEFINITIONS

Concentrated:	Containing less water.
Defecate:	Have a bowel movement.
Digestive Tract:	Body system which digests food.
Elimination:	Removal.
Emesis:	Vomit.
Respiratory:	Body system involved in breathing.
Secretion:	Fluid product released by glands.
Specimen:	Sample of body material.
Sputum:	Fluid coughed up from lungs.
Stool:	Waste material from digestive tract, feces.
Voiding:	Urinating.

BLADDER AND BOWEL CARE

Some of your residents may not be able to get out of bed to use the bathroom. They must use a bedpan or a urinal. A urinal is used by male residents to urinate. The bedpan is used by males to **defecate** and by females for both urination and defecation. The small, flat fracture pan is used for most residents, especially those who have difficulty moving following a hip fracture or for other reasons.

Elimination of waste products is a normal process. In most cultures it is also a very private function. When a resident must ask for assistance for elimination, this can be very embarrassing. You should assist the resident in a matter-of-fact manner, not reacting to the process of elimination or the odors. In this way, the resident's embarrassment will be minimized and his or her dignity preserved. The nursing assistant is responsible for providing maximum privacy for the resident during elimination.

USING THE BEDPAN

The procedure for offering the bedpan to a resident is as follows:

1. Assemble the necessary equipment: the bedpan and a cover or urinal, toilet tissue, wash cloth and a towel.

2. Explain to the resident what you are going to do, wash your hands and put on disposable gloves.

3. Provide privacy for the resident.

4. Lower the side rail.

5. Assist the resident in removing his or her lower clothing or raising it.

6. Ask the resident to bend the knees and place the feet flat on the mattress. Now ask the resident to raise the hips. If the resident needs assistance, slip your hands under the lower back and lift.

7. Place the bedpan under the resident with the seat of the bedpan evenly under the buttocks.

8. If the resident is unable to assist, turn the resident to one side and place the bedpan against the buttocks, pushing it downward into the mattress as you gently turn the resident back onto the bedpan.

9. Raise the head of the bed if this is allowed to help the resident remain in a sitting position. If the resident is not able to sit unassisted, stay with the resident and hold him or her in an upright sitting position.

10. Place a top sheet over the resident to provide privacy.

11. If the resident can be left unattended, place toilet tissue and the call light within easy reach; raise the side rails, and instruct the resident to call you when finished.

12. Dispose of the gloves and wash your hands.

13. When the resident signals, return to the room quickly. If the resident cannot signal, check frequently as the resident should never be left on a bedpan for more than 10 minutes.

14. Wash your hands and put on disposable gloves.

15. Assist the resident to raise the hips. Remove the bedpan and cover it. If the cover is not available, use a paper towel.

16. Assist the resident to wipe from front to back, if necessary, making sure that the area is clean. The resident may be turned to the side for easier cleaning.

17. Remove the bedpan and take it to the bathroom. If a specimen is required or if output must be measured, now is the time to do it.

18. Check feces and urine for blood, dark color, strange odor, mucus, or sediment. If anything abnormal is found, report it to the charge nurse.

19. Empty the bedpan into the toilet and flush it.

20. Clean the bedpan according to the established procedure in your facility.

21. Put the clean bedpan away.

22. Remove and dispose of your gloves.

23. Wash your hands.

24. Assist the resident to wash his or her hands.

25. Record the specimen collected, the output if measured, and any unusual observations.

USING THE URINAL

The procedure for offering the urinal to a resident is as follows:

1. Obtain the urinal. (If the urinal is already in the room, it may be contaminated, and you should wash your hands and put on gloves first.

2. Explain to the resident what your are going to do.

3. Provide for the resident's privacy.

4. Give the urinal to the resident or assist, if necessary, by placing the urinal between his legs with his penis inside the opening.

Chapter 47: Bladder and Bowel Care

5. If the resident can be left unattended, place the signal cord within easy reach and instruct the resident to call when finished.

6. Dispose of the gloves, wash your hands, and leave the resident to urinate in private.

7. When the resident calls, respond quickly. Residents should not be left with the urinal for more than 10 minutes.

8. If the resident cannot be left unattended, stay with the resident until finished.

9. Wash your hands and put on disposable gloves.

10. Remove the urinal, cover it, and take it into the resident's bathroom.

11. Check the urine for any unusual signs. If a specimen or output measurement is required, do it now.

12. Empty the urinal into the toilet and flush it.

13. Wash out the urinal according to procedures at your facility.

14. Replace the urinal in the bedside table.

15. Remove and dispose of your gloves.

16. Wash your hands.

17. Assist the resident with handwashing.

18. Record the specimen if collected, the output if measured, and any unusual observations.

Some residents may not be able to go to the bathroom, but may be able to transfer from the bed to a bedside commode. A commode is a chair with a hole in the seat and a bedpan attached under the hole. It is used just like a toilet, but the pan must be emptied. The procedure for using a bedside commode is as follows:

1. Assemble the necessary equipment: commode next to bed, bedpan and cover, toilet tissue.

2. Explain to the resident what you are going to do.

3. Wash your hands and put on disposable gloves.

4. Provide privacy for the resident.

5. Insert a bedpan under the seat of the commode. Lock the wheels of the commode if they have a lock.

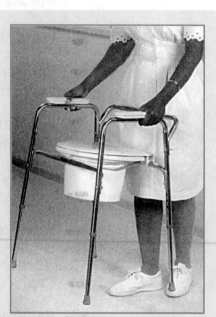

A bedside commode.

6. Help the resident sit on the edge of the bed, help him or her put on slippers, and then transfer the resident from the bed to the commode.

7. If the resident can be left unattended, place toilet tissue and the signal cord within easy reach and instruct the resident to call you when finished.

8. Dispose of your gloves, wash your hands, and leave the room.

9. If the resident cannot be left unattended, stay with the resident until finished. Never at any time use restraints with a resident on a commode.

10. When the resident calls, respond quickly. The resident should not be left on the commode longer than 10 minutes.

11. Wash your hands and put on disposable gloves. If necessary, assist the resident in wiping, using the proper direction. Be sure the area is left clean and dry.

12. Transfer the resident back into bed.

13. Remove the pan from the commode, cover it, and take it into the bathroom.

14. Check the feces and urine for abnormal color or odor, blood or mucus. If a specimen or output measurement is required, do it now.

15. Empty the pan into the toilet and flush it.

16. Clean the pan according to your facility's procedure and return it to the bedside table.

17. Remove and dispose of your gloves.

18. Wash your hands.

19. Assist the resident with handwashing.

20. Record the specimen if taken, the output if measured, and any abnormalities.

SPECIMEN COLLECTION

A specimen is a sample of body material. It can be urine, blood, feces, **sputum**, **emesis**, or wound drainage. A specimen is taken to test for abnormalities. When a specimen is required, it is the nursing assistant's responsibility to collect it.

Testing urine is a good indication of kidney function. Ideally the urine specimen should be taken in the morning from the first *voiding* of the day. This is when the urine is the most *concentrated* and abnormalities are most obvious. The amount of urine needed for a specimen is approximately 75 to 100 cc's (2-1/2 to 3-1/2 ounces).

Routine Urine Specimen

The procedure for collecting a routine urine specimen is as follows:

1. Assemble the necessary equipment: a bedpan and cover or urinal, a graduate measure, a specimen container and lid, label, disposable gloves and a paper bag.

2. Explain to the resident what you are going to do and why the specimen is necessary.

3. Wash your hands and put on disposable gloves.

4. Provide for the resident's privacy.

5. If the resident is able, have him or her collect the sample unassisted.

6. Instruct the resident to urinate in the bedpan or urinal. Ask the resident not to put toilet tissue in the bedpan, but to put it in the paper bag provided.

7. Fill in the label with the resident's name, room number, date, and the time of specimen collection.

8. Take the bedpan or urinal into the bathroom. Pour the urine into the graduate.

9. Pour urine from the graduate into the specimen container, filling it three-fourths full, if possible.

10. Place the lid and label on the container.

11. Pour the leftover urine into the toilet and flush it.

12. Wash the bedpan or urinal and graduate and put them in their proper place.

13. Remove and dispose of your gloves.

14. Wash your hands.

15 Assist the resident with handwashing.

16. Take the labeled specimen to the charge nurse or directly to the refrigerator used for lab specimens in your facility and report to your charge nurse.

17. Record the specimen collection and any abnormalities observed.

Midstream, Clean-Catch Urine Specimen

When the specimen must be free from contamination, a special method is used to collect the urine. This method is the midstream, clean-catch method. The object is to collect urine between the beginning and end of the stream, but NOT to collect urine from the first flow or the last flow. The procedure is as follows:

1. Assemble the necessary equipment: a bedpan and cover or urinal, a graduate measure, a specimen container and lid, label, disposable gloves and a paper bag.

2. Explain to the resident what you are going to do and why the specimen is necessary.

3. Wash your hands and put on disposable gloves.

4. Provide for the resident's privacy.

5. Thoroughly cleanse the genitals of a male or female resident with soap and water or an antiseptic solution.

6. Ask the resident to start voiding. After the stream has started, place the collection container under the stream and catch the necessary amount. It is better not to interrupt the stream.

Now complete the procedure by following steps seven onward from the routine urine collection procedures.

Catheter Urine Specimen

Obtaining a urine specimen from a urinary catheter is the best means of collecting a sterile sample. The urine collection container is emptied into the graduate following the instructions for Daily Catheter Care in Chapter 46. The urine is then poured into the specimen container, and the lid and label are put on. *At no time is the drainage tube to be disconnected from the catheter by the nursing assistant.*

STOOL

Stool, or feces, is waste material from the *digestive tract*. Stool specimens are taken to be examined for abnormal changes. Following is the procedure for obtaining a stool specimen:

1. Assemble the necessary equipment: a bedpan with cover, toilet tissue, a wooden tongue depressor, a specimen container with lid, a label, plastic bag and disposable gloves.

2. Explain to the resident what you are going to do and why the specimen is necessary.

3. Wash your hands and put on disposable gloves.

4. Provide for the resident's privacy.

5. Have the resident use the bedpan to have a bowel movement.

6. Write the resident's name, room number, date and the time of specimen collection on the label.

7. When the resident has finished, remove the bedpan and use the tongue depressor to transfer about two to three tablespoons of the stool to the specimen container.

8. Put the lid on the container. Wrap the soiled tongue depressor in a paper towel and discard it in a plastic bag.

9. Empty the bedpan in the toilet and flush it.

10. Wash the bedpan and put it away.

11. Remove and dispose of your gloves.

12. Wash your hands.

13. Assist the resident in handwashing.

14. Take the specimen to the charge nurse or store it until it is taken to the lab.

15. Record the taking of the specimen and any abnormalities observed in color, consistency, odor, or amount.

SPUTUM

Sputum is the substance coughed up from the lungs. It is not a **secretion** from the mouth. Sputum is collected and studied when the resident is suspected of having a **respiratory** disease. The first sputum of the morning is usually the best specimen. The amount necessary for lab tests is about four cc's (about one teaspoon). Although it is not done often, the nursing assistant may be asked to collect a sputum specimen.

The resident should be instructed to cover the mouth and nose when coughing up sputum to prevent the spread of germs. Following is the procedure for collecting a sputum specimen:

1. Be sure you have a specimen container with a lid and a label with the resident's name, room number, date, and time of specimen collection.

2. Explain to the resident what you are going to do and why the specimen is necessary.

3. Wash your hands and put on disposable gloves.

4. Provide privacy for the resident.

5. Assist the resident to sit up.

6. Instruct the resident to breathe deeply several times and then cough into the specimen container.

7. To avoid contamination, do not touch the inside of the specimen container or the inside of the lid. Cover the container and label it. Put it into a plastic bag for transportation.

8. Dispose of your gloves and wash your hands.

9. Deliver the container to the charge nurse or the refrigerator used for that purpose.

10. Record the taking of the specimen and any abnormalities observed, such as blood, thick and sticky sputum, or green color.

11. If the resident is unable to cough up sputum, notify the charge nurse.

A lot of information can be obtained from specimens regarding a resident's state of health. Proper collection of these specimens is an important function performed by the nursing assistant.

BOWEL AND BLADDER TRAINING

Sometimes it is possible to help residents regain bladder and bowel control. This not only helps the residents with a bodily function, but it also helps to restore their sense of control and good feelings about themselves.

The resident's physician and the charge nurse will develop a plan for bowel and bladder training. This plan will be in the resident's chart. Bowel and bladder training usually consists of scheduled toileting. For example, a resident might be scheduled for toileting every two hours. The most important ingredient in a bowel and bladder training program is consistency. The plan must be followed 24 hours a day by everyone providing care for the resident.

The nursing assistant can help the resident with bowel and bladder training by doing the following:

1. Encourage the resident to drink fluids. Fluid intake of approximately eight cups (about two quarts or 2000 cc's) daily provides adequate hydration for an average adult.

2. Be sure the resident eats the prescribed diet and that amounts are recorded. High fiber foods should be encouraged, if permitted.

3. Keep a log of when the resident is incontinent to help establish a toileting schedule.

4. Help the resident be as active as possible.

5. Respond immediately to the resident's call light or request to use the toilet or bedpan. DON'T MAKE THE RESIDENT WAIT.

We know that people tend to repeat behavior which is rewarded. Rewards feel good. Rewarding the incontinent resident for every positive step toward control will help the resident repeat the behavior. Positive rewards can be:

- ▶ Praise and positive reinforcements.

- ▶ Smiles.

- ▶ Hugs.

- ▶ Extra attention.

Rewards must be given immediately following the behavior to have a positive effect. Rewards must also be consistent. It is important to remember to reward the resident who is making progress. NEVER punish, shame, or scold the resident who is not making progress.

*Circle the correct answer. There is only **one** correct answer.*

1. **What is a urinal used for?**

    a. Both male and female residents urinate into it.

    b. Male residents with a hip fracture urinate into it.

    c. Female residents urinate into it.

    d. Male residents urinate into it.

    e. All residents use it for defecation.

2. **Privacy when using a bedpan or urinal is the responsibility of the resident.**

    a. True   b. False

3. **A resident can safely be left on a bedpan or commode for at least a half hour.**

    a. True   b. False

4. **Specimens you may be asked to collect include:**

    a. Tissue.

    b. Blood.

    c. Sputum.

    d. Lymph.

5. **It is best to take urine and sputum specimens**

    a. At bedtime.

    b. Before the evening meal.

    c. First thing in the morning.

    d. At noon.

6. When should you use the midstream, clean-catch method to collect urine?

   a. Every time you need a urine specimen.

   b. Every other day.

   c. When the specimen must be free from contamination.

   d. Only with residents confined to bed.

7. When obtaining a urine specimen from a urinary catheter, you should always disconnect the drainage tube from the catheter.

   a. True   b. False

8. Abnormalities observed in stool specimens include color, consistency, odor and amount.

   a. True   b. False

9. What is sputum?

   a. A substance coughed up by the lungs.

   b. A secretion from the mouth.

   c. A type of stool sample.

   d. A disease found only in elderly males.

10. Consistency and a regular schedule are important in helping a resident regain bladder and bowel control.

    a. True   b. False

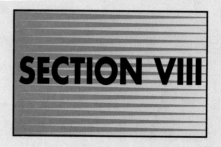

SECTION VIII

PSYCHOSOCIAL ISSUES

Chapter 48

UNDERSTANDING BEHAVIOR

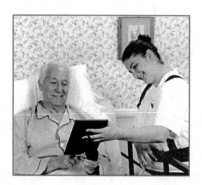

In this chapter... you will learn about:

▶ What affects a resident's behavior.

▶ How you can influence a resident's behavior.

DEFINITIONS

Behavior:	Action that can be observed and measured.
Depression:	Feelings of sadness, dejection, worthlessness, helplessness, or hopelessness. Depression may be symptomatic of a mental or physical condition, or part of syndrome of related symptoms associated with a particular disease, such as diabetes or thyroid abnormalities.
Economic Depression (the Great Depression):	A period in the 1930s when banks failed and many families lost their homes, jobs and possessions.
Hierarchy:	A form of order in which items are arranged from lower to higher.
Hoarding:	Gathering and saving things in a guarded or hidden place.

Behavior refers to the actions of people that can be observed or measured. There are many reasons why people conduct themselves as they do. Some of these reasons are:

▶ *Self-esteem.* How worthwhile a person feels.

▶ *Beliefs.* What a person believes in.

▶ *Patterns of behavior.* The ways a person learned to behave as a child.

▶ *Personal value system.* What a person sees as important, based on beliefs about what is proper or decent behavior.

▶ *Judgement or Ethics.* What a person sees as right and wrong.

▶ *Culture.* How people in the person's national or ethnic background expect the person to act.

▶ *Life experience.* Everything that has happened to the person.

▶ *Needs.* The person's need for approval, independence, and a sense of belonging.

▶ *Motives.* What the person hopes to gain.

Behavior is rarely simple. At any one time several or all of these factors are interacting to cause a resident's behavior. No two people are alike. Older people are especially different from one another. They have lived a long time and have had many different experiences. All these experiences affect behavior.

The person who lived through the **economic depression** of the 1930s may view money and security very differently from a younger person who did not have this life experience. What appears to be stinginess and **hoarding** may be a logical response to memories of the past and fears of another economic depression. In order to influence your residents' behavior, you must first try to understand why they act as they do.

＊ acaparamiento

You should get to know the residents as people. Learn about their beliefs, cultures, and personal value systems. Learn about their life histories and what they want now, and learn what will make them happy. Sometimes if you offer a simple greeting or show interest in a resident's past, you can change the resident's entire outlook and make him or her much happier.

Maslow's Hierarchy of Needs

In order to help understand behavior, a psychologist named Abraham Maslow developed a simple order, or **hierarchy**, of human needs. He divided our needs into five broad groups, and he argued that people had to satisfy the most basic needs first—physical needs for food, water and air. Only then could they try to satisfy higher needs.

- ▶ *Basic needs.* The physiological needs for food, water, air, and shelter. → Refugio
- ▶ *Security and Safety.* The need to feel safe and have enough money to go on living.
- ▶ *Love or belonging.* The need to love or to be part of a friendly social group.
- ▶ *Self-esteem.* The psychological need to respect yourself and have others respect you.
- ▶ *Self-actualization.* The psychological need to feel successful, to be all that you can be.

Dealing with Loss

One of the life experiences of all people who live to old age is loss. It may be the loss of health, independence, job, friends, or a spouse. One normal reaction to loss is anger. Losing something you value or someone you love makes you angry. The resident needs to be able to express this normal anger without being made to feel guilty. Another normal reaction to loss is sadness or grief. You mourn for what is lost. **Depression** is a part of grief. Depressed residents may lose interest in the world around them. They may experience a loss of appetite, lack energy and motivation, have difficulties sleeping or sleep for extremely long periods of time. New residents in long-term care are often angry and or depressed over the loss of their independence.

* duelo → grief
   Llorar → mourn.
   Faita → lack

Dependence

Overly dependent behavior may be the result of the culture's expectation of dependence in old people. By being dependent, the older person is doing what is expected. Dependent people may also be afraid that no one will be there to help them if they appear to be independent. This may be their way of asking for affection or trying to keep someone caring for them.

The resident's relatives may be encouraging the resident to behave in a dependent manner. They may feel guilty about placing the person in a long-term care facility. This guilt may cause them to try to do too much for the resident and may be reinforcing tendencies to dependent behavior. They expect the resident to be dependent.

Refuerzo

elogiar

One way to respond to this is to point out and praise the resident's independent behavior when the relatives are present. This will gently reinforce the importance of letting the resident be more independent, and it may serve as a "model" they can follow for their own behavior. It is also important to reinforce and compliment the family on their positive attention and help to the resident, such as coming to visit, gifts, and telephone calls.

Stubbornness

Stubbornness may really be a fear of doing things differently. The fear of not being able to handle changes is common as the resident feels less able to cope. Familiar routines feel safer.

Hacer frente a
enfrentar

Low Self-esteem

Residents with low self-esteem, who don't see themselves as important any more, may become extremely demanding. The response to these demands tells the residents they are important enough to receive attention. These residents need constant reinforcement to feel worthwhile. -) Vale la pena

Expectations

Expectations also influence behavior. People tend to behave in ways that others expect them to behave. This is often referred to as a "self-fulfilling prophecy." This means that by expecting a certain kind of behavior, even if we don't like it, we may actually end up encouraging a person to behave that way. We communicate our expectations by what we say, how we say it, facial expressions, touch, and attitude. If you always expect positive behavior from your residents, that is what you will usually get.

Coping with Losses

Residents in long-term care facilities may be coping with many losses: the loss of health, mobility, or independence. They focus most of their energy and interest on themselves. This may make them appear selfish and self-centered; however, this focus is often necessary in being able to cope with these changes. As the residents becomes more secure and adapted to this new environment, the nursing assistant can help them direct some of this focus outward toward others and other activities.

Making an effort to know your residents and trying to put yourself in their place will help you understand their behavior. Always remember that the residents are just people, like yourself, who may have been through many severe losses and painful experiences. Coming to a long-term care facility can be very frightening. Many residents are facing the fact that they have entered the last stage of their lives, and they may never be able to leave the facility again.

When you understand these fears and how they affect behavior, you can begin to help your residents behave in more positive, productive ways.

*Circle the correct answer. There is only **one** correct answer.*

1. **Self-esteem, culture, and patterns of behavior are some reasons why people behave as they do.**

    ⓐ. True   b. False

2. **In order to influence residents' behavior, you must first ignore the reasons for the behavior.**

    a. True   ⓑ. False

3. **An experience that is common among older residents is:**

    a. Stubbornness and rage.
    b. Extreme dependence.
    ⓒ Loss.
    d. Happiness.

4. **Anger and depression are common reactions to loss.**

    ⓐ. True   b. False

5. **Overly dependent behavior may be the result of the culture's expectation of older people.**

    ⓐ. True   b. False

6. **Residents who have just entered a long-term care facility are usually happy and rarely angry or depressed.**

    a. True   ⓑ. False

7. **Stubbornness could really be a fear of doing things differently.**

    ⓐ. True   b. False

8. **How are expectations communicated?**

    a. By what we say and nothing else.

    b. By the way we say things but not what we say.

    c. By our facial expressions but not what we say.

    d. By our whole manner and what we say.

9. **Mr. Howell's daughter and son-in-law are constantly doing things for him, so much so that he is dependent on them and everyone else in the care facility. What can the nursing assistant do to encourage Mr. Howell's independence?**

    a. Praise his dependent behavior in the family's presence.

    b. Discourage the family from visiting or calling.

    c. Reinforce the importance of letting him be more independent in the family's presence.

    d. Never doing anything for Mr. Howell.

10. **Because they may be coping with many losses, residents in long- term care facilities focus most of their energy and interest on _____.**

    a. Their families.

    b. Themselves.

    c. Staff members.

    d. Visitors.

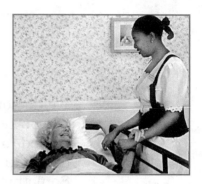

Chapter 49

REMOTIVATION

In this chapter... you will learn about:

▶ What remotivation is.

▶ How to help remotivate a resident.

DEFINITIONS

Motivated:	Having a reason for doing something.
Positive Reinforcement:	Compliments or rewards for doing something.
Remotivated:	Give a reason for doing something again.
Self-esteem:	Feelings about oneself.

We do something because we are **motivated** to do it. We have a reason for doing it. Motivated means urged on or moved to do something. If what we do makes us feel good or produces a reward, we are motivated to do it again. Something extra done for a resident is often rewarded with a smile and sincere thanks. When you feel good about what you have done and want to do it again, you are remotivated.

Residents who have lost the strength and ability to do many of the things they used to do easily will often feel this loss as failure. They will be reluctant to do things. They will not be motivated to do things because failure doesn't feel good. When these residents again have the desire to do things, we say they are **remotivated**, or motivated again.

Helping Remotivate Residents

The resident care plan will list the remotivation goals for each resident. The entire healthcare team should become aware of these goals so that everyone can strive toward the remotivation of the resident.

The nursing assistant has many opportunities each day to remotivate residents. The goal may be for the resident to attend the activity program at the facility. This is a big goal for a resident who appears not to be interested in even talking to others. The nursing assistant should think in terms of smaller goals which would lead toward accomplishing the larger goal.

How you feel about yourself is called **self-esteem**. Residents cannot be motivated to interact with others until they feel good about themselves. Many times during the day, the nursing assistant has the opportunity to raise a resident's self-esteem with compliments. Compliments must always be sincere. This should not be difficult as everyone has accomplishments, traits, and objects worthy of a compliment. A resident may have beautiful eyes, a new hair style, a colorful robe, a caring family, some fresh flowers. Noticing and commenting on these things helps make the resident feel worthwhile and important. Attention and approval are powerful motivators.

Get to know your residents. You may find much about their past that interests you, and this in turn will help you find new ways to compliment them. Your interest and concern by itself may help remotivate someone who feels cut off from life.

Positive reinforcement means noticing and praising each step toward a goal and ignoring failures. All of us respond to praise. Praise motivates us to keep trying. On the other hand, being scolded or shamed makes us not want to try again. A resident should never be scolded, shamed, or made to feel worthless. To motivate, praise the positive and ignore the negative.

Setting Goals

Set small goals that lead to bigger ones. A small goal may be simply to get the resident to smile. A smile is a sign of a good feeling even if just for that moment. If you are interested in the resident and convey this interest with positive comments as you go about the daily routine, the reaction from the resident may be a smile. The resident will feel better and so will you when you see a small goal being met.

The next small goal may be for residents to express a positive comment about themselves. If you express positive comments about them, they will begin to see themselves in a more positive way and may express this.

A further small goal might be to have the resident express interest in another resident. By routinely mentioning other residents in a positive way, you may stimulate some interest in others. The next step may be assisting a resident to visit with another resident. Eventually, you may be able to remotivate the resident to attend an activity.

The big goal, at the end of all your small goals, may then be to get the resident to participate in the activity.

It is important to remember that remotivation takes place in small steps and cannot be rushed. You must be patient in your efforts to remotivate residents. Appreciating and celebrating each small step taken are the rewards for progressing toward a bigger goal. They are also what motivates the resident and yourself to continue the process.

It is important to realize that the goals of remotivation may begin with the smallest of tasks, such as brushing the teeth or learning to comb the hair again, and progress to very large goals, such as relearning to ambulate.

*Circle the correct answer. There is only **one** correct answer.*

1. **A resident who has lost the strength and ability to easily perform everyday activities may be reluctant to attempt tasks independently.**

    a. True   b. False

2. **How can the nursing assistant help improve the resident's self esteem?**

    a. With compliments and praise.
    b. By insisting the resident talk to other residents.
    c. By scolding the resident.
    d. By setting very large goals immediately.

3. **In order to motivate a resident, it's okay for the nursing assistant to point out the resident's mistakes.**

    a. True   b. False

4. **Success in small goals motivates the resident to continue to strive for larger goals.**

    a. True   b. False

5. **Which of the following is an example of a large goal of remotivation?**

    a. Giving a smile.
    b. Relearning to ambulate.
    c. Saying hello to another resident.
    d. Opening the eyes.

6. **Everyone has accomplishments, traits, and possessions worthy of a compliment.**

    a. True   b. False

7. **How is remotivation best accomplished?**

    a. Quickly.
    b. In big steps.
    c. In small steps.
    d. When unassisted.

8. **Remotivation is the sole responsibility of the nursing assistant.**

    a. True   b. False

9. **When a resident has the desire to do things again, the resident is**

    a. Weak.
    b. A failure.
    c. Motivated.
    d. Remotivated.

10. **Positive reinforcement means ignoring failure and noticing and praising one's steps toward goals.**

    a. True   b. False

Chapter 50

PSYCHOSOCIAL NEEDS

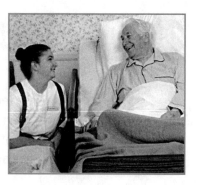

In this chapter... you will learn about:

▶ The resident's psychosocial needs.
▶ Your responsibility in meeting these needs.

DEFINITIONS

Anxiety: A feeling of worry or uneasiness.

Depression: Feelings of sadness or hopelessness.

Orient: Helping the resident to become familiar with people, place and time.

Psychosocial: An individual's mental or emotional processes which are used to interact with others.

Reminiscences: Recalling past experiences or events.

PSYCHOSOCIAL NEEDS

Basic needs are common to all of us, including residents in long-term care facilities. We have discussed physical needs in Chapter 30. Everyone also has **psychosocial** needs. These include needing to feel:

▶ Loved and appreciated.

▶ Approved of and respected.

▶ A sense of accomplishment.

▶ Recognized as an individual.

▶ Worthwhile and important.

At every age these needs have to be filled. When older people enter a long-term care facility, they face many losses and changes which may make it difficult to fulfill these needs. For example, most residents are losing the role of being an independent person. They may no longer have a job or a function. The ability to come and go at will is lost, and the familiarity of home and family is gone. The residents must often share a room and bathroom with strangers, depend on others for daily functions, and eat and sleep when told. The purpose and direction of their lives have changed.

Anxiety and Depression

Most residents go through a period of **anxiety** and **depression** after being admitted to a long-term care facility. The nursing assistant can help the resident overcome these feelings by being understanding, helping the resident become comfortable in the new surroundings, and respecting and appreciating the resident as an individual.

Some ways the nursing assistant can help the resident overcome feelings of anxiety and depression and fill psychosocial needs are:

- **Orient** the resident to the facility. Explain the schedule, introduce staff and other residents, and help new residents find their way around the facility. Particular care should be taken to help roommates become acquainted.

- Give the resident your full attention when giving care. Listen and respond to the resident. Take the resident's comments seriously and do not pass them off lightly. Ask questions, but do not pry into anyone's personal life if this makes a resident uncomfortable.

- Accept the resident's feelings even if they are negative. The resident may have good reason to feel negative. You can respond with statements which accept the resident's feelings as real. For example: "You must feel rather lost right now. I'll help you get to know your new neighbors here." Accept the feelings, but then offer some hope.

- Don't respond with phrases such as "You shouldn't feel that way," or "Everything is going to be just fine." Also, don't say "I understand," because you cannot understand unless you have been an older person and have lived in a long-term care facility.

- Always address the resident by name. Use Mr. Smith or Mrs. Jones unless the resident has given permission to use the first name, and never use nicknames such as "honey," or "sweetie." This shows you recognize and respect the resident as an individual. Remember the resident's personal interests, likes and dislikes, and the names of family members. You can then make your conversation with the resident more personal and individualized.

- Respond quickly to the resident's requests for assistance. Making a resident wait suggests that the resident is unimportant.

- Encourage steps toward increased independence and trying new things. The more independent residents are, the greater their self-esteem will be. Praise each success, no matter how small, and overlook failures.

- Help the resident be well groomed each day. A good appearance will help the resident feel worthwhile.

- Whenever possible, allow residents to make their own choices and decisions. This increases a sense of control over their own life.

- Give care in a calm, caring manner. Remember that it can be difficult to become dependent on someone else for your activities of daily living. Make the situation as comfortable as possible with a kind, considerate, matter-of-fact manner.

- A gentle voice and a gentle touch convey a sense of warmth and care. Holding a resident's hand and a gentle hug convey affection and caring. But be sensitive to personal and cultural feelings. Some residents may not want to be touched or may not feel comfortable being touched by someone they have just met.

- Respect the resident's privacy. Closing the door or pulling the curtains whenever you are going to provide care shows respect.

- Listen to and be interested in a resident's *reminiscences*. These memories are saying that he or she was once independent and important. Reminiscing helps older people come to terms with their life experiences.

- Encourage residents to form friendships and to participate in appropriate activities. Being interested in others and in activities is a sign that depression and anxiety are lessening.

These are just some of the ways to meet the psychosocial needs of your residents. You will find many more as you strive to understand each residents and his or her particular needs. If you treat all resident as you would like to be treated, you will be meeting their psychosocial needs to the best of your ability.

*Circle the correct answer. There is only **one** correct answer.*

1. **We all have psychosocial needs for love and appreciation, approval and respect, and recognition.**

    a. True   b. False

2. **Very few residents go through periods of anxiety and depression after being admitted to a long-term care facility.**

    a. True   b. False

3. **Mrs. Goodwin is a new resident in a long-term care facility. What can the nursing assistant do to help her feel comfortable in her new surroundings?**

    a. Introduce her to staff and other residents.
    b. Keep her waiting for care.
    c. Address her by a nickname.
    d. Tell her you understand how she feels.

4. **Pointing out a resident's failures helps him or her become more independent.**

    a. True   b. False

5. **A resident entering a long-term care facility _____.**

    a. Should not feel depressed.
    b. Should not be allowed to make choices and decisions.
    c. Has lost the familiarity of home and family.
    d. No longer needs be concerned about personal appearance.

6. **Care should be taken to help roommates become acquainted.**

    a. True   b. False

7. **Residents should be talked out of any negative feelings.**

    a. True   b. False

8. **When assisting a resident who is being difficult, the nursing assistant should maintain a kind, considerate manner and give full attention.**

    a. True   b. False

9. **Residents should be discouraged from reminiscing and should focus instead on what's going on now.**

    a. True   b. False

10. **If you treat all residents as you would like to be treated, you will be meeting their psychosocial needs as best you can.**

    a. True   b. False

Chapter 51

SOCIALIZATION NEEDS

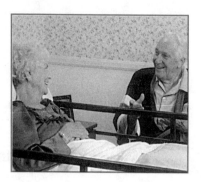

In this chapter... you will learn about:

▶ The resident's socialization needs.

▶ Your responsibility in caring for the resident's socialization needs.

DEFINITIONS

Gregarious:	Outgoing and talkative.
Initiate:	Start.
Socialization:	Interacting with people.

We all have a need to interact with other people every day. This is called **socialization**. Socialization provides us with:

▶ Information.

▶ Ideas.

▶ Support.

▶ Affection.

▶ Stimulation.

Talking with other people helps us stay aware of what is happening around us and in the world and exposes us to new ideas to think about. This stimulation helps keep minds active and relieves boredom.

Giving and receiving affection and appreciation is an important part of socialization. Concern for someone else and having the concern returned makes us feel good. This good feeling helps us like ourselves and feel good about who we are. When a resident is interacting with and helping someone else, that resident will feel better.

How Socialization Needs are Met

In long-term care facilities, the need to interact with others can be met in many different ways. It can be met with family and friends who visit and with staff and other residents who share the resident's environment. The interaction can be simply a conversation or friendly visit, or it can be sharing a hobby or craft project, a TV program or a book read, or just a quiet moment. Socialization doesn't have to be an action; it can also mean just being together.

Everyone has a different way of socializing. This depends on personality, life experiences, interests, age, and state of health. Entering a long-term care facility means the person's life is changing in many ways. The person no longer lives among family and friends, but among strangers. The relationships with family and friends can remain, but they are changed. The resident must wait for visits and is no longer able to **initiate** them.

The physical changes that often occur with age may affect a resident's ability and opportunity to socialize. A decrease in the ability to ambulate limits a person's opportunities for socialization. A hearing loss may prevent normal conversation or the noise from a group may be irritating. The ability to participate in projects and programs may be decreased by a vision loss. These physical changes may necessitate finding new ways to meet socialization needs.

Role Changes

Our roles in life provide many rewards such as affection, appreciation, and admiration. Remember that the role of spouse, parent, or grandparent is lost or greatly changed when a person becomes a resident. With this change, some of the rewards are lost. New ways must be found to fulfill socialization needs. We will discuss role changes in more detail in the next chapter.

How the Nursing Assistant Can Help

In order to help the residents, the nursing assistant will need to get to know the residents, their previous lifestyles, occupations, family names and relationships, interests, and hobbies. Only by understanding the residents can the nursing assistant plan the care to meet their needs.

There is no one right way to meet socialization needs. Residents who have always been quiet and private will usually not find their socialization needs met in large groups of people, while the more **gregarious** residents may find the group just what they need. When you know your residents, you can help develop plans to meet their socialization needs. Following are some ways you can encourage appropriate social interaction among residents:

- Encourage socialization, but don't insist on it or push it. Introduce residents who are sitting together. Even if they have met before, mention their names in case they have forgotten. Suggest visits with other residents. Offer to take residents to social functions or group activities in the facility. Tell residents they may leave the activity if they wish. Then be sure someone is there to assist them if they do wish to leave and they need assistance.

- Support family relationships. Show interest in and make positive comments about the resident's family. This is the resident's major support system. If residents are able, encourage them to call or write to family members. When families visit, a friendly greeting and a positive comment about the resident are important.

- Encourage residents to keep previous friendships. Remind the residents of friends who visit or write. Help the residents call or write to friends.

- Preserve as much as possible of the resident's previous lifestyle. Family pictures and familiar objects help residents preserve their identity and provide opportunities for conversation.

- Help roommates get to know each other. It is very difficult to share a room with a stranger, but sharing with a friend can be very rewarding. Help them to find common interests and experiences.

Although we all have many of the same needs for socialization with family and friends, we fulfill them in many different ways. The nursing assistant's responsibility is to know the residents and then help them fulfill their socialization needs. The goal is to make each resident feel appreciated, needed, and worthwhile.

*Circle the correct answer. There is only **one** correct answer.*

1. **Socialization provides information, affection and stimulation.**

    a. True   b. False

2. **Socialization does not require other people.**

    a. True   b. False

3. **How can the need to interact with others in a long-term care facility be met?**

    a. By doing hobbies or crafts.
    b. By watching TV alone.
    c. By reading alone.
    d. By staying in bed.

4. **When residents enter a long-term care facility, changes in roles and relationships may affect their socialization.**

    a. True   b. False

5. **What physical changes that may occur with age could affect the resident's way of socializing?**

    a. Hearing loss.
    b. Vision loss.
    c. Decreased ability to ambulate.
    d. All of the above changes.
    e. None of the above changes.

6. **It is helpful for socialization if the nursing assistant knows**

    a. A resident's blood pressure.
    b. A resident's family names and relationships.
    c. A resident's pulse rate.
    d. None of the above.

7. There's only one right way to meet a resident's socialization needs.

    a. True   (b.) False

8. In order to help residents socialize, the nursing assistant should not encourage the maintenance of previous relationships.

    a. True   (b.) False

9. Which of the following describes an appropriate way to encourage socialization among residents?

    a. Try not to talk about resident's families.
    b. Insist that residents learn a new skill that they have never tried.
    (c.) Suggest that residents visit with other residents.
    d. Tell residents to forget about their previous lifestyles.

10. Unless the nursing assistant understands the residents, it will be difficult to help develop care plans for their socialization.

    (a.) True   b. False

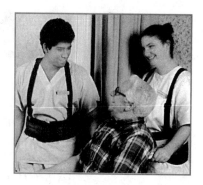

Chapter 52

INTERVENTION AND SUBSTANCE ABUSE

In this chapter... you will learn about:

▶ Some resident behaviors that cause problems.
▶ How to intervene to change these behaviors.

DEFINITIONS

Alcoholism:	A condition in which a person cannot stop drinking alcohol.
Apathy:	A feeling of indifference or lack of emotion.
Hallucinations:	Seeing things, such as monsters, that aren't there.
Manipulative:	Trying to manage another's behavior.
Oriented:	Able to accurately describe who you are, and the time and place.

PROBLEM BEHAVIORS

It is normal for you to have different feelings about individual residents. Some residents may make you angry, some may make you happy, while others may hurt your feelings. These are natural feelings, but it is important not to let them interfere with quality care for every resident. It is never appropriate to express your anger or hurt feelings, either verbally or physically, to the resident. If you cannot control your feelings, you should leave the room until you can. Talking with a coworker may help you regain control.

As a nursing assistant you can help your residents change inappropriate behavior by the way in which you respond to them. Once you understand why residents behave in a certain way, you can begin to help them change their negative behaviors into positive ones. The way in which you respond to the resident will either reinforce the behavior and cause it to happen again or help eliminate the behavior. We all tend to repeat actions which produce the results we want. If stomping your foot always gets the attention you want, you will continue to stomp. If everyone ignores the stomp, you will soon look for another way to get attention.

INTERVENTION

Following are some characteristic problem behaviors of residents and ways in which you can respond in order to help the resident change the behavior. Some other behaviors that are characteristic of residents with dementia or Alzheimer's Disease will be discussed in Chapter 54.

Apathy

The resident who wants to stay in bed or sits alone and stares at the wall is said to be withdrawn or suffering from **apathy**. These residents are quiet and easily overlooked. This resident needs a great deal of love. The best approach is one of active friendliness. Seek these residents out and give them attention. Praise each small step toward independence. Sincere compliments and attention help to rebuild confidence and trust.

Anxiety, Suspicion

Fear causes some residents to be anxious and suspicious. Being actively friendly with a frightened or suspicious resident may only increase the problem. A feeling of security needs to be established. This is best done by letting the person know you care and offering help, but not pushing things on the resident. Let the resident request your help.

Manipulation

Some people have lifelong patterns of **manipulative** behavior. They have found this gets them what they want. The manipulative person usually uses your desire to help, making you feel guilty to achieve his or her goals. Matter-of-factness is the best approach for this type of behavior.

Some residents who are capable of propelling themselves in their wheelchairs may prefer to be dependent because it is easier and it gets attention. They may sit in their wheelchairs looking helpless, hoping someone will push them. Since most people want to be helpful, someone will probably come along and push them where they want to go. They have manipulated that person. The nursing assistant should encourage the residents to propel their wheelchairs on their own and reward this independent behavior with praise.

You must make it clear what you will do and what you will not do. It is best not to reward manipulative behavior by letting yourself be manipulated.

Depression

Depression is the most common mental illness among older residents. It is often justified considering the extent of loss as one ages. However, when it interferes with a resident's daily activities, firm kindness must be used. You must be willing to listen to a depressed resident's negative feelings but be firm in insisting that he or she get up, get dressed, and eat. Depressed residents often need you to take the initiative.

Uncooperativeness

Some residents refuse to do what you ask. Saying no may be the only way they have of exerting some control over their lives. Rather than arguing and insisting, find other ways for these residents to make decisions about their care, such as what clothes to wear, or whether the drapes are open or closed. Gaining some control over small areas of their lives may make these residents more cooperative.

Combativeness

The resident who strikes out is expressing fear and anger at the situation. Insisting that the combative resident do something will only increase the fear and anger. The best approach is one of making very few demands. If the resident strikes out at you, move away. Attempting to restrain the resident may only make things worse. Speak in a calm voice to sooth the resident. Attempts to restrain should only be made if residents might harm themselves or others. If the resident feels no pressure, the fear and anger may disappear.

The only demands that are absolutely necessary are the following:

- Residents cannot be allowed to harm others or themselves.

- Residents must take their medications.

- Residents cannot leave the facility.

Confusion may be temporary or permanent. Often, the trauma of becoming a resident causes temporary confusion. After a period of adjustment, the resident will again be alert and **oriented**. Other residents may be suffering from chronic or permanent confusion. The confused resident may appear absentminded, and forgetful, and may tend to wander. The resident's conversation may make no sense to you. Most confused people are anxious and frightened. A calm, friendly approach works best with confused residents. You will learn more about dealing with confusion in Chapter 54.

Residents act the way they do for many reasons--not just to frustrate you. Don't take the behavior personally, but adapt your response to help the resident learn appropriate behavior. None of these changes will occur in one day; but if you consistently respond appropriately, change will happen. For all residents, kindness, respect, and courtesy are always appropriate responses.

SUBSTANCE ABUSE AND ALCOHOLISM

You may find any kind of substance abuse in residents of any age. It is probably most common, however, to find younger residents using illegal drugs such as marijuana and cocaine, and older residents abusing alcohol. Many different substances can be abused. Some substances, such as alcohol, barbiturates, tranquilizers or heroin, cause relaxation and drowsiness. Other substances, such as cocaine and Methedrine, tend to cause excitement and agitation. Still other substances, such as marijuana and LSD, can cause disorientation and **hallucinations**. Even over-the-counter medications such as antihistamines can be abused, as can simple substances such as the caffeine in coffee, tea, or medications.

You should stay alert for any signs of substance abuse. Some of these signs are:

- ▶ Sudden changes in behavior or sleeping habits

- ▶ Unexplained drowsiness

- ▶ Rapid speech or behavior

- ▶ Mood swings or angry outbursts

- ▶ The odor of alcohol

- ▶ Forgetfulness

Many of these signs can also indicate a medical condition, or a change in psychological health. If you notice any sign of possible substance abuse, you should report it to the charge nurse or physician immediately.

Drug Abuse

About 25% of all teenagers admit trying an illegal substance at some time. You shouldn't assume that because a teenage resident is in an institution, illegal drugs are impossible to get. Friends or family members can easily sneak illegal substances into the facility for the person.

If you suspect substance abuse in a resident or a coworker, you must report it to your supervisor. Try to remain sympathetic and helpful, even if you have had bad experiences with substance abuse by a friend or someone in your family. Help is available for the person.

It is especially important to discover substance abuse quickly because many substances can cause dangerous reactions when mixed with prescribed medications that the resident may be taking. For example, alcohol can increase the effects of anticonvulsants, anticoagulants, and antidiabetic drugs. You should watch carefully for extreme reactions to any of those medications.

About two-thirds of the population over 65 use alcohol in some amount, and about 15% of them are subject to **alcoholism**. Something in the person's brain or nervous system makes it nearly impossible to stop drinking once they start. Because so many people use alcohol in small amounts to relax, some people do not take alcohol abuse seriously. However, it can be a very serious problem.

If you suspect that a resident or a coworker is abusing alcohol, report it to your supervisor. As with other forms of substance abuse, help is available. Organizations such as Alcoholics Anonymous can help a person stop abusing alcohol. And you can take steps to make sure alcohol is not available to a resident and help the person overcome any depression or fear they experience as they try to quit.

*Circle the correct answer. There is only **one** correct answer.*

1. **It is appropriate to express anger or hurt feelings to your residents.**

    a. True   b. False

2. **Actions that do not get the results we want are usually**

    a. Repeated.
    b. Oriented.
    c. Eliminated.
    d. Reinforced.

3. **Withdrawal, suspicion, and manipulation are some characteristic behaviors of residents.**

    a. True   b. False

4. **In dealing with the manipulative person, what approach works best?**

    a. Let the resident take the initiative.
    b. Reward the resident.
    c. Have a matter-of-fact attitude.
    d. Active friendliness.

5. **Mr. Watson is capable of propelling his own wheelchair, but he is constantly asking you to do it for him. What should you do?**

    a. Push him wherever he wants.
    b. Ignore him.
    c. Ask another resident to push him.
    d. Encourage him to push himself and praise him when he does.

6. **How should the nursing assistant respond when caring for a depressed resident who refused to get up or eat?**

    a. Let the resident take the initiative.
    b. Scold the resident.
    c. Restrain the resident.
    d. Use firm kindness.

7. **What is the best approach in dealing with the combative resident?**

    a. Be very demanding.
    b. Make few demands.
    c. Restraint.
    d. Manipulation.

8. **If you suspect substance abuse in a resident you must:**

    a. Search their belongings.
    b. Tell another resident.
    c. Report it to your supervisor.
    d. Ignore it and let them sleep it off.

9. **Confusion may be either temporary or permanent.**

    a. True   b. False

10. **For all residents, kindness, respect, and courtesy are always appropriate responses.**

    a. True   b. False

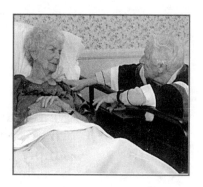

Chapter 53

ROLE CHANGES

In this chapter... you will learn about:

- ▶ Roles in life.
- ▶ How a change of roles can affect a resident.
- ▶ How the nursing assistant can help the adjustment to new roles.

DEFINITIONS

Nurturing:	Caring for others.
Positive Reinforcement:	Noticing and making positive comments about desired behavior.
Role:	The part one plays in relationships with others.
Traumatic:	Shocking and painful.

We relate to others in different ways depending on the **role** we are assuming. This doesn't mean we are playacting; it simply means we are behaving the way we are expected to behave in a certain situation. Each day we play many different roles depending on who we are, what we are doing, and who we are with. For example, a woman may be in the role of mother one minute while she is talking to her child and then she may turn to her husband and play the role of wife and a minute later turn to her sister and play a third role, that of sister.

Roles are determined by:

► *Gender.* Gender roles are changing, but many older people grew up during a time when women were expected to be dependent and **nurturing** and men were supposed to be independent and strong.

► *Age.* Toddlers are expected to be curious, active, and always into things. Adults are expected to be independent, conscientious, and serious. We often expect the older resident to be quiet, slow, and dependent.

► *Relationship.* When we are with our parents, we are children. When we are with our children, we are parents. At the same time we can be brothers, sisters, cousins, aunts, uncles, husbands, wives, and friends.

► *Occupation.* What we do to earn a living or prepare to do so is another role. Right now you are students; hopefully, you will soon be certified nursing assistants.

► *Special Interests.* Many of us are members of organizations and groups, such as church, PTA, Sierra Club, or bowling team. Being a member is also a role. Hobbies and talents can include roles, such as biker, jogger, musician, or artist.

► *Illness.* While illness or good health are physical conditions, based on the presence of disease or other conditions, these facts also affect our psychology. Those who see themselves in the role of a "sick person" will tend to become dependent, weak, feel useless, lack responsibility, and often become passive. Those who see themselves as a "well person" tend to be independent, responsible, feel more useful, and make their own decisions.

Some roles are fixed (female, child, adult) while others are chosen and can be changed (wife, parent, student, swimmer). Knowing how we are to act in each role helps us shift from one role to another quickly and easily. If we had to stop and figure out how a student acts every time we went to class, we would have little time for studying. Roles not only help us know how to act, but roles also tell others how to respond to us. Roles help life move more smoothly.

ROLE CHANGES

Roles constantly change. We get older, change jobs, have grandchildren, try new hobbies. When too many changes occur at one time, confusion often results. And when roles change against our will, sadness and depression can result. This is often what happens when a person enters a long-term care facility.

Relationships change. The resident is no longer the parent who takes care of children, but the elderly parent who must be cared for, often by the children. The roles of spouse, friend, and companion also change. The occupational role has probably ended and many special interests can no longer be pursued.

There is another very important role change for many residents. Many of them may have gone from being people who saw themselves as "healthy and independent" to people who see themselves as "sick" or "handicapped." The role change from independent to dependent is very **traumatic**. This is not a chosen role, and it is one that is difficult to accept. The new resident may be depressed, angry, confused, and disoriented in the new surrounding, trying to fill the new role. It takes much time, understanding, and care to adjust and accept the role of resident.

How the Nursing Assistant Can Help

By knowing each resident and the many different roles that particular resident has had throughout life, you will be better able to understand and help in the new role changes. Stop for a moment and imagine the position of a man who was a good student in high school and then college, a world traveler, then a husband and father, a journalist, then a newspaper editor, then a respected teacher to young reporters, then a grandfather surrounded by loving grandchildren. Now, after that long and eventful life, this man may have lost his wife and home and see himself as little more than a sick, tired, dependent old man. This can be a very traumatic role change.

If you realize how difficult these role changes are, you will be able to understand the confusion or anger that many residents express. The anger is not directed at you, but at the situation over which they feel they have no control. By listening to the anger and frustration the residents express, you will be helping them work through that anger.

The residents who are depressed or lonely can be helped by showing genuine concern and interest. Learn who they are and what they have done in their lives. Sincere compliments, **positive reinforcement**, and encouragement of independence are the best care plan. It is important to reinforce well behavior. Those who are sick receive much care and attention. If we want them to continue toward wellness, we must also give attention and positive reinforcement to well behaviors, such as dressing or shaving themselves, walking, or even smiling. Residents who are disabled but not sick should be treated just like any other well residents within the limits of their disability.

Our behavior is influenced by the varied roles we have. The nursing assistant should help the residents work, as much as possible, toward the well role of independence and control over their own lives.

Circle the correct answer. There is only **one** *correct answer.*

1. **Role playing refers to playacting.**

    a. True   b. False *(circled)*

2. **Gender, relationship, and occupation are some ways roles are determined.**

    a. True *(circled)*   b. False

3. **Which of the following is an example of a fixed role?**

    a. Student.
    b. Mystery reader.
    c. Male. *(circled)*
    d. Well person. *(circled)*

4. **The roles of teacher, artist, and nurse are all**

    a. Chosen. *(circled)*
    b. Assigned.
    c. Traumatic.
    d. Nurturing.

5. **Both Mrs. Martin and Mrs. Stewart, who are residents, love to knit and spend hours knitting homemade gifts for family and friends. In their facility these ladies are known as "the knitters." How are their roles determined?**

    a. By age.
    b. By gender.
    c. By occupation.
    d. By special interests. *(circled)*

6. **Roles are constantly changing.**

    a. True *(circled)*   b. False

7. **How would you describe a person's role change from being well to becoming handicapped?**

   a. Occupational.
   b. Fixed.
   c. Traumatic.
   d. Nurturing.

8. **Relationships never change.**

   a. True   b. False

9. **The best way to help an angry residents is to listen to them.**

   a. True   b. False

10. **Noticing and complimenting well behavior is called**

    a. Traumatic.
    b. A disability.
    c. Role playing.
    d. Positive reinforcement.

Chapter 54

DEMENTIA AND CONFUSION

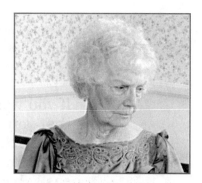

 See additional examples, descriptions and demonstrations of the concepts discussed in this chapter in the Medcom videotape "The Confused Resident: Strategies for Quality Care" (M107R).

In this chapter... you will learn about:

▶ Some causes of dementia.

▶ Degrees of dementia.

▶ How to deal with dementia.

DEFINITIONS

Alzheimer's Disease:	A progressive disease of the brain that very slowly destroys all ability to think or function.
Catastrophic Reaction:	A sudden tantrum or burst of anger.
Dementia:	A mental state in which the mind no longer functions properly.
Progressive:	A condition that slowly gets worse.
Sundowning:	The tendency of persons with dementia to grow more confused in the late afternoon and evening.

DEMENTIA

If you work in a long-term care facility, it is almost certain that you will have to care for some residents with **dementia**. People with dementia are confused and disoriented. They sometimes get frustrated and angry easily because they feel the whole world is becoming unfamiliar. They can wander aimlessly and even try to slip away from the facility when you are not watching. They can hurt themselves with simple objects. And they can lose the ability to communicate or perform even simple functions.

Dementia can have many causes. About half the cases of dementia are caused by **Alzheimer's Disease**. This is a **progressive** disease of the brain that slowly destroys all ability to think and function. It is not curable. The resident with Alzheimer's can slowly grow worse for 20 years or more before dying.

Dementia can also be caused by mental illnesses such as schizophrenia. And it can be caused by a stroke that has destroyed parts of the brain.

Dementia can also be caused by thyroid problems, severe vitamin deficiencies and depression. Unlike Alzheimer's, these conditions are treatable. If you notice any new signs of dementia in a resident, inform the nurse. It is possible that the resident has a treatable condition.

DEGREES OF DEMENTIA

How you care for a resident with dementia will depend to some degree on the severity of the condition. Some residents may have a permanent form of one of these types of dementia. Other residents, particularly those with Alzheimer's, will steadily move through the stages and grow worse.

Mild Dementia

In this type you will see confusion, loss of memory for recent events (short-term memory), loss of attention span, disorientation and carelessness. The residents with mild dementia can still do many things for themselves with your help.

Moderate Dementia

In this type you will see more memory loss, even loss of old memories (long-term memory). You will also see complete disorientation, wandering, speech problems, particularly repeating words over and over, incontinence, and the inability to use simple objects like a comb or a spoon.

There are two common reactions of people with moderate dementia that you should know about:

1. *Sundowning.* It is very common in this stage for residents to grow much worse in the late afternoon or early evening. No one knows why this happens.

2. *Catastrophic reaction.* A resident can suddenly snap and start shouting or have a tantrum. This is probably because life is becoming increasingly frustrating, and the resident just can't cope with the changes. To avoid this, you should try not to make demands or force residents to do anything. Remain calm, slow and patient.

Severe Dementia

In this type, the residents are bed-ridden and helpless. They have usually lost the power of speech and may not even focus. They sometimes have seizures.

In caring for people with dementia, you should try to put yourself in their position and imagine how frightening and frustrating the world is. Things are not the way they remember them.

It's as if you were dropped into a foreign country, and everyone speaks a language you don't understand. All the objects look strange and people speak nonsense to you. People expect you to do things, but you can't figure out what they want.

In general, you need to be slow and patient and only ask them to do one thing at a time. There are a number of other helpful suggestions you can follow for other problems associated with dementia:

Arguing and Aggression

- Stay calm.

- Always explain what you are doing.

- Avoid bad times of day for difficult tasks.

- Offer diversions or entertainment.

- Be agreeable. (Does it really matter if they are wrong about something.)

- Keep to a simple routine.

Clinging and following

- Offer simple tasks or entertainment.

Depression

- Tell your supervisor. This may need psychological care.

- Offer reassurance and affection.

- Offer entertainment.

Hoarding (this is very common)

- Make regular checks in drawers and other places for perishable foods.

- Reduce clutter and temptations to hoard.

- Create a dedicated place in plain sight for storing things.

- Accept it with good humor. (It is not a tragedy if a hidden sandwich goes moldy.)

Incontinence

- Ask the nurse if there is any bladder infection.

- Schedule regular visits to the toilet.

- Point out how to use the toilet, if necessary.

- Watch for nonverbal signals that a trip to the toilet is needed.

- Use clean-up time to express affection and overcome any lingering sense of shame.

Non-recognition (they may not recognize you or family members)

- Announce who you are.

- Show a photo of a family member immediately before a visit and explain who it is.

- Just keep giving affection. They will respond to memories and feelings of kindness even if they don't recognize you.

Paranoia (and thinking things are being stolen)

- Try using diversions.

- Make a written list of where objects are stored.

- Help them hunt for an object.

- Attach objects to furniture with string.

- Make regular searches of hiding places.

Personal Hygiene

- Help the resident maintain as much independence as possible.

- Suggest one step of a task at a time.

- Never scold.

Safety

- Keep all dangerous implements (scissors, etc.) out of reach.

- Keep medications and cleansers out of reach.

- Carefully check water temperature.

- Don't leave objects on the floor that could cause slipping or tripping.

- Beware of small objects that could go into the mouth.

Sexuality (and undressing)

- Ask the nurse if medications may be causing a problem.

- Offer activities and diversions.

- Offer someone with "busy hands" something to hold.

- Try not to overreact.

Stealing

- If the resident persistently goes into other resident's drawers, set aside a "rummage drawer" full of things.

- Learn the obvious hiding places.

- Don't scold. This is a memory problem, not a moral problem.

Sundowning

- Take extra care in late afternoon and evening.

- Turn on more lights.

- Offer activities or entertainment.

- Try not to overstimulate.

Wandering

- Keep familiar objects near the person so it seems like "home."

- Follow all your facility's rules for keeping doors closed and activating door alarms.

- Discuss any necessary precautions with the nurse.

- Sometimes simply covering a doorknob or hanging cloth on it will keep the wanderer from recognizing it as a door.

There are certain simple things you can do to help people with mild to moderate dementia remain oriented to where they are and who they are as long as possible. It can also help to keep the residents as involved as possible in their own personal care.

- ▶ Treat all residents as adults, with dignity.

- ▶ Frequently use your own name and their name.

- ▶ Work the date and location into your conversation.

- ▶ Speak clearly and simply.

- ▶ Don't ask questions about facts. (Do you know who I am? What's your name?)

- ▶ Keep to structures and routines.

At a certain point in the progress of the condition, these techniques will no longer work. Expecting any response at all, may even make the resident more agitated. If you think this time is approaching, talk it over with the nurse.

*Circle the correct answer. There is only **one** correct answer.*

1. **About half of the cases of dementia are caused by Alzheimer's disease.**

    a. True   b. False

2. **No causes of dementia are curable.**

    a. True   b. False

3. **Alzheimer's disease steadily gets worse.**

    a. True   b. False

4. **Which symptom is not characteristic of moderate dementia?**

    a. Complete disorientation.
    b. Repeating words.
    c. Incontinence.
    d. Loss of focus.

5. **People with severe dementia sometimes have seizures.**

    a. True   b. False

6. **In dealing with dementia, it can help to speak loudly and rapidly.**

    a. True   b. False

7. **One particularly bad time of day for many people with dementia is:**

    a. Dawn.
    b. Midnight.
    c. Noon.
    d. Sundown.

8. **Hoarding is one common form of behavior for those with dementia.**

    a. True   b. False

9. **If incontinence is a problem, it can help to schedule regular visits to the toilet.**

    a. True   b. False

10. **Which technique is not a good idea to help keep a resident oriented to reality?**

    a.   Announcing your name.
    b.   Asking the resident's name.
    c.   Keeping to a daily routine.
    d.   Speak clearly and simply.

Chapter 55

SEXUALITY

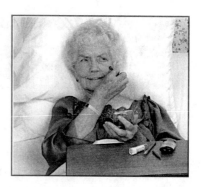

In this chapter... you will learn about:

▶ Resident sexuality.

▶ The nursing assistant's role in coping with these needs.

DEFINITIONS

Inhibiting:	Preventing, limiting.
Masturbation:	Sexual self-stimulation.
Myth:	A popular belief or tradition which may not be true.
Neuter:	Having no sexual characteristics.
Procreation:	Creating new life.
Sexuality:	Interest in sexual activity, physical attraction to others.

Chapter 55: Sexuality

529

SEXUALITY AND THE ELDERLY

Sexuality is often thought to apply only to young people, but we are sexual beings our entire life span. Sexuality is more than sexual intercourse. It includes attraction to someone else, and simple acts of touching, hugging, loving, and caring for someone else. The warmth of a caress is felt at any age, and we all have needs to be physically comforted from birth to death. The need to express these feelings and feel loved and desirable continues throughout life.

Myths About Sexuality And The Elderly

There have been many widely accepted **myths** regarding aging and sexuality. Some of these are:

▶ MYTH: Old people are not interested in sex.

FACT: The interest in and need for love, touching, and sexual release continues for many people into old age.

▶ MYTH: Old people cannot perform sexually.

FACT: For many people, the capacity to engage in and enjoy sexual activity continues into old age unless certain diseases and medications interfere.

▶ MYTH: Sex is for the young, and old people should "act their age."

FACT: Advertising has taught us that only the young and beautiful are sexy, but this is just not true. Sexual attraction is much more than physical appearance.

▶ MYTH: Sex is only for **procreation**.

FACT: Enjoyment is now accepted as a reason for sex, and enjoyment is important at all ages.

▶ MYTH: Sex is too strenuous for old people.

FACT: Physical exercise is good for everyone including older people. Sexual activity reduces tension and feels good.

Many older people may believe these myths and feel shame about their own sexual feelings. They may accept these myths and give up the comfort and joy of a caring relationship.

Accepting sexual needs and activity of older people doesn't mean that those older people who are not sexually active should be seen as abnormal. An older person's sexuality usually follows a lifelong pattern. Those who have always been sexually active will probably remain so. If sex was never a strong desire, it will not become so in old age. While sexual activity should be accepted as normal for people of all ages, it should not be an expectation which all should have to live up to. What is normal is what feels right to the person involved.

Factors Affecting Sexuality

As people age there are changes which can affect their ability to be sexually involved with another person. The greatest *inhibiting* factor is the lack of a suitable partner. Widowhood brings an end to a longstanding relationship, and the opportunity to form a new relationship is often limited. **Masturbation** is a normal, healthy means of sexual release for both men and women who lack suitable partners.

Older people living in long-term care facilities lack the privacy to develop relationships and are often discouraged by staff and families from doing so.

The normal aging process also results in physical changes which affect sexual function. In females, there is less vaginal lubrication and a loss of elasticity of the vagina which may make intercourse more difficult or painful. In males, there is usually a gradual decline in sex drive and erections are less firm and require more stimulation to achieve.

Disease can also affect sexual performance. Diabetes often causes a decline in sexual ability due to decreased circulation. Depression causes a decline in sexual interest. Some drugs and alcohol also have a negative effect on sexual desire and performance.

THE NURSING ASSISTANT'S RESPONSIBILITY

The nursing assistant can help residents understand and cope with their sexuality by:

- Being willing to listen to concerns regarding sexuality without shaming the residents or making them feel guilty.

- Helping residents be as attractive as possible by assisting with clothing, cosmetics, and grooming.

- Treating residents as adult males and females, not as "boys" "girls," or **neuters**.

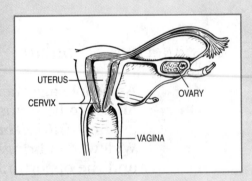

Female sex organs

- Maintaining the residents' dignity by not exposing their private parts unnecessarily, and by remembering to pull privacy curtains and close doors.

- Providing understanding, acceptance, and

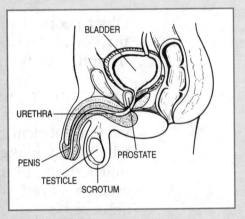

Male sex organ.

privacy for a resident's expression of sexuality. Resident rooms should be respected as private space, and the nursing assistant should always knock before entering.

- Accepting individual expressions of sexuality which do not harm the individual or others and do not intrude upon the rights of others.

Self-esteem increases and people feel better physically and emotionally when some form of sexual activity is part of their lives. As a nursing assistant, you can help your residents feel good about themselves and their sexuality.

*Circle the correct answer. There is only **one** correct answer.*

1. **Sexuality applies only to the young.**

    a. True   b. False

2. **Touching and hugging can be a part of sexuality.**

    a. True   b. False

3. **Sex is too strenuous for older people.**

    a. True   b. False

4. **The interest in and need for love, touching, and sexual release continues into old age.**

    a. True   b. False

5. **What is usually the greatest inhibiting factor to sexuality in residents in long-term care facilities?**

    a. Decreased interest.
    b. Privacy.
    c. Lack of suitable partners.
    d. Disease.

6. **Masturbation is a normal, healthy means of sexual release for people who lack suitable partners.**

    a. True   b. False

7. **Less vaginal lubrication and elasticity in women, and less firm erections in men can affect sexual function.**

    a. True   b. False

8. **Diabetes often causes a decline in sexual ability due to**

    a. Depression.

    b. A decline in interest.

    c. Decreased circulation.

    d. Increased stimulation.

9. **How can the nursing assistant help residents understand and cope with their sexuality?**

    a. Assist residents with clothing, cosmetics, and grooming.

    b. Tell them to act their age and stop worrying about sexuality.

    c. Make them feel guilty.

    d. Treat them as young boys and girls.

10. **Providing privacy for a resident's expression of sexuality is not a responsibility of the nursing assistant.**

    a. True   b. False

Chapter 56

CULTURE AND RELIGION

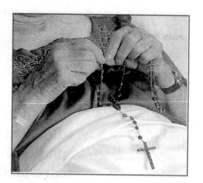

In this chapter... you will learn about:

▶ Differences in cultural background.

▶ Remaining sensitive to different customs.

▶ Differences in religious background.

▶ Being aware of religious needs.

DEFINITIONS

Culture:	A set of customs belonging to a particular nation or people.
Fast:	Period of time without eating.
Geography:	A particular place on the earth.
Halal:	Acceptable to eat, in Moslem dietary laws.
Hanukkah:	A Jewish holiday.
Koran:	The Moslem holy book.
Kosher:	Acceptable to eat, in Jewish dietary laws.
Lent:	The 40 days before Easter in the Christian calendar.
Passover:	A Jewish holiday.
Ramadan:	The ninth month of the Moslem calendar, involving fasting from sunrise to sunset.
Rosary:	Roman Catholic prayer beads.
Spiritual Needs:	Personal needs relating to moral, ethical or religious concerns.
Yarmulke:	Jewish skullcap.

CULTURAL DIFFERENCES

Customs, habits and eating tastes are determined by many different things. They are affected by **geography** (where a person lives), by race, **culture**, and religion. In a long-term care facility, your main awareness of cultural differences among the residents may well be differences in their tastes in food. You should become aware of these, but also remain sensitive to many other cultural differences, too.

Geography, Culture, and Food

Most cultures in the world developed characteristic foods based on their geography, the kinds of vegetables that grew nearby and the kinds of animals or fish that lived in their area. Even within the United States, there are regional differences in tastes. People from the North traditionally eat more beef and people from the South more pork. People who grew up near the oceans eat more seafood than those from the plains states.

Since the United States is a nation of immigrants, many of us are also influenced by the tastes of our parents or grandparents from other countries or of large immigrant groups in the areas where we live. Many people in the West and Northwest, for example, are fond of Asian foods which are based on rice, vegetables, and fish. Mexican foods, based on corn meal and beans with chili peppers as a seasoning are very popular with people from the Southwest. And German and Polish foods are popular in the Midwest.

The development of refrigeration and efficient transportation networks is changing these old habits, but many older people still cling to those foods they find most familiar. You should be aware of the backgrounds of your residents and understand how these affect their tastes.

Regions and cultures affect us all in far more ways than the foods we like. Many people from the South, for example, often seem slow and very relaxed to people from the North. And people from the North, particularly the New York area, often seem too "speedy" to those from the South.

Immigrants from other areas in the world naturally bring the customs they learned with them. The more you learn about these customs, the more sensitive you will be to any cultural differences you will meet in the residents. Below are just a few examples of cultural differences you might encounter:

▶ Many people from Asia and the Middle East remove their shoes whenever they are indoors. Some might be offended if you insisted they wear shoes in their own rooms.

▶ Many Asians do not like to be touched as much as Westerners do. Constant touching, even to show affection, can make them very uncomfortable. If you have Asian residents, you should find out if being touched bothers them.

▶ Many Africans and people from the Middle East are offended if you hand them something with the left hand. You should find out if this is the case. It is just as easy to use the right hand or both hands.

There are many, many other cultural differences. You should not treat any of these as "right," or "wrong." When people grow up doing something a certain way, or eating certain foods, it is only natural that they feel most comfortable continuing to do those things. You should learn about any cultural differences you might find among the residents, and think of them as enriching your own knowledge of the world, the regions of the country, or different cultures.

There are many religions in the world. The United States developed as a land that welcomed all religions and offered everyone the right to practice whatever religion they wished, or no religion at all. Today in North America there are people who follow almost all the world's faiths: Catholic, Jewish, Baptist, Moslem, Buddhist, Presbyterian, Mormon, Jehovah's Witness, Lutheran, Christian Scientist, Seventh-Day Adventist, and many more. You should learn the religious beliefs of the residents at your facility and do what you can to help the residents follow and honor the practices of their religions.

Religion and Foods

Some religions have dietary rules and restrictions which affect people's eating habits. For example:

> The Jewish religion has a great number of eating, cooking, and food handling restrictions, including a ban on eating any pork products. The person who follows these rules eats only *kosher* foods. Kosher food has been inspected and prepared in the way specified by the rules.

> Moslems also have dietary restrictions that are similar in some ways to Jewish rules. They eat only *halal* foods which have been inspected and prepared in the way specified by these rules. Moslems are also not allowed to drink alcohol.

> The Mormon religion does not allow drinking any beverage that contains alcohol or caffeine. Mormons cannot have alcoholic beverages, coffee or tea.

> Many Catholics still honor the custom of eating fish but not red meats on Friday. This is no longer a rule of the Catholic Church, but some older Catholics still follow it as a custom.

- The Hindu religion and some others specify only vegetarian diets. Some strict vegetarians will not even eat milk products or eggs.

- Some religions have **fast** periods when the person is not supposed to eat. Moslems, for example, fast from dawn to sunset in the ninth month of their calendar known as **Ramadan**. This falls roughly during October.

- Some Christians give up certain foods for **Lent**, the 40-day period preceding Easter.

- Some religions have festival periods when they eat particular foods or avoid other foods. During the Jewish **Passover** period, for example, there are many special foods and dietary restrictions.

All residents have the right to practice their own religions and follow their dietary rules and customs. There are long-term care facilities which are administered by particular religious groups. In these facilities, all diets meet the particular religious requirements. Sometimes it is difficult to provide these special diets in a facility which is administered for the general public. However, every reasonable effort must be made to provide an acceptable diet for each resident.

The nursing assistant can assist the resident by being aware of the dietary restrictions and customs of the residents. Every effort should be made to ensure the resident has a pleasant experience at mealtimes.

Religion and Other Customs

Religious needs are very personal, and we all seek the meaning of life in our own way. Beliefs and practices differ, and can dictate:

- When and how a person worships (Saturday, Sunday, daily; at temple, church, or on a prayer mat at home).

- What days are religious holidays and how they are to be observed (Easter, **Hanukkah**, Ramadan).

- Articles of clothing which must be worn (such as, the orthodox Jewish head covering, the **yarmulke**).

- What medical treatments may be accepted (some religions refuse medications or blood transfusions).

- What symbols and objects are appropriate (a cross, a **rosary**, the Bible, the Koran).

A person can have religious beliefs without belonging to any organized religious group. Some people may believe in a supreme being or force and live according to their own personal religious guidelines rather than those of a specific religious group. Some people may doubt the existence of a supreme being and still follow strong ethical and moral guidelines.

Religion is only one way in which people find meaning in life. Other ways are through nature, art, music, relationships with and service to others, and self-awareness. The meaning of life may be found in a sunset, a snow-capped mountain, a symphony, a majestic sculpture, the caring relationship with another, or meditation and self-understanding. There are as many different ways of fulfilling **spiritual needs** as there are people.

Whatever way residents and their families use to meet spiritual needs, they have the right to observe their own beliefs and practices without interference or ridicule.

You as an individual will also have your own spiritual beliefs and practices which are very personal and important to you. Just as you want others to respect your beliefs, you must respect and protect those of your residents and their families.

Most long-term care facilities provide regularly scheduled religious services conducted by local clergy. These are available for those residents interested in attending. Families may also take residents outside of the facility to attend services.

Clergy members often make personal visits to residents.

You must never argue about religion with a resident. If you sincerely believe something very different, or feel that a resident is "wrong" about religion, you must keep it to yourself. Listen politely and honor their beliefs. This is common courtesy, but it is also required by the Resident's Bill of Rights. The nursing assistant can help residents and their families fulfill their spiritual needs by:

- Accepting and supporting residents in expressing their own beliefs.

- Trying to learn as much as possible about a resident's religion or beliefs.

- Helping other residents understand and respect different religious practices.

- Listening with respect when a resident or family shares beliefs.

- Treating religious articles with care and respect.

- Notifying the charge nurse of requests for clergy visits.

- Providing privacy for religious observances and clergy visits.

- Helping residents be ready to attend services.

Spiritual beliefs and practices provide residents and their families with meaning, comfort, and strength, particularly during periods of loss and suffering. Respecting these beliefs and helping residents and their families continue their rituals and practices are an important responsibility of the nursing assistant.

Circle the correct answer. There is only **one** *correct answer.*

1. **Most people eat and enjoy those foods which are familiar to them.**

    (a.) True   b. False

2. **The food eaten in a culture is not influenced by the local geography and the foods that grow there.**

    a. True   (b.) False

3. **The Mormon religion does not allow its members to drink alcoholic beverages, coffee, or tea.**

    (a.) True   b. False

4. **Kosher foods are**

    a. Not inspected.
    (b.) Prepared in specified ways.
    c. Only eaten on fast days.
    d. Never found in vegetarian diets.

5. **Every resident has the right to practice his or her own religion including following the dietary rules and regulations.**

    (a.) True   b. False

6. **You cannot have religious beliefs without belonging to an organized religious group.**

    a. True   (b.) False

7. **Sometimes it is appropriate to argue your own beliefs with the residents.**

    a. True   (b.) False

8. Some people find the meaning of life in nature, self-awareness, art and music.

    a. True   b. False

9. Residents can practice their own religions but they are not allowed to have religious symbols openly displayed.

    a. True   b. False

10. Most long-term care facilities provide religious services conducted by local clergy.

    a. True   b. False

Chapter 57

DEATH AND DYING

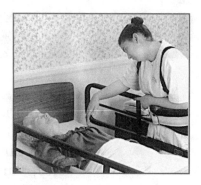

In this chapter... you will learn about:

► Feelings about death.

► Stages in dying.

► The nursing assistant's role as a resident is dying.

► Providing postmortem care.

DEFINITIONS

Advance Directive (Living Will):	Instructions by a resident about what steps to take or not to take to extend life as the resident approaches death.
Imminent	Likely to happen soon.
Inevitable:	Certain to happen.
Glycerine:	A fluid used to keep the mouth soft and moist.
Mortuaries:	Funeral homes.
Postmortem Care:	Care of a body after death.
Reluctant:	Unwilling.
Unique:	One of a kind.

FEELINGS ABOUT DEATH

Death and dying are subjects we seldom discuss. We often use words which try to hide or soften the harsh reality. Words such as "passed away," "taken from us," or "fallen asleep" are used rather than "dead" or "died." Yet death is the natural end to life and will happen to all of us.

In previous generations, loved ones often died at home, and families took care of the body and the burial. The reality of death was a part of life. Now most people die in hospitals and long-term care facilities, and **mortuaries** assume responsibility for the body and burial.

How do you feel about death? Has anyone close to you died? Have you seen and touched a dead body? It is important for nursing assistants to think about these questions and identify their feelings. You will be caring for older people, getting to know them and becoming good friends with some of them. Eventually they will die and you will have to deal with your own feelings of grief, just like the families.

Strong feelings are normal reactions to death. They are experienced by all who lose someone they love. It is important to accept these feelings and work through them. Often we try to push the feelings of grief down inside and pretend everything is all right. We think we are being very brave, but the feelings don't go away, and the next time we suffer a loss, the grief is even greater.

Accepting your feelings and talking about them can help you to work through them. Crying is a natural release for feelings of grief, but often we try hard not to cry and deny ourselves this normal expression of grief.

Your feelings about and acceptance of death will be based on your background, experience, and religious beliefs. These are different for everyone, and your feelings are **unique**.

How you feel about death will influence your behavior when caring for a dying resident. If you fear death, you may be **reluctant** to be near the resident and find yourself spending less time with the dying person. Your own feelings may prevent you from understanding and being sensitive to the dying resident's needs. Talking about your feelings with other nursing assistants and with your charge nurse will help you work through these feelings.

When a resident dies, other residents are affected. They will be concerned and want to know what happened. Sometimes it seems kinder to pretend or avoid the subject, but the residents will know that something has happened, and they deserve an honest explanation. The nursing assistant can simply state that the resident has died and will be missed. Residents may need to talk about the death, and the nursing assistant can help them by being a good listener.

Older people are not preoccupied with death, but they often find that people avoid the subject when they want to talk about it. If you can face your own fears, you will be better able to help your residents deal with theirs.

The Needs of the Dying

In working with residents for whom death is **imminent**, it is important to remember that 1) they are living individuals and 2) the dying residents have needs. The dying resident has the same emotions, needs, and concerns as other residents and should to be treated with respect and dignity.

Until recently, people were not told when they were dying. This information was kept a secret by doctors, nurses, and families to protect the person from the harsh reality of death. It is now felt that people want to know and they have a right to know when they are dying. Even though they want to know, it is very difficult information to cope with.

Emotional Stages in Facing Death

In studying the reactions of dying residents, Dr. Elisabeth Kubler-Ross found five stages or phases which many people go through when faced with their own death.

1. Denial. *The "No, not me!" stage.* This is the initial reaction when the fact of death just cannot be accepted. The denial stage allows the person time to begin to accept the reality of death. The nursing assistant can help by simply accepting this reaction and not trying to correct it.

2. Anger. *The "Why me?" stage.* The resident begins to accept the fact of death and is angry over being singled out. The resident may resent and show anger at anyone who is well. The resident may be angry at God, the doctors, the family, and at you. It is important not to take this anger personally and not to become angry yourself with the resident.

3. Bargaining. *The "Yes, but . . ." stage.* The fact of death is beginning to be accepted, but bargains are struck with God or fate to prolong life. Promises of service to others and goodness are made in exchange for longer life, or goals, such as an anniversary or child's wedding, are set. Often this stage is not obvious because residents do not usually talk about the bargaining going on in their own minds. If bargains are expressed, the nursing assistant should just accept them.

4. Depression. *The "Poor me!" stage.* The reality can no longer be denied or bargained away, and the resident becomes depressed. The resident begins to pull away from interaction with others and may cry and refuse to eat or drink. This is when the resident needs a great deal of care and understanding. Trying to cheer the resident up is not helpful. Rather, the nursing assistant should accept the resident's deep sadness as a normal reaction to impending death.

5. Acceptance. *The "Yes, me" stage.* The resident comes out of depression and waits for death with acceptance and patience. This usually occurs close to the time of death. Death is not always welcomed,

but can be accepted as **inevitable**. The resident will probably interact very little with others and prefer to be with only one or two family members or close friends. The nursing assistant can help the resident by simply being there to provide care and comfort.

No one goes through these stages in perfectly timed order. Some stages last longer than others, and people flow back and forth between stages. Also, not every dying person goes through these stages. Those who die quickly do not have time. No one should be pushed to move on through these phases. They are meant to help you understand the experience of the dying resident. If you understand, you will accept the resident's reactions and will not take the anger and depression personally, but accept them as normal.

How The Nursing Assistant Can Help the Dying

In caring for a dying resident, the following guidelines should be followed:

1. Provide comfort for the dying resident:

    • Change the resident's position every two hours if the resident is unable to do this on his or her own.

    • Keep the resident and the bed linen clean and dry.

    • If the resident's mouth is dry, swab it with **glycerine**.

    • If the nostrils are dry, clean them with Q-tips and swab them with glycerine.

    • Touch conveys caring and securing. Just being with a resident and holding a hand or touching an arm can provide comfort.

2. Be friendly, accepting, and natural in responding to the resident's needs.

3. Don't avoid appropriate human responses such as laughter.

4. Do avoid FALSE cheerfulness. This denies the reality of the dying process and is never appropriate.

5. Keep the resident's room as bright and cheerful as usual. A dark room may be frightening unless specifically requested by the resident.

6. Speak in a normal voice, and don't whisper.

7. Assume the resident can hear and understand everything you say. Don't talk about the resident as though he or she is already dead. Hearing is one of the last senses to fail.

8. Respect the resident's view of death and afterlife even though it may not be your belief. Share your view only if specifically asked to do so by the resident.

9. Report requests for clergy to the charge nurse as soon as possible.

10. Be a willing listener. The resident may want to talk about fears and concerns. You don't have to have any answers, you simply have to listen and accept what the resident says.

11. Be a willing listener to the resident's family. They may need to talk about their fears and grief, also.

12. If the resident has filed an **advance directive** (living will) or some other expression of what steps to take or not to take to extend life as death approaches, you should obey the resident's wishes. A living will, if it exists, should be filed with the resident's chart. If you feel there is any change in these wishes, inform the charge nurse immediately.

We all must live in our own way and die in our own way. There is no one right way to do it. It is not the nursing assistant's responsibility to judge or question the resident's way of dealing with impending death. It is the nursing assistant's responsibility to accept the resident's style of coping and assist the resident in dying with as much comfort and dignity as possible.

Care of the body after death is called **postmortem** care. In some facilities, the nursing assistant provides this care, and in others, mortuary personnel provide postmortem care. You should only begin postmortem care when specifically instructed to do so.

If the resident has a roommate, explain the situation and offer to escort the resident to another area while arrangements are made. If the resident declines or cannot be moved, draw the dividing curtains or place a folding screen between the beds. Do not leave the resident alone in the room with the body.

Remember to treat the body with the same dignity you would a living person. Work quickly and quietly and maintain respect for the body. You should only speak if it is necessary for a procedure. Do not move parts of the body roughly or press on them. You can cause bruising even after death.

To provide postmortem care, use the following procedures.

1. Assemble the necessary equipment: a shroud or clean sheet, basin of warm water, washcloth and towels, disposable gloves, cotton, bandages, pads, any ID tags used in your facility.

2. Identify the resident and provide privacy.

3. Wash your hands and put on gloves.

4. Place the body on the back, with a pillow under the head and shoulders.

5. Close the eyes. If they do not remain closed, place a damp cotton ball on each eye. Do not press down.

6. If dentures are out, replace them in the mouth and close the jaw. Use a light bandage to hold it closed if necessary.

7. Bathe the body as necessary and replace any soiled dressings with clean ones.

8. Put a disposable pad beneath the buttocks.

9. If the family is coming to view the body, take these steps:

   - Groom the hair.

   - Put a clean hospital gown on the body.

   - Cover the body up to the neck with a sheet.

   - Tidy the room and lower the light level.

   - Offer the family privacy as they visit.

10. After any family visit, put the shroud on the body.

11. Fill out the ID cards used in your facility. Usually there will be three:

   - One for the body's right ankle or right big toe.

   - One for the valuables.

   - One for mortuary use.

12. Collect all the resident's property, label it and deliver it to the charge nurse, with one ID tag.

13. If there is another resident in the room, stay with the body until the mortuary personnel arrive. If there is no resident in the room, close the door and wait for the mortuary personnel to arrive. Assist them moving the body if directed by the charge nurse.

Always remember to give the body the same respect and privacy that you gave the living resident.

*Circle the correct answer. There is only **one** correct answer.*

1. **Using words such as "passed away" or "taken from us" to describe someone's death is our way of trying to soften the blow of death.**

    a. True   b. False

2. **How can you work through your strong feelings about death?**

    a. Deny them.
    b. Ignore them.
    c. Accept them, then talk about them.
    d. Forget about them.

3. **When caring for a dying resident, your feelings about death have no bearing on your behavior toward the resident.**

    a. True   b. False

4. **Crying is a natural release for feelings of grief.**

    a. True   b. False

5. **When a resident dies, how should the nursing assistant respond to the other residents?**

    a. Avoid the subject.
    b. Pretend nothing happened.
    c. Listen to the residents who need to talk about death.
    d. Tell the residents not to talk about it.

6. **Most people want and have a right to know when they are dying.**

    a. True   b. False

7. **When dying residents are in the depression or "Poor me!" stage, how should the nursing assistant respond?**

    a. Try to cheer them up.
    b. Become angry with them.
    c. Provide care and understanding.
    d. Ignore them.

8. **Acceptance is usually one of the first stages a dying person experiences.**

    a. True   b. False

9. **It is best to keep the dying resident's room dimly lit.**

    a. True   b. False

10. **In providing postmortem care it is no longer necessary to treat the body with dignity.**

    a. True   b. False

Chapter 58

USING A COMPUTER

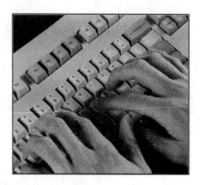

In this chapter... you will learn about:

▶ The parts of computers.

▶ The uses for computers.

▶ How to begin using a computer.

DEFINITIONS

Boot up:	To start up the computer.
CD-ROM:	Compact Disc, Read-Only Memory, a device for storing large amounts of data, usually not erasable. Often shortened to "CD."
CPU:	Central processing unit, the heart of a computer, where the main memory and processing take place.
Cursor:	Usually a small arrow, flashing line or block that appears on the computer screen. It is controlled with the mouse to operate items on the screen.
Disc, Disk:	Terms used for flat, round devices used for storing data, such as, "compact disc," "hard disks," and "floppy disks."
E-mail:	Electronic mail; mail sent from computer to computer.
Floppy Disk:	A small removable, reusable data storage device. Also known as a "diskette."
Icon:	A small drawing on a computer screen that represents a file or a program.

Internet:	The network of linked-up computers all over the world, which holds immense amounts of information.
Keyboard:	The keys used to enter data to a computer, like a typewriter.
Monitor:	The display screen of a computer.
Mouse:	A small device that is rolled on a desktop to move a cursor on a computer screen.
Network:	Computers connected to each other. This can be within a facility, called an internal network, or all over the world, as with the Internet.
Server:	A central computer which has a large amount of memory and where the main body of information is stored.
Software:	Computer programs.
Spreadsheet:	A program for keeping accounts and handling finances.
WWW:	World Wide Web, often "the web." A part of the Internet that allows sharing and viewing of text, graphics, video and audio content.
Web browser:	A program that allows the user to search the Internet and find information.
Word processor:	A program for writing documents.

THE COMPUTER IN HEALTHCARE

Computers are an important part of the long term healthcare field and growing in importance. Reimbursement to nursing facilities is based on resident information often transmitted by computer. Over the next 10 years, it is almost inevitable that you will be required to have some computer knowledge. You should be prepared to welcome computers into your job because they will make providing care easier for you, and safer for residents. Be sure to know and follow your facility's policies as they relate to computer use and resident data.

Computers are not something to be afraid of. Even though a computer may appear complicated at first, today's computer is much simpler to operate than those of just a few years ago. Even if you have never used a computer before, after learning a few simple steps, you will discover just how easy it is to use one, and how much it can help you on the job.

In the long term care facility, as in most other facilities in the healthcare field, computers and computerized records will be used more and more to make providing care easier, safer and more accurate. This is for the benefit of residents as well as all the members of the healthcare team.

Computers have many benefits over other forms of data storage and communication. A few of these advantages are:

- Computer terminals can make complete medical records available immediately for resident care.

- Medical tests and other records can become a permanent part of the resident's record, and there is no chance, for example, of test results or prescriptions on slips of paper to become lost.

- All caregivers can communicate easily and accurately from shift to shift, day to day, and department to department.

- Resident care can be ordered and documented without errors made from sloppy handwriting.

- Passwords can be used so casual visitors cannot view records, as they might when a chart file is left open at a desk.

- Administrators can check certain data across many residents to assure consistent and appropriate resident care.

- Training programs can be made available on the computer to help you in career advancement.

First we will look at the main parts of most computers.

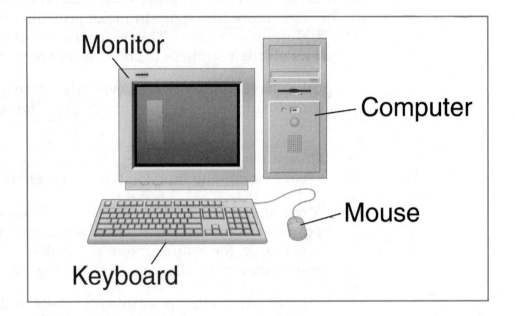

► ***The Monitor:*** This is like a television set. You can read information on the monitor's screen, and it shows you the words you type into the computer.

► ***The Keyboard:*** This is where you enter information by pressing keys with your fingers, just like a typewriter. There is a Backspace key, which is a good one to remember because it erases the last character you typed. The Enter key is also an important one to know. The computer also has some extra keys such as Control (CTRL) and Alternate (ALT). These can have special uses, depending on the program you are using.

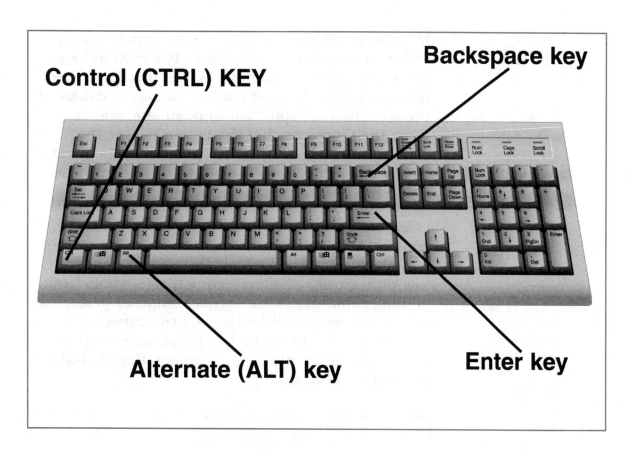

Control (CTRL) KEY

Backspace key

Alternate (ALT) key

Enter key

▶ *The Mouse:* Most modern computers have a mouse, which is a small device that you roll around on an area of the desk or a rubber pad to control the cursor on the monitor. In a document, the cursor is a small flashing line or block that shows you where your typing will go. If you move the mouse to the left or right, the cursor will move left or right on the screen. You can also move the cursor to the right and up and down using the arrow keys on the keyboard. If you click the left button on the mouse, the cursor will stay in the new position you have chosen.

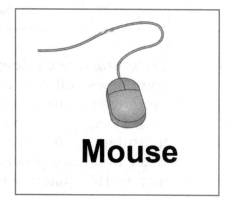

Mouse

In some programs the cursor is an arrow or other shape. In these programs you will see what look like images of push buttons on the monitor. These images of push buttons control various activities of the computer. If you wish to push one, you can move the mouse so that the cursor is over the button and then click the left button on the mouse.

▶ *The Computer:* This is where the computer's Central Processing Unit *(CPU)* is located. The CPU is like the computer's brain and memory, and it controls everything the computer does. The memory is usually a "hard disk," which can store large amounts of information, as much as a whole bank of filing cabinets. All the other computer parts, the mouse, monitor, and keyboard, are connected to the computer. It usually has an on-off switch, a restart (reboot) button, and slots for *floppy disks* and *compact discs*.

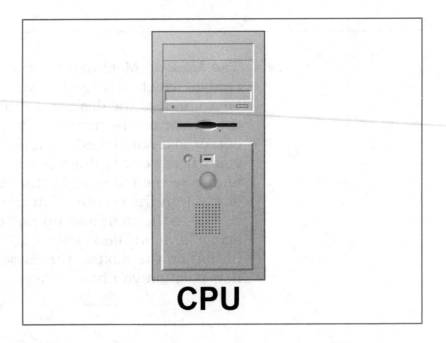

CPU

▶ *Data storage devices:* A 3 1/2 inch "floppy disk," sometimes called a "diskette," can store about 1.4 megabytes of data, which is about the same as a long novel. (A byte is a very small amount of information. It takes about 10 bytes to make one letter in a word processing program. 1.4 megabytes means 1.4 million bytes, or about 20,000 words.)

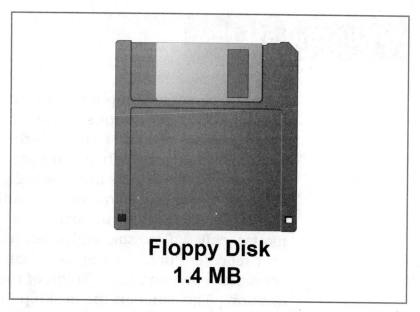

**Floppy Disk
1.4 MB**

Files you put on a floppy disk can be erased, and it can be reused many times.

A Compact Disc Read-Only Memory (**CD-ROM** or CD) is very similar to CD music discs, except it holds 700 megabytes of data. This is about the same as a small encyclopedia. A CD is usually used for more permanent storage and often the CD-ROM drive is designed only to read information from the CD. Some drives can also write to a special type of recordable CD.

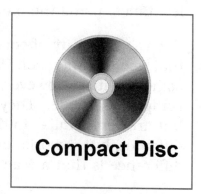

Compact Disc

▶ *Other devices:* The computer may also be connected to a printer, for printing out information, a scanner for copying documents, and speakers to give voice messages or make various noises to warn you about errors.

On most personal computers, the operating system is some form of Microsoft Windows®. The operating system is the basic program you use to control the computer and other computer programs. When you turn the computer on, the operating system starts automatically and creates pictures on the monitor that allow you to control the computer. These pictures include an arrow that you move with the mouse, called a **cursor**, and small pictures, called **icons** that represent programs or files that you can make the computer open and use. Think of the entire screen as a desktop. The icons on the desktop are different things you can make the computer do, and you use the cursor to choose them.

For example, there is an icon for a wastebasket or recycle bin. If you move the cursor over the icon of a file you want to erase, you can click and hold down the button of the mouse to grab onto the file. Then keep holding the button down and move the mouse to drag the file over the trash can icon. Let go of the button to "drop" the folder into the trash, which will erase it. This action is called drag-and-drop. It may sound complicated, but if you practice this a few times, using the mouse will become automatic to you.

The vast majority of computers in use in healthcare are PCs that use the Microsoft Windows® operating system. At some facilities, however, you might find Macintosh® computers in use. They use their own operating system, but are very similar to the PCs. A Macintosh® may look different, but it works in much the same way. The main difference is that a Macintosh® mouse has only one button.

Computer programs are called "**software**." Some of the main types of software are:

- **Word processors** – programs for typing documents.

- **Data management programs** – for storing and arranging large amounts of data.

- **Graphics programs** – for drawing or working on photographs.

- **Communications programs** – for sending and receiving **E-mail**.

- **Web browsers** – for finding information on the Internet.

- **Spreadsheets** – for keeping accounts and handling finances.

- **Desktop publishers** – for making newsletters and leaflets.

The programs that you will probably use in your work, such as a medical records data entry program, or a **word processor**, will each be represented by an icon. The icons will either be on the "desktop," (on the screen) or in what is called the Start Menu. To open the Start Menu, use the mouse to click on the Start Button at the bottom left of the screen. A menu with several icons will appear. To start any program, move the **cursor** over the icon that represents that program and double click the left button on the mouse. Click rapidly twice without moving the mouse. This may take a moment of practice. The program you want to use will then open, or appear on the screen so you can use it.

Most program functions can be chosen from the "menu bar" at the top of the screen. The menu bar will list words like "file," "edit, "view," etc. across the screen. Moving the cursor arrow over these words, then clicking and holding down the mouse button will make a list of options drop down to perform actions such as saving or printing your work. The specific words in the menu bar and available options will differ from program to program.

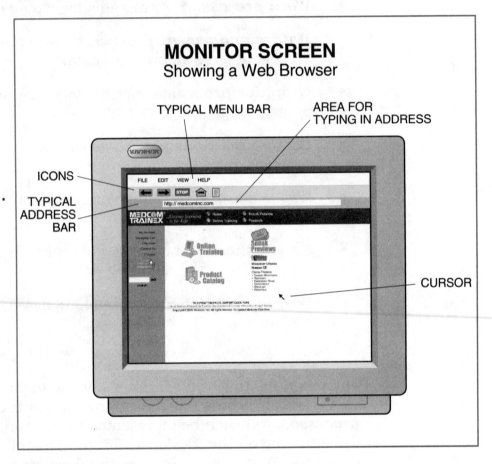

As you get more experienced using the computer, there might be programs you use all the time. You can learn "keyboard shortcuts" for common actions you do in these programs to become more efficient and work faster.

Common Keyboard Shortcuts

Common actions, like saving and printing files, can be done quickly using keyboard shortcuts. To use them, hold down the "control" key in the lower left corner (it may say "CTRL") and press the key for the shortcut. On Macintosh computers, hold down the "command" key.

- ▶ **Save:** CTRL+S

- ▶ **Print:** CTRL+P

- ▶ **Cut:** CTRL+X

- ▶ **Copy:** CTRL+C

- ▶ **Paste:** CTRL+V

NETWORKS

The computers you use in your facility will probably be connected to other computers in the facility. This is called a **network**. Networks allow computers to share information and messages. There may be one central computer, called a **server**, which has much more memory and where the main body of information is stored.

Networks can be just within a facility, called an "internal network," or they can extend outside the facility, like the Internet. We will discuss the Internet in more detail later.

Because networks can allow access to programs and files on other computers, you will need to know and follow your facility's policies regarding the use of computers on a network.

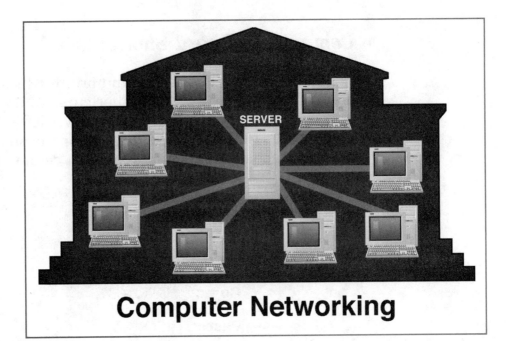

Computer Networking

▶ *Internal E-mail.* You may have an internal e-mail program on your network. This can be handy for leaving important messages for healthcare workers in your facility working on other shifts, or who happen to be away from their desks. You should learn how to start the program, how to compose a message, and how to select who you want to receive the message and any copies of the message.

▶ *File sharing.* In most networks, you can use any computer in the network to read and enter information to stored files, such as medical records. This is a great convenience in healthcare, since you can double check physician's orders at any location and you can document care provided at any location. Access to the computers and to certain records may be controlled by a special password that will be issued to you. You may only be able to access certain information in the resident record using your password.

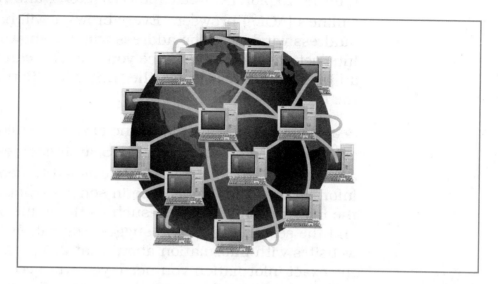

The Internet is like a huge network that includes just about all the computers in the world. Many people and organizations around the country and all over the world have set up their computers with permanent displays of information that anyone can enter and read or download. For example, you can go to the American Medical Association website and read pages and pages of medical information. You must be careful of information you read on the Internet, however, because people can display anything they want, or pretend to be something they are not. For example, a person who wanted to cause harm could set up a website called AllMedicalFacts.com* and fill it with false and dangerous information. If you use the Internet, especially for medical information, you should only rely on names of organizations you know and trust.

Using the Internet

To use the Internet your computer must have two things: an Internet connection, and a program called a **web browser,** or "browser." The Internet connection can be **dial-up**, which means it uses the regular telephone lines and connects you temporarily to the Internet when you need it. Dial-up systems are relatively slow. It is more likely that you will have a permanent connection in what is called **broadband**. This is a connection by permanent telephone line or cable that allows a lot of information to move very fast. You can move from site to site quickly.

* No website named "AllMedcialFacts.com" exists at the time of publication of this text.

A browser allows you to access and move to different places on the Internet. Some popular browsers are Microsoft Internet Explorer®, Netscape Navigator®, and America Online's (AOL®) browser. Every browser will have an "address window." The address window shows you the Internet address of the place you are. You can also type in an Internet address, push the "Enter" or "Return" key, and the browser will take you there.

Searching for information is one of the most common activities done on the Internet. "Search engines" like Yahoo® and Google™ are Internet sites designed to help you find information. You simply type in some keyword relating to the information you need—such as the name of a drug—and the search engine will suggest several, or hundreds, of websites with information about that drug. In order to get the exact information you need, you will need to learn how to limit your search using extra words. For example, if you wanted to find out about reactions to Inderal® you could just type in the single word "Inderal," but you would get many thousands of suggested websites, including places where it is sold, short stories containing the word and even people with that name. If you specify "Inderal reactions," that will probably lead you to a drug information sheet from a manufacturer with a section on reactions.

Using the Internet efficiently to find information requires practice, and it also requires a certain amount of caution. Beware of false information, tricks and cheats. In general, you should rely only on organizations and people you know and trust.

DATA SECURITY

The Health Insurance Portability and Accountability Act (HIPAA) requires that all resident information be kept private and out of view to casual visitors. One form of data security will be the use of a password. You will be issued a password in order to open and look at files in your facility. You should only open files that you have a direct need to read or add information to. Follow the policies of your facility.

Computers are having more and more uses in the modern world. The more you know about computers and especially the different types of software, the better equipped you will be for changes that may happen in your job. You will also be equipped to take advantage of opportunities to train for newer jobs that may interest you. And, you will be able to use computers at home, to write letters, sort digital photographs, store recipes, send e-mail and search the Internet for your own purposes.

*Circle the correct answer. There is only **one** correct answer.*

1. **Circle below the statement that is NOT a benefit of using computers.**

    a. Medical records can be made available immediately for resident care, wherever there is a computer terminal.

    b. Resident care can be ordered and then documented without errors made from sloppy handwriting.

    c. A large number of records can be destroyed at once with a single click of a button.

    d. All caregivers can communicate easily and accurately from shift to shift and day to day and department to department.

2. **With which part of the computer, do you enter data?**

    a. The monitor.
    b. The keyboard.
    c. The mouse.
    d. The central processing unit.

3. **Which part of the computer displays data?**

    a. The monitor.
    b. The keyboard.
    c. The mouse.
    d. The central processing unit.

4. **Which data storage device is most common for erasing files and adding new files?**

    a. CD.
    b. Printer.
    c. Floppy disk.
    d. Scanner.

5. **What is an icon?**

    a. A storage device.

    b. A small drawing that represents something.

    c. A key that erases the last character typed.

    d. A kind of hard disk.

6. **A computer mouse is used primarily to**_____

    a. Erase documents.

    b. Move the cursor.

    c. Add data.

    d. Make copies.

7. **A web browser is used for** _____.

    a. Finding information on the Internet.

    b. Sending e-mail.

    c. Erasing files.

    d. Managing finances.

8. **A spreadsheet program is primarily used for** _____.

    a. Finding information on the Internet.

    b. Sending e-mail.

    c. Erasing files.

    d. Managing finances.

9. **When computers are networked, it means** _____.

    a. They are connected so they can communicate.

    b. They are right next to each other.

    c. They are in the same room.

    d. They are portable.

10. **The Internet includes computers** _____.

    a. Throughout a facility only.

    b. Throughout one state only.

    c. Throughout the world.

    d. Throughout the USA only.

Chapter 59

YOUR HEALTHCARE CAREER

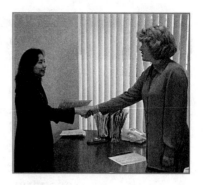

In this chapter... you will learn about:

- ▶ How to Apply for Your First Job.
- ▶ Continuing Your Education.
- ▶ Choosing Your Career Path.

DEFINITIONS

Resume:	A short written summary of your education and work history.
Career Path:	A group of positions in the same field with each requiring more training and offering more responsibility and more pay than the preceding one.

FINDING YOUR FIRST

Once you have completed your training and any certification required in your state, you are ready to begin looking for a CNA position. Unless the situation changes dramatically, there will probably be several positions available in the area where you live. The healthcare field is growing daily and Certified Nursing Assistants are in demand in many facilities.

In fact, you may have your choice of different shifts, which can be of great assistance in child care and working out your schedule with other family members. You should not, however, expect to have all your wishes met. Healthcare is a demanding 24-hour-a-day profession, and you will be working on a team that must accept the need to work on holidays or work extra shifts to fill-in for absent employees. Remain flexible and keep in mind that you are performing a service to those who are ill or weak or may desperately need your help.

Where to Look

If you have just completed a course at a community college or training facility, the institution may have a placement service to help their students find work. If not, you should ask your instructors for their recommendations. Other places to check include:

▶ Friends and other nursing assistants or healthcare workers you know.

▶ Visit local nursing homes, hospitals and other likely facilities. Many of these facilities post job openings on signs or bulletin boards or on their websites. If not, you can ask to speak to a nursing supervisor and inquire if there are any openings.

▶ Check the newspaper's classified ads under the healthcare or nursing section.

▶ Check the Internet for job search websites.

► Check with employment agencies. Some of these require that you pay a fee. Be sure to ask before you register with an agency if they require a fee. Many agencies will not take persons who do not have a specified amount of work experience.

You may not want to take the first job you find. Talk to a few employees at the facility first and see if they like their jobs. Does the facility have a good reputation for providing care? Does it treat its employees well? Is the facility properly accredited?

How to Appy

Once you have located a few likely opportunities, you will need to apply for the job. Call the facility and ask for an appointment for a job interview. Ask what you will need to bring with you. For a Certified Nursing Assistant position it is unlikely that the facility will ask for a **resume** (see box), especially if you have no job experience yet. But there may be other information that you will need to have with you to fill out their application form. Some of these may include:

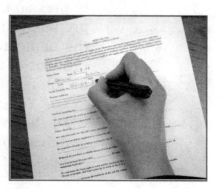

► Your own address and telephone number.

► Social Security Number.

► Certificate of Completion of a Nursing Assistant Course or State Certification Course.

► Places and dates of your education.

► Other verified work history.

► Contact information for anyone you are using as a reference. Be sure to ask the person in advance if they are willing to act as a reference for you. If you have worked at unrelated jobs, you may still be asked for your supervisor's contact information to see if you were a reliable, punctual and honest employee.

The Job Interview

First impressions are important. To make a good impression, you must be prepared. Be sure you know the name and telephone number of the person who will be interviewing you, and where to go. You should also know what the job is and how it

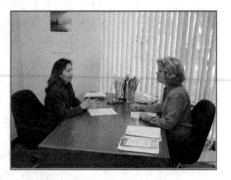

matches your skills and training. If you can, talk to someone at the facility before the job interview.

You should be a few minutes early for the interview and look your best. Dress professionally and wear clean clothing. Keep jewelry, cosmetics, perfumes, colognes and after shaves to a minimum. Come prepared with two working pens, in blue or black, and all the information you will need for the job application.

Be friendly and offer to shake hands. Stand until the interviewer invites you to sit down. Do not sit in a sloppy manner or cross your legs casually. Offer truthful and positive answers to all the questions you are asked. Most job interviewers will ask some or all of the following questions. Prepare your answers in advance, but try to answer naturally.

- Why did you choose to become a certified nursing assistant?

- Have you enjoyed your training?

- What was your greatest strength during training?

- What was your greatest weakness?

- Did you have trouble with any of your instructors or fellow students?

- Why do you want to work here?

- Why should we hire you and not someone else with more experience?

- Is there anything you would like to know about this facility?

Be prepared to use the interview time to find out about the facility—just as they are finding out about you. Be curious but positive about the job. Some of the questions you might want to ask include:

- Salary.

- Hours you might be working.

- Benefits.

- If there are dress requirements.

- If they have any in-service education or other opportunities for career growth.

During the interview, if you are asked something you do not understand, do not try to fake an answer. Ask for clarification. Always be honest.

One final hint: If you need to say something very positive about yourself, it is usually best to attribute it to one of your instructors or supervisors, but only if this is truthful. For example, it can sound like bragging if you say:

"I am always cheerful, even when I am exhausted."

But it is different if a supervisor once said it about you:

"In my last evaluation at the county job, the supervisor said I was always cheerful, even when I seemed exhausted."

At the end, the interviewer will usually tell you when you can expect to hear if you have been hired. Getting a job on the spot is very rare. Before you leave, offer to shake hands again and say something upbeat about wanting to work at this facility.

When you get home, write a short thank-you note to the interviewer, thanking him or her for giving you the time and for considering you. This will help the interviewer remember you if many people are being considered for the job.

CONTINUING YOUR EDUCATION

Your learning does not end the minute someone hands you your certificate or gives you your first job. The healthcare field is always changing and growing and you will need to remain curious and ready for new learning experiences throughout your career. Even if you do not change jobs, there will always be new procedures and equipment that you will need to learn. Remain curious on the job and learn all you can about the conditions of the patients and participate actively in team conferences.

Many facilities provide opportunities for you to attend in-service training, continuing education and other forms of staff development. You can also subscribe to professional journals and magazines that provide continuing education. Many companies provide courses on the Internet. Ask your supervisor what opportunities are available and seek out learning along career paths that interest you. You can also attend night schools, opportunity programs, and use correspondence courses and access Internet training directly, if you have your own computer.

In order to decide which educational path to follow, you should think about which aspects of the job interest you most. Over the first year on the job you should observe other technicians and healthcare workers to see if you would enjoy doing what they are doing. The most obvious path of career advancement is from CNA to a lead or advanced CNA, and then, through more education and certification to, LPN/LVN or RN, but there are many other paths available in healthcare.

YOUR CAREER PATH

If you refer back to Chapter 1, on page 4 you will see a list of some of the members of the healthcare team. Many of these, such as occupational therapist and speech therapist, represent different careers in healthcare that you might consider as you gain more experience and desire a path to a higher skilled job, a better paid job, or simply a different job. In a large facility, such as a hospital, there are also many technical careers, such as x-ray technician and laboratory technician that offer different **career paths**.

The reason it can be important to choose early is that each one of those paths can have many steps and can involve years of learning. For example, in a clinical laboratory the career path might look like this:

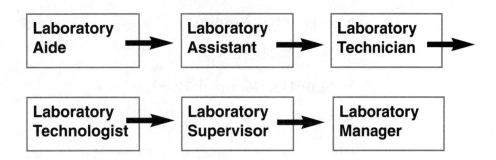

Any path you choose will have a different place to start your education, so you should begin thinking about this today.

Here are some of the healthcare fields that provide positive career paths:

- Central Supply Work
- Clerical Work
- Clinical Laboratory Work
- EEG Services
- EKG Services
- Environmental Services
- Food Service
- Home Health Care
- Licensed Vocational Nursing
- Medical Assisting
- Medical Coding and Billing
- Nutritional Care
- Phlebotomy
- Physical Therapy
- Physician
- Radiology Services
- Registered Nursing
- Speech Therapy
- Staff Development Teaching
- Surgeon

You have just set out on what can become a long and rewarding career in healthcare. Congratulations! All around you, you will find opportunities to learn and grow and advance your career.

*Circle the correct answer. There is only **one** correct answer.*

1. **Today job opportunities for CNAs are _____.**

    a. Very rare.
    b. Non-existent.
    c. Very common.
    d. Only in large states.

2. **All of the following are places that might provide leads to a job except one. Mark the one that will most likely NOT provide a good lead to a CNA opening.**

    a. Friends.
    b. Telephone book white pages.
    c. Placement service.
    d. Classified advertising.

3. **A resume is _____.**

    a. A summary of your education and work history.
    b. A blank job application.
    c. A copy of your CNA certificate.
    d. An oral job interview.

4. **For a job interview you should arrive _____.**

    a. A few minutes late.
    b. Exactly on time.
    c. A few minutes early.
    d. Several hours early.

5. **To make a good first impression for a job interview you should wear _____.**

    a. A borrowed nursing uniform.
    b. Tidy professional attire.
    c. A lot of make-up and perfume.
    d. Blue jeans and a sweater.

6. **In an interview, if you are asked a difficult question you should
    _____.**

    a. Fake an answer.
    b. Ask for clarification.
    c. Call a friend.
    d. Lie.

7. **One question you should NOT ask in a job interview is
    _____.**

    a. How many coffee breaks do you get?
    b. How many hours you might be working?
    c. What are the dress requirements?
    d. Are there opportunities for career growth?

8. **Only one of the paths below is a logical career path. Select
    that one.**

    a. Radiology aide ⟶ Medical assistant ⟶ Food dervice worker.
    b. Laboratory technician ⟶ Laboratory aide ⟶ Radiologist.
    c. LVN ⟶ Environmental Services Supervisor ⟶ Speech Therapist.
    d. Radiology Aide ⟶ Radiology Technician ⟶ Physician Radiologist.

9. **Continuing education can be found in all of the following
    places except one. Mark the one where it is most likely NOT
    found.**

    a. Broadcast television.
    b. The Internet.
    c. Clinical journals.
    d. Community Colleges.

10. **At the end of a job interview, you should_____.**

    a. Say that it is all right if you aren't hired.
    b. Insist on knowing if you got the job.
    c. Thank the interviewer and say something positive.
    d. Ask for money to cover your transportation home.

APPENDIX A: ABBREVIATIONS

The following are some of the more common abbreviations you may see on a physician's order or the resident's chart. You can use these to help you write brief, concise, but complete chart entries. As you study and use these abbreviations, they will become familiar to you and you will become comfortable using them.

ā:	Before	CHF:	Congestive heart failure
abd:	Abdomen	c/o:	Complains of
a.c.:	Before meals	cont.:	Continuously
ADL:	Activities of daily living	CPR:	Cardiopulmonary resuscitation
ad lib:	As desired	CS:	Central supply
adm:	Admitted	CVA:	Cerebral vascular accident (stroke)
a.m.:	Morning		
amb:	Ambulate	d/c:	Discontinue, stop
amt:	Amount	DOA:	Dead on arrival
ap:	Apical	Dr.:	Doctor
approx.:	Approximately	drsg:	Dressing
assist:	Assistance	Dx:	Diagnosis
ax:	Axillary	ECG (or EKG):	Electrocardiogram
b.i.d.:	Two times a day		
BP:	Blood pressure	EEG:	Electroencephalogram
bm:	Bowel movement	ER:	Emergency Room
BR:	Bathroom	F:	Fahrenheit
BRP:	Bathroom privileges	FBS:	Fasting blood sugar
C:	Centigrade, Celsius	F/C:	Foley catheter
c̄:	With	FF:	Force fluids
cc:	Cubic centimeters	fld:	Fluid
cap:	Capsule	ft:	Foot or feet
cath:	Catheter	g:	Gram
CBC:	Complete blood count	GB:	Gallbladder
cc:	Cubic centimeter	GI:	Gastrointestinal

gm:	Gram	PRN:	As necessary
gr:	Grain	q.d.:	Every day
GU:	Genitourinary	q.h.:	Every hour
gyn.:	Gynecology	q2h, q3h, etc.:	Every 2 hours, every 3 hours, etc.
h (or hr):	Hour	q.i.d.:	Four times a day
H$_2$O:	Water	q.o.d.:	Every other day
hi-cal	High caloric	q.s.:	Quantity sufficient
H.O.H.:	Hard of hearing	(R):	Rectal
hr:	Hour	Resp:	Respirations
H.S.:	Hour of sleep (bedtime)	RLQ:	Right lower quadrant
ht:	Height	ROM:	Range of motion
HTN:	Hypertension	RUQ:	Right upper quadrant
IM:	Intramuscular	Rt:	Right
I&O:	Intake and output	Rx:	Prescription
IV:	Intravenous	s̄:	Without
kg:	Kilogram	shwr:	Shower
KUB:	Kidney, ureter, bladder	S.O.B.:	Short of breath
L:	Liter	spec:	Specimen
lb:	Pound	ss:	One half
LLQ:	Lower left quadrant	SSE:	Soap suds enema
LP:	Lumbar puncture	stat:	Immediately
Lt:	Left	Supp:	Suppository
LUQ:	Left upper quadrant	Tab:	Tablet
mg:	Milligram	tbsp:	Tablespoon
M.I.:	Myocardial infarction	t.i.d.:	Three times a day
NKA:	No known allergies	tsp:	Teaspoon
ml:	Milliliter	TPR:	Temperature, pulse, respirations
min:	Minimum	TWE:	Tap water enema
no:	Number	TX:	Traction
noc:	Night	u/a:	Urinalysis
N/V:	Nausea/vomiting	vag:	Vaginal
NPO:	Nothing by mouth	VS:	Vital signs
N/S:	Normal saline	WBC:	White blood cell count
O$_2$:	Oxygen	W/C:	Wheelchair
O.D:	Right eye	wt:	Weight
O.S.:	Left eye	<:	Less than
os:	Mouth	>:	More than
O.U.:	Both eyes	Δ:	Change
oz:	Ounce		
p̄:	After		
p.c.:	After meals		
p.m.:	Afternoon, evening		
P.T:	Physical therapy		
pt.:	Resident (patient)		

APPENDIX B: UNDERSTANDING MEDICAL TERMS

Medical terms often sound like long, confusing foreign words because, in a way, they are. Many medical terms are based on ancient Latin and Greek words or parts of words combined together. By understanding a few of these frequently used words, you are able to unlock the meaning of many medical terms.

Medical terms can be broken into three parts: a prefix, a root word, and a suffix. Some terms will be made up of a prefix and a root word, or a root word and a suffix, or all three together. For example:

pre / natal /	appendic / itis /	peri / vascul / itis /
(prefix) (root)	(root) (suffix)	(prefix) (root) (suffix)

Prefixes

Prefixes always come before the root word. In fact, "pre-" is a prefix that means "before." Common prefixes you should know include the following:

Common Prefixes

Prefix	Meaning	Prefix	Meaning
a-, an-	not; without	inter-	between
ab-	away from	intra-	within
ad-	toward	peri-	around
ante	before	post-	after; behind
bi-	double; two	pre-	before; in front
brady-	slow	semi-	half
dys-	abnormal; difficult	sub-	under; beneath; less
hemi-	half	super-	above; better quality
hyper-	high; above	supra-	above; on top of
hypo-	low; below	tachy-	fast

Root Words

The root word is the thing or object that prefixes and suffixes give more specific information about. For example, "febril" is the root word meaning "fever." The prefix "a-" means "without." Put them together and "afebril" means "without fever." Root words usually have a combining form of the word that ends in an "o" or sometimes an "i" that is used to combine the root word to another root word or to a suffix. Common root words you should know include the following:

Root Words

Root Word	Meaning	Root Word	Meaning
arthro	joint	glyco	sugar
angio	blood vessel	hem, hema, hemo, hemato	blood
arterio	artery		
cardio	heart	myo	muscle
cranio	skull	neuro	nerve
colo	colon	osteo	bone
dent, denti, dento	teeth	pneumo	lung, air
derma	skin	psycho	mind
entero	intestines	pulmo	lung
febrile	fever	pyo	pus
gastro	stomach	veno	vein

Suffixes always come after the root word. Common suffixes you should know include the following:

Suffixes

Suffix	Meaning
-algia	pain
-asis	condition
-ectomy	removal by surgery
-emia	in the blood
-genic	producing
-ism	a condition
-itis	inflammation
-lysis	destruction of
-ology	study of; science of
-opathy	disease

Suffix	Meaning
-ostomy	a created opening
-penia	lack of
-phasia	speaking
-phobia	fear
-plegia	paralysis
-pnea	breathing
-ptosis	sagging; dropping
-rrhage, -rrhagia	flowing excessively
-rrhea	flowing freely
-urea	urine

GLOSSARY

Abuse:	Causing physical or emotional harm to someone in your care.
Abduction:	Moving an arm or leg away from the center of the body.
Abnormality:	Condition different from the normal.
Active neglect:	Failing to provide needed care on purpose.
Active Range of Motion:	Range of motion exercises performed by the person himself or herself.
Activities of Daily Living (ADL):	Common daily tasks such as dressing, eating, grooming, or bathing.
Activity Coordinator:	Staff member responsible for planning and carrying out social activities for the residents.
Acute Pain:	Sudden onset not long lasting.
Adduction:	Moving an arm or leg toward the center of the body.
Admission:	Steps followed when a resident is first brought to the facility.
Advance Directive (Living Will):	Instructions by a resident about what steps to take or not to take to extend life as the resident approaches death.
Aligned:	Formed into a straight line.
Allergy:	Hypersensitive reaction of the body to a specific food or substance called an allergen.
Alveoli:	Tiny air sacs in the lungs.
Alzheimer's Disease:	Chronic degenerative brain disease resulting in loss of memory, personality, and judgment.
Ambulation:	To walk in upright position, or assist someone to walk.
Ambulation Device:	A device used to assist in walking; a cane, crutch, walker, physical therapy bars, or quad cane.
Ambulatory:	Able to walk in an upright position.
Amino Acids:	Units of protein structure.
Anatomy:	Parts of the body.
Angina:	Acute pain in the chest from low blood supply to the heart.
Anterior:	Front.

Anus:	The opening of the rectum located between the buttocks.
Anxiety:	A feeling of worry or uneasiness.
Apathy:	A feeling of indifference or lack of emotion.
Aphasia:	Loss of the ability to use language effectively.
Apical (Apical Pulse):	Heart rate measured with a stethoscope near the heart.
Appendage:	An attachment.
Arrhythmia:	An abnormal rhythm in the heartbeat.
Arteries:	Blood vessels which carry oxygenated blood away from the heart.
Arterioles:	Tiny arteries which carry blood from large arteries to capillaries.
Arteriosclerosis:	Hardening of the arteries.
Arthritis:	Chronic disease of the joints resulting in stiffness and pain.
Asepsis:	Preventing the growth and spread of dangerous microorganisms.
Aspiration:	Inhaling of food, liquid, mucus, or vomitus into air passages.
Assault:	Physical violence or a threat to use violence against someone
Asthma:	A disease of the bronchi, causing narrowing of air passages and difficulty breathing.
Atrium:	Upper chamber of the heart.
Atrophy:	Wasting away of muscle with muscle becoming smaller and weaker.
Autoclave:	A machine used to kill all microorganisms on medical instruments or supplies.
Axilla:	Armpit.
Axillary:	Relating to the armpit.
Baseline Assessment:	First observations made on a new resident.
Base of Support:	The area on which an object rests. Relating to your body, the base of support is your feet when standing and your hips when sitting.
Battery:	Actually using violence against someone.
Behavior:	Action that can be observed and measured.
Bifocal:	Two different prescriptions in one eyeglass lens.
Bile:	Substance manufactured by liver, stored by gallbladder; aids in the digestion of fats.
Bladder:	Urinary organ which retains urine until it is excreted.
Blood Pressure:	Force of blood against artery walls.
Body Language:	Communicating through posture or facial expression or actions.
Boot up:	To start up the computer.
Bowel:	The intestines.

Brachial:	On the arm.
Bronchi:	Tubes which connect trachea to lungs.
Bronchitis:	Inflammation of the bronchi.
Bulb:	End of thermometer containing mercury.
Bursa:	A pad of cartilage that keeps bones from rubbing together.
Bursitis:	Inflammation of the bursa at a joint.
Capillaries:	Small blood vessels which carry nutrients to individual cells.
Carbohydrates:	Sugars and starches, the chemicals in foods that supply quick energy.
Calorie:	Unit for measuring the amount of energy the body can get from a food.
Cardiovascular:	Refers to heart and blood vessels.
Career Path:	A group of positions in the same field with each requiring more training and offering more responsibility and more pay than the preceding one.
Cataract:	Clouding of the lens of the eye.
Catastrophic Reaction:	A sudden tantrum or burst of anger.
cc:	Cubic centimeter, a metric unit for measuring fluids; 1000 cc's = roughly 1 quart.
CDC:	See Centers for Disease Control.
CD-ROM:	Compact Disc, Read-Only Memory, a device for storing large amounts of data, usually not erasable. Often shortened to "CD."
CPU:	Central processing unit, the heart of a computer, where the main memory and processing take place.
Celsius:	The system of temperature measurement used in the metric system.
Center of Gravity:	Place where the mass or weight of an object is centered (for example, your center of gravity is higher when you are standing up then when you are lying on the ground).
Centers for Disease Control (CDC):	The government agency that investigates outbreaks of diseases and sets standards to try to prevent the spread of diseases.
Centigrade:	A former name for Celsius.
Centimeter:	Metric measurement of height; 1 cm = 1/100 of a meter. About 0.39 inch.
Cerebral Palsy:	Chronic disease of the nervous system resulting in uncontrolled movement.
Cerebral Vascular Accident or CVA:	See Stroke.
Chart:	The chart contains the healthcare plan, the physician's orders, and all the health information on one particular resident. It is a legal document and must be maintained properly.

Chronic:	Ongoing, lasting a long time.
Chronic Brain Syndrome (Alzheimer's Type Dementia):	Large areas of the brain stop functioning, causing memory loss, fear and poor judgment.
Chronic Obstructive Pulmonary Disease (COPD):	A lung condition arising from repeated injury of the tissue, with tissues becoming less elastic and breathing becoming difficult.
Chronic Pain:	Constant, long lasting and on-going, lasts over six months.
Chronological:	Written in the order in which the events occurred.
Cilia:	Microscopic hair-like appendages that sweep foreign matter out of the trachea and bronchi
Clean:	Considered to be free from pathogens.
Client:	A person receiving nursing assistant care in his or her own home instead of a long-term-care facility.
Closed Urinary Drainage System:	The complete catheter drainage unit which connects the catheter, drainage tube, and collection container.
CNA:	A Certified Nursing Assistant who has successfully completed an approved certification training program including a written and/or manual skills test, and who has received a certificate by the state.
Coccyx:	The tailbone.
Code of Ethics:	An agreed-upon set of moral principles or values.
Coercion:	Use of force.
Colon:	The large intestine.
Communication:	Exchange of information or opinions.
Compassion:	Sorrow for the suffering of others with the desire to help.
Concentrated:	Containing less water.
Confidentiality:	Not revealing information about residents except within the healthcare team.
Confrontation:	Argument.
Contracture:	Shortening of muscle due to inactivity.
Contraindicated:	Not acceptable for treatment of a condition.
Culture:	A set of customs belonging to a particular nation or people.
Cursor:	Usually a small arrow, flashing line or block that appears on the computer screen. It is controlled with the mouse to operate items on the screen.
Cutlery	Knives, forks and spoons used for eating.
Cyanosis:	Bluish color of skin due to lack of oxygen.

Cystitis:	Infection of the bladder.
Decubitus Ulcer (Pressure Sore):	An open sore on the skin caused by tissue breakdown due to pressure and reduced blood flow.
Defecate:	Eliminate fecal waste, have a bowel movement.
Defecation:	Eliminating fecal matter through the anus.
Degeneration:	Worsening condition.
Dehydration:	Condition in which fluid output is greater than fluid intake.
Dermis:	Inner layer of skin.
Dementia:	Mental deterioration, loss of ability to think clearly.
Depression:	Feelings of sadness, dejection, worthlessness, helplessness, or hopelessness. Depression may be symptomatic of a mental or physical condition, or part of syndrome of related symptoms associated with a particular disease, such as diabetes or thyroid abnormalities.
Diaphragm:	Muscle which separates the chest cavity from the abdomen.
Diastolic:	Blood pressure when the heart relaxes.
Digestion:	Breaking down food substances.
Digestive tract:	Body system which digests food.
Disaster:	Any event that disrupts the normal activities of a community and causes casualties.
Disc:	Cushions of tissue between the bones of the spine.
Disc, Disk:	Terms used for flat, round devices used for storing data, such as, "compact disc," "hard disks," and "floppy disks."
Discharge:	Steps followed when a resident is released from the facility.
Disinfection:	Process of killing microorganisms.
Discrimination:	Act of treating someone unfairly based on age, sex, race, religion, or ethnic origin.
Dislocation:	A change in the normal alignment of bones at a joint.
Documentation:	Written information in the medical record.
Dressing:	Clean, cloth covering for a wound or sore.
Drip Chamber:	The small area under the IV bag or bottle that the fluid drips into. From the drip chamber the fluid goes down through a tube to the resident.
Duodenum:	First loop of small intestine where most of digestion occurs.
E-mail:	Electronic mail; mail sent from computer to computer.
Economics:	Amount of money available.
Edema:	Swelling due to increased fluid in the tissues.
Elasticity:	Ability to expand and contract.

Elder Abuse:	Mistreatment of elderly people.
Electrolyte:	A fluid that conducts electricity.
Elimination:	Process of removal of waste products from the body.
Embolism:	Blockage of a blood vessel, often by a blood clot.
Emesis:	Vomit.
Emesis Basin:	Small, curved basin placed under resident's chin and used for resident to expectorate into.
Empathy:	Ability to experience the feelings and thoughts of another person.
Enema:	Insertion of fluid into the rectum and colon.
Endocrine System:	System of glands which secrete hormones into the blood.
Enriched:	Vitamins added to a product.
Environment:	The world around you.
Epidermis:	Outer layer of skin.
Epiglottis:	Tissue that closes during swallowing to cover the top of the trachea.
Equilibrium:	Balance.
Erythema:	Redness of skin.
Ethnic Origin:	Referring to a certain cultural group such as race or national origin.
Evaporate:	Give off moisture.
Excretion:	Eliminating or expelling from the body, such as waste or harmful materials.
Exocrine System:	System of glands which secrete hormones into a body cavity or directly outside the body.
Expectorate:	To spit.
Extension:	Straightening an arm or leg.
External Respiration (Breathing):	The exchange of gases between the body and the outside world.
Fahrenheit:	A system of temperature measurement used mainly in North America.
Fallopian Tubes:	Tiny tubes connecting the ovaries with the uterus.
Fast:	Period of time without eating.
Fat Soluble Vitamin:	A vitamin that dissolves in fat rather than water.
Feces (Fecal Matter):	Solid or semi-solid body waste.
Feeding Pump:	A small machine used for tube feeding. It pumps liquid food slowly from a container to a resident.
Flexion:	Bending a joint.

Financial abuse:	Taking money or possessions from those in your care.
Floppy Disk:	A small removable, reusable data storage device. Also known as a "diskette."
Flow Sheet:	A graphic chart that is commonly used in long-term care to record resident information over time.
Fluctuate:	To change continually from one condition or position to another.
Follicle:	Tube holding hair root.
Foot Drop:	Contracture of the muscles in the calf, so that the foot falls forward and cannot be returned to a normal position.
Fortified:	Having vitamins and minerals added.
Gait Belt (Transfer Belt):	A belt placed around the resident's waist to assist in transfer.
Gangrene:	Death of body tissue due to a lack of blood.
Gastric Juices:	Digestive fluids secreted by the stomach.
Gastrointestinal (GI):	Referring to the stomach and intestines.
Gauze:	Thin, mesh-like cloth.
Genetic:	Inherited.
Geography:	A particular place on the earth.
Glaucoma:	Increased pressure in the eye, due to the inability of the fluid in the eye (vitreous humor) to circulate properly.
Glucose:	Simple sugar to which food is converted.
Glycerine:	A fluid used to keep the mouth soft and moist.
Graduate:	See Measuring graduate.
Gregarious:	Outgoing, talkative.
Halal:	Acceptable to eat, in Moslem dietary laws.
Hanukkah:	A Jewish holiday.
Heart (Myocardial Infarction):	Death of tissue in the heart due to a lack of blood supply.
Hazard:	A danger that may cause an injury.
Heimlich Maneuver:	Application of abdominal thrusts to clear an obstruction from the airway.
Hemiplegia:	Paralysis on one side of the body.
Hemisphere:	Half of a round mass of tissue.
Hemoglobin:	Red substance in blood.
Hierarchy:	A form of order in which items are arranged from lower to higher.
Highly Transmissible:	Easily spread through the air or by contact.
Hoarding:	Act of gathering, saving a supply in a guarded or hidden place.

Home Care:	Care provided in a person's home.
Home Health Assistant (Home Healthcare Aide):	A nursing assistant who goes to the patient's home to provide care.
Hormones:	Fluid which starts a set of reactions within the body.
Hypertension:	High blood pressure.
Hypotension:	Low blood pressure.
Icon:	A small drawing on a computer screen that represents a file or a program.
Imminent:	Likely to happen soon.
Immobile:	Unable to move.
Immune:	Protected against infection.
Immune System:	System of the body which protects from invasion of certain diseases.
Incapacitate:	Disable.
Incontinence:	Inability to control functions of bowel or bladder.
Incontinent:	Unable to control the bowel or bladder.
Indwelling:	Staying inside the body.
Indwelling Catheter:	A tube inserted into the bladder and remaining to drain the urine.
Inevitable:	Certain to happen.
Inflamed:	Red, swollen.
Inflammation:	Tissue reaction to disease or injury displayed by redness, heat, swelling, and pain.
Infection:	Invasion of the body by disease-producing organisms.
Informed Consent:	Obtaining permission to perform a procedure on a resident, only after explaining all the risks.
Inhibiting:	Preventing, limiting.
Initiate:	Start.
Inspiration:	Breathing in.
Insulin:	Hormone secreted by pancreas, needed to turn carbohydrates into energy.
Integumentary:	Outer covering of body; skin, hair, nails.
Intensity:	The strength or power of a feeling, such as pain.
Interaction:	Conversation, communication relating to others.
Internal Respiration:	The exchange of gases between the blood and the cells of the body.

Internet:	The network of linked-up computers all over the world, which holds immense amounts of information.
IV (Intravenous Infusion):	Putting fluids directly into a resident's body through a vein.
Kardex:	A card file kept at a convenient place that summarizes the nursing care plan for each resident.
Keyboard:	The keys used to enter data to a computer, like a typewriter.
Kidneys:	Two organs in the lower back which filter the blood.
Kilogram:	Metric measurement of weight; 1 kg = 1,000 grams. About 2.2 pounds.
Koran:	The Moslem holy book.
Kosher:	Acceptable to eat, in Jewish dietary laws.
Labia:	Folds of skin surrounding the female genital area.
Larynx:	Voice box.
Laxative:	A substance that aids defecation.
Learned Helplessness:	Belief that you have no effect on what happens to yourself.
Legal:	According to the laws of community, state, and/or nation.
Leg Bag:	A urine collection bag attached to a catheter and worn on the leg.
Lent:	The 40 days before Easter in the Christian calendar.
Libel:	False, damaging written statement.
Limbs:	Arms and legs.
Linear:	Following in order along a line.
Living Will:	See Advance Directive.
Lubricate:	To oil or grease.
Lungs:	Two organs in the chest cavity responsible for exchanging gases with the blood.
Lymph Vessels:	Structures which collect body fluid.
Lymph Nodes:	Small glands which filter body fluid.
Macrominerals:	Nutritional minerals used by the body in relatively large quantities.
Malpractice:	Neglect or wrong treatment of a resident by a licensed professional person.
Manipulative:	Trying to manage another's behavior.
Masturbation:	Sexual self-stimulation.
Measuring Graduate:	Container with markings to measure fluids.
Menstruation:	The monthly loss of blood and some tissue from a woman of sexual age who is not pregnant.

Metabolism:	Breakdown of food and oxygen in the cells, process by which energy is made available for use by the body.
Microorganism:	Tiny living objects seen only with a microscope (germ).
Mobility:	The ability to move about.
Monitor:	The display screen of a computer.
Mortuaries:	Funeral homes.
Motivate:	Give a reason for doing something.
Mouse:	A small device that is rolled on a desktop to move a cursor on a computer screen.
Mucus:	Secretion from the mucous membrane.
Mucous Membrane:	Moist tissue that lines the mouth, nose, eyes, rectum, urethra and vagina.
Muscular Dystrophy:	A progressively crippling disease of the muscles.
Multiple Sclerosis:	Chronic degenerative disease of the nervous system resulting in decreased ability to move.
Myocardial Infarction:	See Heart attack.
Myopia:	Difficulty seeing things that are far away.
Myth:	A popular belief or tradition which may not be true.
Nasogastric Tube:	Tube inserted through the nose and into the stomach.
Negligence:	Failure to perform one's duty, resulting in physical or emotional harm to a resident.
Nephron:	A microscopic filtering unit in the kidneys.
Nephritis:	Infection of the kidney.
Network:	Computers connected to each other. This can be within a facility, called an internal network, or all over the world, as with the Internet.
Neurons:	Specialized cells of the nervous system.
Neuter:	Having no sexual characteristics.
Nursing Assistant:	Member of the healthcare team who provides care to a resident, meeting his or her physical, psychosocial and individual needs.
Nursing Care Plan (or Resident Care Plan):	The complete plan of care for each resident.
Nurturing:	Caring for others.
Nutrients:	Substances in food that the body uses to provide energy and build tissue.
Nutrition:	The science of foods and how they affect health.
Objective Observation:	Observation based on facts you can see.
OBRA (Omnibus Budget Reconciliation Act):	A federal program that focuses on giving quality care to the elderly in long-term care facilities.

Observation:	Noticing a fact or event (activities, looks, speech, behavior).
Occupational Safety and Health Agency (OSHA):	The government agency that investigates and promotes safety and health issues in the workplace.
Ombudsman:	A guardian who is assigned to look out for the rights of others.
Optimum Level of Health:	The most favorable level of health and well-being possible.
Oral Hygiene:	Care of mouth, teeth, gums, and tongue.
Organism:	Any form of life.
Oriented:	Able to accurately describe who you are, and the time and place.
Orientation:	Knowing the month, day, year, your name, and where you are.
OSHA:	See Occupational Safety and Health Agency.
Osteoarthritis:	Deterioration of cartilage in the joints with age, causing pain and stiffness.
Osteoporosis:	A condition that causes a decrease in the size and strength of the bones.
Outpatient:	The care of a patient who comes to a facility, rather than staying at the facility.
Oxygen:	The gas in the air we breathe that supports fire.
Pacemaker:	A part of the heart that initiates and transmits electrical impulses to cause the heart to contract.
Paralysis:	Loss of voluntary movement.
Parkinson's: Disease:	Disorder of the nervous system resulting in body stiffness and shakiness.
Passive neglect:	Failing to provide needed care, unintentionally.
Passive Range of Motion	Range of motion exercises, as performed with the assistance of someone else.
Passover:	A Jewish holiday.
Pathogen:	A microorganism that is harmful and can cause an infection (for example, a bacteria or virus).
Perineal Area:	In a female, the area between the vagina and anus. In a male, the area between the scrotum and anus.
Peripheral:	Away from the center of something.
Peripheral Vision:	Vision seen to the side while looking straight ahead.
Peristalsis:	Rhythmic contractions of the intestine that help move food along.
Perspiration:	Sweat.
Personal Hygiene:	Grooming which includes oral hygiene, nail care, care of the hair, shaving, make-up, and dressing.
Pertinent:	Important information related to the observation.

Pharynx:	Throat.
Philosophy:	General beliefs and attitudes of a person or a group.
Physical abuse:	Causing harm with a blow, a slap, or rough handling.
Psychological abuse:	Causing emotional harm by humiliating, insulting, or isolating someone.
Physiology:	How the body parts work.
Pigment:	Substance that provides color.
Plaque:	A film made up of saliva and microorganisms that sticks to the teeth.
Platelets:	Elements of blood which form clots.
Pleura:	Lining of chest cavity.
Pneumonia:	A disease caused by a virus or bacteria in which the lung tissue is inflamed and the airways fill with fluid.
Podiatrist:	Foot doctor.
Policy:	Statement that describes what will be done.
Positive Reinforcement:	Noticing and making positive comments about desired behavior.
Posterior:	Back.
Postmortem Care:	Care of a body after death
Posture:	Alignment of the skeletal body as a whole.
Postural Support:	Soft protective device used to protect a resident from injury.
Prehypertension	Blood pressure higher than normal, but below hypertension.
Prejudice:	Preconceived, unreasonable judgement or opinion.
Presbyopia:	Decrease in ability of eye to focus.
Presbycusis:	Hearing loss for high-pitched sounds.
Procedure:	Description of how something will be done.
Procreation:	Creating new life.
Progressive:	A condition that slowly gets worse.
Pronation:	Turning palms down.
Prone:	Face down.
Prostate:	A small gland that surrounds the urethra in men.
Prosthesis:	Artificial body part.
Protein:	Nutrients derived from animals and some plants.
Psoriasis:	Reddish scaly patches, usually on elbows and knees.
Psychosocial:	Individual's mental or emotional processes combined with ability to interact with others.

Puberty:	The age when boys and girls become capable of sexual activity and reproduction, usually from age 11 to 13.
Pulse (Pulse Rate):	The rate the heart is beating.
Pulse Deficit:	A condition where the pulse measured at the wrist is lower than the pulse measured at the heart.
Radial (Radial Pulse):	Heart rate measured at the inner wrist.
Radiate:	To spread outward from a source.
Ramadan:	The ninth month of the Moslem calendar, involving fasting from sunrise to sunset.
Range of Motion:	Moving a joint through its normal range of activity.
Rectum:	The lowest part of the large intestine that connects to the anus.
Rehabilitation:	Process of assisting the individual to the highest level of functioning.
Reluctant:	Unwilling.
Reminiscences:	Recalling past experiences or events.
Remotivate:	Give a reason for doing something again.
Reprisal:	Injuring someone because he or she injured you.
Resume:	A short written summary of your education and work history.
Resident Care Plan:	See Nursing care plan.
Respiration:	The act of breathing.
Respiratory System:	Organs involved in the transfer of gases between the body and the environment.
Restraint:	Device that holds back or limits movements, which the resident cannot remove.
Rheumatoid Arthritis:	Inflammation of the joints, causing limitation of movement.
Role:	Part one plays in relationships with others.
Rosary:	Roman Catholic prayer beads.
Rotation:	Moving joint in circle.
Sacrum:	The rear pelvic bone.
Secondary sexual characteristics:	Breasts, pubic hair, and other traits that develop during puberty.
Secrete:	Give off.
Secretion:	Fluid product released by a gland.
Sediment:	Material which settles to bottom of liquid.
Segment:	A part into which something naturally separates or is divided.
Self-Esteem:	Feelings about oneself.

Senses:	Sight, hearing, smell, taste, touch.
Sensory System:	Eyes, ears, nose, tongue, skin.
Septum:	Tissue dividing heart in half.
Server:	A central computer which has a large amount of memory and where the main body of information is stored.
Sexuality:	Interest in sexual activity, physical attraction to others.
Skin Integrity:	Good skin condition.
Slander:	False, damaging spoken statement.
Socialization:	Talking with and listening to others.
Software:	Computer programs.
Spasm:	Involuntary muscle contraction
Spatial:	Oriented in space.
Specimen:	Sample of body material.
Sphincter:	A muscle that contracts to close a body opening.
Sphygmomanometer:	The instrument for measuring blood pressure.
Spiritual Needs:	Personal needs relating to moral, ethical or religious concerns.
Sprain:	A torn or stretched ligament or tendon.
Spreadsheet:	A program for keeping accounts and handling finances.
Sputum:	Fluid coughed up from lungs.
Standard Precautions:	Standards set by CDC to decrease disease transmission through body fluids.
Stasis:	Stoppage of the flow of body fluids.
Stethoscope:	The instrument for listening to sounds in the resident's body such as heart beat.
Sterile:	Free from all microorganisms.
Stimulus:	Action that causes a response.
Stool:	Waste material from digestive tract, feces.
Stress:	Tension and nervousness that build up in a person.
Stroke (Cerebral vascular accident or CVA):	Sudden stoppage of the blood supply to an area of the brain.
Subjective Observation:	Observation based on what you think.
Sundowning:	The tendency of persons with dementia to grow more confused in the late afternoon and evening.
Supination:	Turning palms up.
Supine:	Face up.

Systolic:	Blood pressure when heart contracts.
Taut:	Tight.
Temperature:	Balance between the heat produced by the body and the heat lost by the body.
Therapeutic:	Pertaining to or useful in treatment of a disease.
Tinnitus:	Constant ringing in the ear.
Toxins:	Waste products released by disease-producing organisms.
Trace Minerals:	Nutritional minerals used by the body in tiny quantities.
Trachea:	Windpipe.
Transfer:	Steps followed when a resident is moved to another unit. The move may be to another room inside your facility or to another building.
Transfer belt:	See Gait belt
Trauma:	A wound or injury.
Traumatic:	Shocking and painful.
Tremor:	A rapid shaking or trembling, often noticeable in the hands or face muscles.
Triage:	Screening a number of disaster victims to determine who has the most severe injuries and needs to be treated first.
Tube Feeding:	Putting liquid food directly into a resident's body through a tube inserted into the nose or a tube into a surgical incision into the stomach.
Tympanic:	Measured in the ear (body temperature.)
Type A fire extinguisher:	A fire extinguisher used for paper, wood or cloth.
Type B fire extinguisher:	A fire extinguisher used for liquids.
Type C fire extinguisher:	A fire extinguisher used for electrical fires.
Umbilicus:	Navel.
Unconscious:	Unaware of surroundings and environment.
Unique:	One of a kind.
Ureters:	Tubes that carry urine from the kidneys to the bladder.
Urethra:	Tube that carries urine from the bladder out of the body.
Urethral Meatus:	Opening at the end of the urethra to the body surface.
Urine:	Fluid waste formed by the kidneys and excreted from the body.
Urinalysis:	Laboratory analysis of the urine.

Varicose Vein:	Weakened swollen vein, usually seen in the legs.
Veins:	Blood vessels which carry unoxygenated blood back to the heart.
Ventricle:	Lower chamber of heart.
Venules:	Tiny veins which carry blood from capillaries to large veins.
Vertebrae:	Bones of the spine.
Villi:	Tiny fingerlike projections in the duodenum which absorb digested food particles and release them into the bloodstream.
Vital Signs:	Temperature, pulse, blood pressure, respiration.
Void:	Urinate.
WWW:	World Wide Web, often "the web." A part of the Internet that allows sharing and viewing of text, graphics, video and audio content.
Walker:	A portable frame that a person can move along as he or she walks to provide support.
Water Soluble Vitamin:	A vitamin that dissolves in water instead of fat.
Web browser:	A program that allows the user to search the Internet and find information.
White Blood Cells:	The white-colored cells in the blood that fight infection.
Will:	A legal document that defines what happens to a person's property after the person's death.
Word processor:	A program for writing documents.
Yarmulke:	Jewish skullcap.

INDEX

Congestive heart failure, 113, 120, 197
Constipation, 156, 343, 451
Contact lenses, 288
Contact precautions, 180
Continuing education 580
Contractures, 87, 94, 223, 231, 339, 340, 351
Coping with loss, 479
Cornea, 143
Cough, 198, 343
Crafts, 274, 275
Crutches, 319, 331
Cubic centimeters (cc), 443, 451
Culture (social), 476, 537-539
Cutlery, 263, 267
Cyanosis, 105, 109
Cystitis, 97, 100

Dandruff, 387
Data storage devices, 562
Death and dying, 547-554
Decubitus ulcers, see Pressure ulcers
Defecation, 151, 154, 457, 458
Degeneration, 339, 340
Dehydration, 443, 451
Dementia, 159, 165, 191, 197, 517-525
Denial, 550
Dentures, 384-385
Dependence, 478
Depression, 475, 476, 477, 489, 490-492, 504, 521, 550
Dermis, 105, 107
Diabetes mellitus, 133, 137, 197
Diabetic diet, 434
Diagnosis related groupings (DRGs), 17
Diaphragm, 125, 127, 128
Diarrhea, 156
Diastolic pressure, 235, 248
Dietary supplements, 437
Diets, 433-439
Dietitian, 4, 14, 434
Difficult resident, 209
Digestion, 151
Digestive system, 152-156
Digital thermometer, 238-239
Dining room, 424-425
Director of nursing, 4
Dirty, 175
Disasters, 67, 68-73
Disc, 87, 89
Discharge, 77, 78, 81

Discrimination, 21, 22
Disease management, 17
Disinfection, 171, 174
Dislocation, 87, 90
Disorientation, 518-519
Diverticulitis, 156
Dizziness, 343
Documentation, 51-55, 438-439
Drainage from wound, 174, 178
Dressing and undressing, 263, 264-265, 267, 390-392, 404-405
Dressings and bandages, 395-399
Drip Chamber, 403, 404
Droplet precautions, 180
Duodenum, 151, 153, 154, 155

Ear, 141, 142, 145-146
Eardrum, 145
Eating habits, 217
Eczema, 105, 109
Edema, 120, 347, 351, 443, 451
Elastic bandages, 395-396, 398-399
Elasticity, 105, 108
Elder abuse, 21, 26, 37-42
Electrolyte, 133, 136
Elimination, 279, 280, 281, 457, 458
E-mail, 557, 568
Emesis, 457, 463
Emesis basin, 381, 383, 384
Empathy, 3, 8
Emphysema, 125,129-130, 198
Employer, 7, 33
Endocrine system, 133-137
Enema, 151, 156
Enriched, 411, 414
Environment, 141, 142
Enzymes, 153
Epidermis, 105, 107
Epiglottis, 126, 127
Equilibrium, 159, 161
Erythema, 105, 109
Esophagus, 152, 153, 155
Ethics in nursing, 31-35
Ethnic origin, 21, 22
Evacuation (disaster), 71-73
Evaporate, 105, 107
Excretion, 97, 99
Exercise, 196, 198, 248, 274, 275, 276
Exocrine glands, 133, 136
Expectorate, 381, 384
Expiration, 235, 251

Peripheral nerves, 160, 162
Peripheral vision, 141, 144
Peristalsis, 152, 153
Personal belongings, 286
Personal care, 6, 14
Personal hygiene, 381-392, 522-523
Personal cleanliness (of nursing assistant), 180
Perspiration, 105, 107
Pertinent, 215, 218
Pharynx, 126, 127
Physical examination, 237
Physical needs, 280-282
Physical therapist, 4, 14
Physician, 4
Physical abuse, 37, 38
Physical needs, 184, 279-282
Physical therapy, 265
Physiology, 88
Pigment, 411, 416
Piles, see Hemorrhoids
Pituitary, 134, 135
Pivot transfer, 312
Plaque on teeth, 381, 382
Plasma of blood, 114, 118, 119
Platelets, 114, 118-119
Pleura, 126, 127
Pneumonia, 126, 129, 199, 351
Podiatrist, 105, 108
Policy, 3, 4, 5
Policy and procedure manual, 4
Polio, 173
Positioning, 344, 347-355
Positive reinforcement, 483, 485, 514
Posterior, 88, 91
Postmortem care, 553-554
Posture, 305-306
Postural support, 327, 333
Preferred provider organization (PPO), 17
Prejudice, 45, 46-47
Prehypertension, 236, 248
Presbyopia, 141, 144
Presbycusis, 141, 145
Pressure relief devices, 350, 351
Pressure ulcers (pressure sores), 105, 109,
    199, 344, 347-355, 360
Privacy, 371, 372,373, 374, 377
Procedure, 3, 4
Procreation, 529, 530
Progressive, 517, 518
Prone, 347
Prostate, 97, 101
Prostate disease, see Benign prostate
    hypertrophy
Prosthesis, 285, 286-289
Proteins, 411, 412, 413
Psoriasis, 105, 109

Psychiatrist, 4
Psychologist, 4
Psychological abuse, 37, 38
Psychosocial issues, 3, 5, 185, 489,
    490-492
Puberty, 191, 192
Pulse rate (pulse), 235, 243-247
Pupil of eye, 143
Pureed diet, 436

Radial pulse, 236, 244-245-246
Radiate, 255, 258
Ramadan holiday, 537, 543
Range of motion exercises, 281, 339, 340-342
Rash, 200, 217
Reality orientation, 525
Recreation, 14
Rectal thermometer, 238, 241-242
Rectum, 152, 155, 156, 198, 446
Red blood cells, 114, 118-119
Reflex, 160, 162
Registered nurse, 5
Religion, 537-543
Reminiscences, 489. 492
Remotivation, 483, 484-486
Reporting emergencies, 70
Reprisal, 21, 22
Reproduction, 135, 136
Resident care plan, 51, 52-53
Resident chart, see Chart
Resident rights, 21-27
Resident's "Bill of Rights," 22
Resident unit, 61-62
Respiration, 126, 235, 236, 251-252
Respiratory system, 125-130 457, 467
Respiratory therapist, 199
Restraints, 38, 327, 329, 332-336
Resume, 577, 578
Retina of eye, 143
Rheumatoid arthritis, 88, 90, 148
Rib cage, 89
Role changes, 497, 511-514
Rotation, 339, 341
Roughage in food, 156

Sacrum, 347, 353
Safety, 293-299, 327-336, 371, 523

Order Form
Order your books and videos today

BOOKS	Product #	Preview	Purchase	Qty.	Price
The New Nursing Assistant Textbook	CNA530T	☐	☐	_____	_____
The New Nursing Assistant Student Workbook and Skills Checklist	CNA533T	☐	☐	_____	_____
The New Nursing Assistant Instructor's Manual	CNA531T	☐	☐	_____	_____

VIDEO PROGRAMS enter your selections here.	Product #	Preview	Purchase	Qty.	Price
1. _____		☐	☐	_____	_____
2. _____		☐	☐	_____	_____
3. _____		☐	☐	_____	_____
4. _____		☐	☐	_____	_____
5. _____		☐	☐	_____	_____
6. _____		☐	☐	_____	_____
7. _____		☐	☐	_____	_____
8. _____		☐	☐	_____	_____
9. _____		☐	☐	_____	_____
10. _____		☐	☐	_____	_____

Medcom collects and remits sales tax on sales in the states listed here. Tax applies in the state where our product is delivered. Calculate the amount of tax using the product cost except in CT, FL, GA, MI, MO, NY, PA, TX, WA where you must use the product cost plus shipping charges.

Subtotal $ _____

CA, CT, FL, GA, IL, KY, LA, MD, MO, NJ, NY, OH, PA, TX, WA add sales tax $ _____

Call for shipping cost $ _____

TOTAL $ _____

ORDERED BY: _____

TITLE: _____

DEPARTMENT: _____

PURCHASE ORDER #: _____

If required for payment processing, P.O. Number MUST be supplied.

FACILITY: _____

ADDRESS: _____

CITY: _____ STATE: _____ ZIP: _____

PHONE NUMBER: _____

EMAIL: _____

SIGNATURE: _____

I attest that I will use the training materials provided in their original video format and not permit these materials to be duplicated or altered without consent from Medcom, Inc.

VIDEO FORMAT - All programs are 1/2" VHS unless specially ordered at additional cost.

PREVIEWS - 10-Day free preview for purchase consideration to qualified educators. Previews are not to be duplicated, used for teaching or for general viewing. You must return the preview after 10 days or you will be invoiced the full purchase price. Medcom pays for shipping to customer. Customer is responsible for charges for return shipping by insured carrier.

ALL SALES ARE FINAL - If a program is defective, return it within 45 days for a replacement.

THE QUALITY OF ALL MEDCOM TRAINEX PROGRAMS IS GUARANTEED!

THANK YOU FOR YOUR ORDER!

Four Easy Ways to Order
1. Call: 800 877-1443
2. Fax: 714 891-3140
3. Mail to: Medcom, 6060 Phyllis Drive, Cypress, CA 90630
4. Go to: www.medcomRN.com